More advance praise for
*The Yale Guide to Careers in Medicine
and the Health Professions*

"Students will love these first-person accounts of how practitioners found their particular niche in the broad realm of medicine. . . . A great tool for pre-med advisors as well."—Cynthia Parker, Colby College Career Services

"This collection of essays reads like a fireside chat with a team of distinguished medical professionals. Every person who counsels young people on the high school or college level and beyond ought to have this book on the shelf."—Susan Paton, Director of College Counseling, Hopkins School, New Haven, Connecticut

"*The Yale Guide to Careers in Medicine and the Health Professions* is a wonderful collection of essays. The *Guide* is personal enough to keep the readers captivated, drawing them into the world of health and medicine, yet informative and educational. I would recommend this book to anyone looking for a more intimate reflection on why one should pursue a career in health care."—Jennifer Lewis, Health Professions Advisor and Coordinator of the Women & Health Initiative, Brandeis University

"*The Yale Guide to Careers in Medicine and the Health Professions* is the first book I have read which really puts a human face to the medical school experience. I found myself identifying with many of the personal anecdotes and enjoyed reading the experiences of real people facing both medical school and a career as a physician."
—John M. Yost, Bowdoin College, Class of 2002

"The pearls of wisdom [in this book] provide excellent advice to people of all ages in an academic or career search. The practical and comprehensive messages reach beyond the field of medicine into all careers requiring high levels of education."—Michael A. Murphy, Headmaster, Pace Academy

"A most valuable collection of essays. [The authors] address most of the questions I am asked routinely by pre-meds and their par-

ents. I wouldn't hesitate to recommend it to my advisees."
—Anthony E. Hilger, Health Professions Adviser, University of
North Carolina

"A wonderful assortment of satisfying essays where students of diverse educational backgrounds, physicians, professors, minorities, pharmacologists, moralists, and others share personal experiences that help illuminate the obscure trail we all walk as we back into our careers."—Michael Caro, Guidance Counselor, Darien (Connecticut) High School

"As a former physician assistant and current medical resident, I can honestly say that this book is a gold mine of forthright, insightful, and beautifully articulated thoughts on entering the medical profession. I wish I'd had a copy at my side during all my points of decision-making. Truly, what more is there to say about a book that compels you to keep turning its pages after thirty-six sleepless hours on call?"—Jinnah A. Phillips, M.D., MMSc, University of Pittsburgh Medical Center

The Yale Guide to Careers in Medicine and the Health Professions

The Institution for Social and Policy Studies
at Yale University

THE YALE ISPS SERIES

THE YALE GUIDE

to Careers

in Medicine

& the Health

Professions

Pathways to Medicine in the
Twenty-First Century

EDITED BY **Robert M. Donaldson, Jr.,** M.D.

Kathleen S. Lundgren, M.DIV.

Howard M. Spiro, M.D.

Yale University Press   New Haven & London

Designed by Sonia Shannon.
Set in Galliard & Gill Sans types by Achorn Graphic Services.
Printed in the United States of America by R.R. Donnelley & Sons.

Library of Congress Cataloging-in-Publication Data

The Yale guide to careers in medicine and the health professions : pathways to medicine in the twenty-first century / edited by Robert M. Donaldson, Kathleen S. Lundgren, and Howard M. Spiro.
        p. cm. — (Yale ISPS series)
Includes bibliographical references and index.
    ISBN 0-300-09542-2 (cl.); 0-300-10029-9 (pbk.)
    1. Medicine—Vocational guidance. 2. Medical personnel—Vocational guidance. I. Donaldson, Robert M., 1927– II. Lundgren, Kathleen S., 1952– III. Spiro, Howard M. (Howard Marget), 1924– IV. Series.
    R690 .Y35 2003
    362.1′023—dc21

                                                                2002009648

A catalogue record for this book is available from the British Library.

The paper in this book meets the guidelines for permanence and durability of the Committee on Production Guidelines for Book Longevity of the Council on Library Resources.

10 9 8 7 6 5 4 3 2 1

CONTENTS

Preface   xiii
Acknowledgments   xvii

PART ONE
CONTEMPLATING A CAREER IN MEDICINE

A History Major: *Why I Wish to Attend Medical School*   5
BJÖRN HERMAN

An English Major: *Coming into Medicine*   8
LYDIA PACE

A Science and Humanities Major: *Listening*   13
MARLYNN WEI

A Pre-Med Major: *Tackling the Pre-Med Decision*   18
MIKE MANN

A Science and Humanities Major: *The Inspiration
of Purpose*   22
JULIE JUNG KANG

PART TWO
PREPARING FOR MEDICAL SCHOOL

A Hospital Chief of Staff: *The Medical School Decision*   31
PETER N. HERBERT

A Premedical Advisor: *On Applying to Medical School*   38
STANLEY H. ROSENBAUM

The Chairman of an Admissions Committee: *Preparing
for Medical School*   43
THOMAS L. LENTZ

The Director of an M.D./Ph.D. Program: *The Purpose of M.D./ Ph.D. Programs*   49
JAMES JAMIESON

A Conscious Evolution in Medical Education   55
VIVEK MURTHY

A Surgical Resident: *In Service to Nation and Medicine*   59
CHRISTOPHER P. COPPOLA

A Medical Resident: *Preparing for Medical School— The Four-Year Plan*   64
STEFAN C. WEISS

A Psychiatrist: *Becoming a Psychiatrist*   69
RICHARD BELITSKY

A Cardiologist: *Character Counts*   74
STEVEN WOLFSON

A Former Medical School Dean: *Learning in the Twenty-First Century*   78
GERARD N. BURROW

PART THREE

TRAINING TO BECOME A DOCTOR

Medical School

An Overview of Medical School Education   89
HERBERT CHASE

Beginning Medical School   95
JULIE CANTOR

Choosing the M.D./Ph.D. Program   99
D. A. ROSS

The First Clinical Year   105
DENA RIFKIN

Teaching Medical Students   110
PEGGY BIA AND FRANK BIA

Advising Medical Students   115
NANCY R. ANGOFF

Residency and Graduate Study
The Ups and Downs of Residency   121
ROSEMARIE FISHER

A Resident's Night in the ER   127
BOBBY KAPUR

A Chief Resident Reminisces   134
MIKHAIL KOSIBOROD

The Inspiration of Medicine and Research   137
JULIE ROTHSTEIN ROSENBAUM

Balancing Research and Medicine   142
JONATHAN A. DRANOFF

PART FOUR
PROFESSING MEDICINE

Medicine as a Profession   153
ROBERT M. DONALDSON, JR.

A Physician's Character   159
ALBERT R. JONSEN

Faithful Physician   166
ALAN C. MERMANN

The Humanities and Medicine   170
THOMAS DUFFY

Medicine as a Calling   176
GERALD FRIEDLAND

International Health and Human Rights   181
RAMIN AHMADI

Women in Medicine   186
DYAN GRIFFIN AND LAURA R. MENT

Embracing Diversity, Overcoming Adversity   193
JUANITA MERCHANT

Civil Rights, Civil Medicine   199
JOHN BLANTON

Transitions in Medical Life   205
VINCENT DELUCA

Growing Old in Medicine   210
HOWARD M. SPIRO

PART FIVE
PRACTICING MEDICINE

The Future of Internal Medicine   219
DAVID B. MELCHINGER

Coming to Surgery from Many Directions   226
CYNTHIA A. GINGALEWSKI AND DANA K. ANDERSEN

Surgery: *High Stakes, High Rewards*   230
CHARLES MCKHANN

Practicing Pediatrics   235
MORRIS WESSEL

A Day in the Life of a Woman in Medicine
(The "XX Files")   242
ANN SKOPEK

The World of Obstetrics and Gynecology   248
MARY JANE MINKIN

Practicing Psychiatry 254
MALCOLM B. BOWERS, JR.

The Future of Diagnostic Imaging 261
BRUCE MCCLENNAN

The Role of the Pathologist in Clinical Medicine 265
BRIAN WEST

Genetics and Medicine 271
MAURICE J. MAHONEY

PART SIX
PRACTICING IN THE HEALTH PROFESSIONS

Nursing: *One Field, Many Arenas* 283
FLORENCE WALD AND CATHERINE GILLISS

A Man's Experience in Nursing 293
DOUGLAS P. OLSEN

Modern Midwifery 298
DEBORAH CIBELLI

How I Became a Physician Assistant 303
ANGELA DELISLE

The Art of the Apothecary 307
SANDRA ALFANO

A Lawyer in a Medical Environment 312
ANGELA R. HOLDER

Applied Ethics in Medicine: *Faith and Process* 316
KATHLEEN S. LUNDGREN

Mental Health at the Margins of Society 321
MICHAEL ROWE

Three Rules of the Road: *A Social Worker's Lessons*   327
EVIE LINDEMANN

My Life in Medical Social Work   332
GAIL KORRICK

A Career in Public Health   337
SUSAN S. ADDISS

Coming to Medicine Through Anthropology   343
NORA GROCE

Lessons from the History of Medicine   349
D. GEORGE JOSEPH

Coming to Medicine Through Health Psychology   359
PETER SALOVEY AND KELLY D. BROWNELL

Why I Chose Chiropractic   364
MICHAEL COCCO

Some Musings About Complementary and Alternative
Medicine   369
HOWARD M. SPIRO

PART SEVEN
CONDUCTING BIOMEDICAL RESEARCH

On Being and Becoming a Physician-Scientist   379
LEON ROSENBERG

A Bioethicist Concerned with Research Involving
Humans as Subjects   384
ROBERT J. LEVINE

Conducting Patient-Centered Research   389
HARLAN KRUMHOLZ

A Career as Physician-Scientist: *Is It Worth
the Effort?*   394
JEFFREY R. BENDER

The Path to Laboratory Research   401
FRED GORELICK

Medical Informatics: *Computers and Patient Care*   407
PERRY L. MILLER

The Rewards of a Life in Science   412
SUSAN HOCKFIELD

PART EIGHT
BECOMING A PHYSICIAN-EXECUTIVE

The Role of the Physician-Executive in Health Care
Management   421
ATTILIO GRANATA

The Role of Physician-Executive in the Pharmaceutical
Industry   426
E. PAUL MACCARTHY

PART NINE
THINKING ABOUT MEDICAL WRITING

Excerpts from *How We Die*   435
SHERWIN B. NULAND

Excerpts from *The Exact Location of the Soul*   441
RICHARD SELZER

Contributors   447
Index   465
Credits   473

PREFACE

Many of you considering a career in medicine and the health professions realize how much change occurred in the last years of the twentieth century and how much change lies ahead. Physicians and other health professionals can help others more than ever, thanks to remarkable advances in the biomedical sciences and in technology. These advances have dramatically enhanced understanding of human biology, the ability to diagnose and treat human disease, and the capacity to prolong human life and to improve its quality. But these very advances have also led to excessive specialization, heightened expectations of patients and their families about what medicine can and should do, overly aggressive treatment of disease, and a disruption of the patient-physician relationship.

We have seen that modern medicine can prolong life but that it does not always improve the quality of the life prolonged. The growth of specialization and expertise within narrow areas has created tensions, difficulties, and dilemmas. Specialists, it seems, look only at the patient's organ systems and often ignore the person. Care has become impersonal as these practitioners concern themselves more with disease than with illness, attuned as they are to biomedical mechanisms more than with whole patients. Moreover, staggering increases in the costs of health care have led to burdensome inequalities and injustices in access to medical care, to the intrusion of managed care, and to a general distrust of physicians and the health care system. Care by health care "providers" tends to be episodic rather than continuous, in part because of the increasing number of health practitioners involved in any one patient's care, because of geographical moves, or because managed care always seems to be changing who can be seen by whom.

It is no wonder that you may have many questions as you contemplate a career in the health professions. We intend this book to address as many of these questions as possible.

Some of our writers consider matters that are as immediate as preparing for entrance to medical, graduate, public health, or nursing schools. Others examine topics as far-ranging and speculative as the emerging science and ethical issues likely to affect a life in the health professions during the twenty-first century. Along the way, they consider and describe the training for these careers, the satisfactions experienced and the perils encountered, and the many opportunities within this broad field. You will read about varied experiences, interests, and decisions leading to a career, but the careers they describe share one theme—caring for patients.

Caring for patients can involve a range of careers—from bench scientist to pharmacologist to ethicist to physician. Our contributors not only provide authoritative information about these topics but share their experiences and aspirations as well. Some have provided a pragmatic guide to a career, and others have recorded their introspection in unique and personal ways. All remind us that there is a life to be lived in and through the professions.

Much in this world is connected with science, medicine, health care, and ethics, as these are elemental to human existence—life and death, sickness and health, and pain, suffering, and joy—and the care of patients is connected with all of these. An interest in biology, chemistry, mathematics, physics, ethics, psychology, sociology, politics, economics, or arts and letters all can lead to careers in medicine and the health professions. But the question remains, *is this for you?* You may feel uncertain or doubtful about what you're best suited for and what to do; many of the essayists have felt this way too. Professional growth includes an element of self-reflection and honest self-appraisal. Some of the writers describe their struggles with the uncertainties in their lives. But they approached these uncertainties with thoughtful introspection, and the result has been satisfaction and even joy in their fields.

We asked the contributors, all of whom have studied or worked at Yale, to explain what it's like to train for their various careers—to describe the nuances, the hurdles, the benefits, the difficulties. We asked that they write in a personal way so that readers get to know them. You will read about their parents, their children, their friends, their mentors, their teachers, their advisors. It is our hope that the contributors will allow you to see what their careers are like and how you may best develop your own talents and interests. And perhaps you will see something of yourself or someone you know in them.

We have tried to ground the book in real-life experiences, with all their varying details. In asking the essayists to write about their own life experiences we have tried to convey a sense of how professionals in the health sciences really grow and develop.

This book began as a pamphlet to be distributed by the Institution for Social and Policy Studies at Yale. As it grew from pamphlet to book, we discovered that the authors indeed, a kind of alpha to omega in age and experience, have found much happiness and satisfaction in the work they've chosen. We want others to enjoy their career choices as much as the authors here have. Our hope is that you will find some of the answers to the question, "Is a career in medicine or the health professions for me?"

ACKNOWLEDGMENTS

We are most grateful to the manuscript editorial team of Yale University Press: Heidi Downey, Margaret Otzel, Jenya Weinreb, Dan Heaton, Nancy Moore Brochin, and Jeff Schier. Our editor, Jean Thomson Black, believed, early on, in the value of our book. Her support has been invaluable and deeply appreciated. We also thank Donald Green, A. Whitney Griswold Professor of Political Science and Psychology and Director of the Institution for Social and Policy Studies (ISPS), for his confidence in what we were doing, and for the same confidence and helpful support of Carol Pollard, Manager, ISPS, and Coordinator, Yale University's Bioethics Project. We also thank our assistant at ISPS, Christiana Peppard. Finally, we thank Toby Appel, John Forrest, Katherine Krauss, and Michael Marsland of Yale University, for providing the photos used in this book. Their generosity, and Mike's photojournalistic talents, have added another dimension to the guidance we hope readers will gain here.

Not least, we thank the authors for providing essays which contain such honest and persuasive accounts of their lives in the health professions. They shared much of themselves, and together with them, allowed us to influence future generations of health care professionals.

I am endlessly grateful to my sons, John and Rob, my grandchildren, Malcolm and Rosa, my step daughters Katie McKee and Susan Garvey, my step son John Garvey and most of all to my wife, Ellen. You have kept me going and made my own life in medicine a very happy and lucky one. R.M.D.

My warmest thanks to Shep Nuland for his reading of "Applied Ethics in Medicine: Faith and Process," and to my dear friends Wanda Needleman and Jan Wohlberg for their reading and friendship. To my daughter, Lydia, my son, Matthew, and my husband, Ken, my deepest love and appreciation—you give depth to the structure of my life. K.S.L.

Times change, but students remain everlastingly young and enthusiastic and eager to learn. I am grateful for the chance to have known so many, and to have learned so much by having to tell them what I knew. The old "Yale System" begun by Dean Milton Winternitz in the 1920s had created a school where learning was more important than teaching, and I owe much to him—whom I never knew—for a school where we faculty could enlarge on our own interests. Marian, my wife of 51 years, made it all possible, in the days before women worked, by putting on hold her own teaching skills until our children had grown.   H.M.S.

PART ONE

Contemplating a Career in Medicine

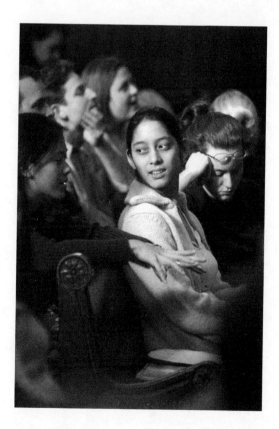

Why some people choose to become physicians is often very personal, even idiosyncratic. Some go along with their parents' desires, others are driven by internal impulses, inscrutable even to themselves, and some just seem to think that they are destined for a life in medicine, especially when a parent is a physician. More than a few, it is said, choose medicine because they fear death and hope to delay its inevitability by staving off disease; such would-be doctors hope to have a pact with the Creator in which they care for the sick, and, in return, receive special attention—and good health.

In this section, five college students tell how they made their choices. At the time of writing, none had yet received that, to them, all-important letter of acceptance to medical school, though we have included brief notes describing what they are doing at the time of printing.

Björn Herman tells a common story: although undecided as a high school senior over whether he wanted to go to medical school, he nevertheless made application to an eight-year medical program along with his other college applications. He was accepted to the program but chose instead to pursue liberal arts studies at Yale University. He writes reassuringly about his uncertainty, even his ambivalence, and his clarity.

A skiing accident confirmed for Lydia Pace how "astonishingly right" she had been to pursue medical school, and it erased any doubts about the validity of a medical profession. But her experience as patient made concrete what, for her, the practice of medicine can be.

Marlynn Wei found the experience of caring for her sick mother, once a nurse now reduced to an anxious passivity by high blood pressure, the major factor in her decision, a choice made lovingly, if slowly and tortuously.

Mike Mann depicts the quandary of indecision. He wants to become a doctor, but he wants to do it for the right reasons. His uncertainty will resonate for more than a few readers, but a decision forged out of such doubt may well strengthen with the reinforcement of experience.

Julie Jung Kang, torn between science and humanities, writes that the solipsistic nature of science was most useful to her when she could apply it to a life of helping. A dual career in law and medicine seems to her the best way to merge the intellectual and emotional streams in her life.

These stories all seem open and honest, yet no narrative can ever give the whole story. One of the editors (HMS) has a different story to relate:

> I usually tell undergraduates that I went to medical school after majoring in English (seventeenth-century American literature) because my father and grandfather told me that is what I should do, and in the 1940s, we listened to our elders. Some years ago, however, a time-capsule, a sheet-metal box put together in junior high school that had been forgotten somewhere in my father's house turned up. In it I found a questionnaire I had filled out around age 13. My ambition then was to be "a teacher in a medical school." Tears of joyful gratitude came at such fulfillment of a boy's ambition until I remember my mother had wanted to become a physician, which in the 1920s was a most unlikely ambition for a young woman. Had I fulfilled my mother's ambition? Or my father's and grandfather's instructions? Still, I have had a rewarding life, justified—if you will—by two children who chose medicine (psychiatry), a third who is a nurse-practitioner, while a fourth started but could not finish medical school. Two daughters are in medicine: my mother would have been proud. Such mysteries of life and generation are beyond my grasp. Some readers will object, I know, that I pushed my offspring into medicine, but that is not what they tell me.

Perhaps as our five writers look back on their lives some years from now they also will see revealed more of the mysteries of hope, generative love, and parental guidance—and the ways in which these mold our circumstances and shape our places in life. But, for now, as students, they look forward and offer to our readers their insights.

BJÖRN**HERMAN**

A History Major
Why I Wish to Attend Medical School

I decided to go to medical school perhaps five different times while in high school and college, but I don't think that any one of those decisions was critical until my junior year in college. So, from my experience, medical school is something to keep in mind early on but not something to worry about too soon if you're uncertain. I am so enthusiastic now about going to medical school because I did not limit myself in college, and because I gave myself time to be sure that a career in medicine is what will most likely make me happy.

During high school I thought frequently that I had made my decision, once and for all, to attend medical school. When I applied to colleges, I was accepted into the University of Rochester Early Medical Scholars program (REMS), an eight-year college and medical school program. But when the commitment date came, I chose Yale University and its liberal arts program of study. Looking back, I realize that I didn't *really* know even then that medical school was the right choice for me. All I had to go on were good grades in my high school science courses, encouragement from my family, and some volunteer work in the radiology department of a local hospital. Clearly that was something; but I was apprehensive about making medical school a foregone conclusion without even having started a pre-medical curriculum.

In college I have had a number of experiences that have allowed me to conclude that attending medical school is the right choice for me. First, I generally enjoyed my pre-medical courses, although during my first two years I changed my mind several times because various classes interested me or discouraged me. I liked one semester of chemistry and biology but not the other semester. I liked organic chemistry, but I didn't like physics as well. It really took two upper-level biology courses (biochemistry and biological reaction to injury) to convince me that I would like a medical school curriculum.

To my surprise, studying for the MCAT was actually encouraging because I saw how the courses I'd taken had prepared me for what lies ahead.

My major is in history. Although I took the science courses necessary for medical school, I wanted to be sure that I wasn't forcing myself into a medical career and away from any opportunity to attend graduate school or law school. If you have other interests it is probably wise to pursue them while in college. This will allow you to keep options available, provide you with a more rounded education, and give you time to get to know yourself, your talents, and your interests. I know medicine is what I want to study not because I have taken only science courses but because I like it *best* of all my options.

The greatest impetus to attend medical school has come from my work-study job. I work in the department of surgery for a laparoscopic surgeon. I've had the opportunity to spend a great deal of time observing in the operating room, as well as just watching medicine at work, learning what the life of a doctor is on a daily basis. A lot of physicians in the department complain about having to deal with paperwork and bureaucracy, but I am still attracted to medicine, and especially to surgery. It has been incredibly beneficial to work in the research and clinical setting of a medical school for nearly four years: it gives one a chance to see how medical students, residents, fellows, and attending physicians must deal with the day-to-day pressures and responsibilities of medicine.

My reasons for wanting to go to medical school are not based entirely on school and work, though. My brother, Jens, has cystic fibrosis, and throughout the past few years I have spent a significant amount of time, during vacations and summer months, keeping him company in the hospital at the University of Pennsylvania, when he has to go for lengthy treatments. This experience with him has shown me what a difference good doctors can make in a person's life. A doctor must be willing to put up with insurance companies and other bureaucracy for reasons other than monetary compensation. Having grown up watching doctors care for Jens, I have found some of those reasons and I hope to have the same impact on people someday as the doctors treating my brother have had on my family and me.

Although it wasn't until my third year in college that I decided to attend medical school, I felt that I made that decision with enough experience to really make it final. If you are unsure about medical school, leave your options open. Chances are that if medicine is right for you, you won't need convincing. When the time comes to apply, you'll know.

N.B.: Björn Herman graduated from Yale University in 2001 and is now doing a research fellowship at Beth Israel Medical Center's Advanced Medical Technology Institution in New York City. He plans to enter medical school in 2003, and aspires to be a surgeon.

LYDIA**PACE**

An English Major
Coming into Medicine

I am writing with my leg propped up on a stool, a bag of frozen peas balanced on top of the high-tech, hinged, and Velcroed brace that encases my swollen knee. Tearing my anterior cruciate ligament (ACL) in my knee a few weeks ago was a painful experience in obvious ways, but it was also an important one. It has made many aspects of medicine real to me in a way that until now I mostly understood in terms of philosophical abstractions, or simply from the point of view of an observer. And it has made me feel astonishingly right about my four years of being pre-med.

The most disorienting aspect of this ACL experience has been my adoption of the identity of a victim. For the first couple of weeks after the accident I hopped down the street on my crutches, waited for the Special Services van, or hobbled into my classes feeling terribly aware of being seen as a disabled person. I *am* a disabled person—I became one in the split second that my knee "popped" on the ski mountain. It's a strange feeling, especially at this fast-paced institution, which values strength and independence so much, and for someone who has difficulty asking for help with the most ordinary tasks. It has been hard for me to accept my inability to change my situation, to accept the fact that I can't run, dance, or ski for the rest of the season. It is hard to confront the mysteriousness of my body's workings and the fact that my ligaments failed. It's hard to look at my knee and have only a vague idea of what is going on there.

Two years ago, when I read Oliver Sacks's memoir *A Leg to Stand On*, I thought a great deal about the effects of injury on identity, and the elusive and complex relationship between our physical and emotional states. After reading the book I felt more legitimate in considering medicine as a career. I had sometimes questioned my place in the world of natural science; I felt surer of my place in the world of poetry and human emotion. But it is only during these past few weeks that I have felt for myself, keenly and constantly, the way that physical ill health can dominate every aspect of our lives and selves. And I understand in a much deeper, more personal way the effects of injury and treatment on identity. It has become impossible for me to doubt a doctor's involvement in the deepest parts of a person's experience.

My recent encounters with health care professionals and institutions have driven home some of my vague notions about the way medicine does work, as well as the way it should work. We all know the importance of connecting as human beings with our doctors and nurses; we know the incalculable value of a kind word or sincere question. But when confronted with what has probably (and thankfully) been the most serious health crisis of my life so far, I found that each real human interaction that I had—in the clinic, at the ski mountain, in the radiology department, in the brace shop, in the orthopedic surgeon's office—felt comforting and restorative to me as the person I know myself to be rather than only as the injured person I'd become. And each rushed or impersonal encounter felt deeply jarring.

Just as significantly, I realized again, at first hand, how crucial it is that doctors make their patients feel a part of their treatment or diagnosis. I have read a bit about medical ethics, and I have talked a fair amount to disadvantaged people in emergency rooms and shelters who feel mystified and terrified about their health and their experiences in the hospital. I have felt strongly, for a while now, about the necessity of empowering individuals in their own health care—both in order to enhance quality of care and promote prevention and as an acknowledgment of a patient's dignity and humanity, of a doctor's own limits and humility, and of the importance of fostering a doctor-patient dialogue rather than a power game between doctor and patient. Yet it wasn't until I felt my own huge frustration with not knowing exactly what and where my knee's ligaments and meniscus *were* that I realized that these efforts toward educating patients about their bodies or ailments are not mere gestures. I felt like hugging the first doctor who pulled out a rubber model of the knee to show me how it works. I've learned that the education of the patient, along with compassion, connection, and communication, is an essential part of health care, for both practical and psychological reasons. And these elements are not simply what differentiates a good doctor from a bad doctor: they are components, I think, of any doctor's true calling. I feel strongly that these are *any* patient's essential rights. Granted, I feel this way with the self-righteousness of the patient and the student who has not yet felt the demands of medical school, the all-consuming and compelling nature of the technical aspects of medicine, the unpleasantness of the "nightmare" patient, or the harrying elements of managed care.

Finally, becoming aware of the possibility that my health insurance might not cover all my costs, particularly my $735 brace, and encountering the ferocity of the stressed secretaries in each office, I was forced to imagine what it would be like to have no insurance at all. I thought about what it would be like to live in dread that a health crisis could occur that would quickly overwhelm my financial resources. I felt for myself (though, because I am lucky, only for a few moments) what it really means to have one's basic right to health care dictated by economics and ability to pay.

Throughout these revelations (most of which came together in my mind while I was lying prostrate in the magnetic resonance imaging [MRI] tunnel listening to that shocking jackhammer sound), I tried to remind myself that my experience had to be one of the easiest ones anyone can have. I am a white, English-speaking, upper-middle-class student from the same sort of ethnic, cultural, socioeconomic, and educational background as many of the doctors I encountered. I am an easy patient who nods trustingly at my doctors, who can understand the idea behind the surgery, and who can be counted on to ice my knee, do my leg lifts, and take my Vioxx. All of my past experiences had taught me to see doctors as my allies. And yet to do that in this experience has been far from easy.

My exposure to the other side of the doctor-patient dyad has intensified my desire to work with people who typically have the hardest experiences with health care—whether because of cultural differences or a lack of resources (money, education, technology, at home or in their hospitals). The only jobs I've ever held have involved working with people with AIDS, inner-city children, or homeless women. "Social service," or "social justice," the only career fields I've ever investigated, became my angle into medicine. I want medicine to be my way to connect with people, to reach them at moments of crisis, to make them feel safe without making them feel utterly dependent on the expertise of doctors, to make them feel as if they can help themselves be healthy. These parts of health care are what make medicine meaningful for me. They are the thoughts that I have held onto as I've made my way through premed-ness at Yale, when transcripts acquired disturbing and inauthentic significance, when my career sometimes seemed to depend entirely on my performance in a fifty-minute midterm or when I spent sunny summer days studying organic chemistry under fluorescent lighting.

I have often doubted my decision to be pre-med, a decision I didn't really make until sophomore year in college. I have questioned the motivation of my sense of justice (doesn't it just make me feel good?); I have wondered whether I picked medicine just because it provided direction, because it feels good to be able to say "I'm premed." I have always been a poetry person, an art person, a flaky person—what was I doing thinking I could do medicine? If I can get stressed out over an English paper, how will I possibly make it through medical school? How will I deal with the stress of a busy day at the clinic, let alone the responsibility for human lives? I want to have a family, too; I want to go rock climbing in the summers; I want to read and write. How will I do those things as a doctor? Aren't there other ways to work with people, to advocate for them, to empower the poor or travel to developing countries? When it comes down to it, will these words really mean something? Will I put them into action? Or will I just burn out?

And I question the probability of my ideals. A doctor reading this might wonder at my naiveté, my assumption that I can make my career what I want it to be, and that medicine can retain its meaning for me even in the complications of the twenty-first century and the assembly-line nature of modern health care. Maybe I'm wrong to criticize the way things are—or often are. My visions give little room to practical concerns like money, and I never think that perhaps I won't be able to support a family while working at a clinic in South Africa or the South Bronx.

Throughout these past few years of being pre-med, it has been most important for me to see medicine as something I can truly envision myself doing, something I have a right to be doing, to have a place in, and to have a vision for. Once it had become a part of me, despite those inevitable doubts, I found that it was harder to imagine *not* being a doctor. Tearing my ACL (like each minor health problem or worry that I've had) has been important in making me feel the truth behind my thoughts about medicine and health, behind the meaning that I have found in medicine. I still have a long way to go before I'll be able to really imagine myself on the other side of the examining table, let alone before I'm ready to be there. But I hope that even as I approach that point I don't forget what it has been like to be the patient, and that whatever ideals I have now don't fade before the reality of twenty-first century medicine. I have a feeling that if I don't let them they won't have to.

N.B.: After graduating from Yale, Lydia Pace spent eight months abroad, working in various clinical and research settings in Nepal and South Africa. She is now applying to medical schools and working for the Public Health Program at the Open Society Institute in New York.

MARLYNN**WEI**

A Science and Humanities Major

Listening

M y ears strain to hear the sound of my mother's heart, my eyes on the falling column of mercury. I turn the knob of the instrument during our nightly ritual, as familiar and regular to me as playing an old piece on the piano. I feel close to my mother yet removed from the rest of the world, enveloped by the muffled silence of the stethoscope. I glance at my mother. Her eyes are closed. I hold my breath when the line passes 150. I listen closely and hear the familiar throbbing in my ears. The silver line drops smoothly past the numbers. I hope silently that it will fall lower. The throbbing disappears, and I breathe again. I hear the familiar throbbing in my ears until it falls silent, feeling as if I am back in the womb. I remove the stethoscope from my ears and return to the familiar world. My mother searches my face with anxious eyes.

"The diastolic is still high, but it is better than yesterday," I say. My mother sighs a mixture of relief and resignation as she sinks against the pillow, almost disappearing into the folds. I store the instrument in the box and set it on her nightstand. I mumble goodnight as I bend down to hug her. I walk quietly to the other side of the bed. I squeeze my father's hand and turn to go. As I leave, I look back once more. I watch the gentle rise and fall of the sheet on their chests, and I feel reassured. I turn the lights off and gently shut the door behind me.

I remember listening to the sound of my mother's cough at

night. I would climb out of bed and walk blindly through the dark hallways to bring her a glass of warm water, feeling inadequate that I could not offer more. Some nights I could not sleep. I would stare into the darkness with fear, listening to the silence, seeing nothing and wondering what I could do to help my parents.

My mother was diagnosed with hypertension when I was thirteen. She taught me how to listen to her heart, how to take her blood pressure, and how to cook low-sodium meals. It was familiar because I had seen my mother do the same for my grandmother.

When I took care of my mother I felt strange, like an actor cast for the wrong role. Some nights I lingered by her side, like a child expecting her to smile and say that this would pass soon. I resented the illness that had gradually transformed her from an energetic, protective mother who made sure I took my vitamins and finished my milk each morning into a distant, withdrawn stranger. I wanted to find again the mother who had cared for me for so much of my life.

My mother was a registered nurse who demanded diligence and perfection. I was afraid to bring home any grades less than 95 percent. I wanted to play the piano, but she wanted me to play violin. I wanted to practice tennis, but she wanted me to learn ballet. On the one hand, she allowed me to pursue my own goals, but the tension of our opposing ideas separated us as mother and daughter. I brooded over my troubles alone, although I went to her willingly when I was sick or hurt. She bandaged our wounds, cooled our fevers with wet towels, and split large pills so we could swallow them more easily.

One time my mother rushed me to the pediatrician, who diagnosed asthma. I was referred to an allergist for extensive tests. With my mother standing beside me, he pricked my back with over two dozen kinds of allergens and gave my mother some cotton swabs. My back was bare, vulnerable, and swollen with pain. I was lying face down, unable to reach the developing swelters. I felt angry and frustrated at the helplessness of the situation. My mother stood beside me, futilely and silently scratching the reddened skin with the cotton swabs. For the next few years my mother gave me weekly allergy shots. She patiently held ice packs against my arms to relieve the swelling. She often brought me herbal brews, and she arranged the array of inhalers on my nightstand each night. Gradually, with my mother's patience and care, I dealt with my asthma. As I grew older the inhalers remained untouched in my drawers for years, and I soon forgot the frustrations of asthma. When I turned thirteen, the focus shifted from my health to my mother's health.

When my mother became dependent on medication and needed her blood pressure checked daily, I was shocked and confused. My mother had been an invincible, strong figure. I remembered her patience, calmness, and reassuring touch during my illness. I wanted to give her the same love, commitment, and strength.

While I was in college I searched for ways to understand what I thought was medicine and its concept of helping people. However, the more time I consciously spent preparing for a career decision, the more frustrated with myself I became. For example, at the Alzheimer's and Parkinson's disease clinics, I took vital signs and ECGs and interviewed patients. One time I walked slowly down the hallway, supporting a frail elderly woman gripping my arm. We inched toward the bathroom together. I stopped at the door of the cramped stall. Was it appropriate that I help her with such a private function? Would she feel awkward? Was she trusting and leaning on me because she wanted to or had to? I looked at her face. She was calm. I helped her slowly sit down on the toilet, her tense hands trembling and clenching my hands. I felt helpless with the inadequacy of my skills and ability to support or connect with patients.

As a member of an undergraduate Yale organization, I volunteered at the local residential home taking blood pressures and vital signs of healthy elderly residents. I felt that the elderly men and women were nervous and wary around the volunteers, but I did not understand why. One week my blood pressure cuff broke, so I started to play the piano for them instead. During the music they relaxed and began to feel much more comfortable. Talking with them afterward I discovered a grave misunderstanding: they thought that the undergraduate volunteer organization was actually a group of medical students who had come to "practice" on them for personal gain.

At the end of these experiences I felt very disillusioned and wanted desperately to do something meaningful, but I did not understand exactly how. I had begun to see the complexity and difficulty of human relationships formed without trust, knowledge, or strong communication. I started feeling less the need or ability to answer my own career questions and more an increased need to do something real, positive, and substantial.

After years of college activities and summer jobs I thought I had gained enough experience to help me decide if I wanted to enter medicine. However, I was still struggling. Could I ever reach certainty? I began to fear that I would never come to a decision. I was unable to extinguish the lingering doubts as I contemplated careers in finance, business, philosophy, or law. I talked with career counselors but usually left with even more questions in my mind: What could I do with my life that captured all that I wanted to do? Could I live a content and fulfilled life doing something other than being a physician? How does anyone ever find the right answer?

During spring break of my junior year, I returned home. As I walked into my bedroom, the coolness of the air washed over me, carrying with it the hints of memories. The canopy bed next to the window was caked with dust. The times I spent with my mother in the room, the many nights I had stared up at the ceiling, worrying about my parents, were all distant, faded memories. Unforgotten emotions resurfaced, now coupled with questions about my own future.

One night during this visit my mother knocked on my door and walked into my room. I was absorbed with my work on the computer. My hands clicked away at the keyboard. She sat on the edge of my bed, watching me intently. "I know you're really busy with your work," she said. "But I was wondering if you had time to take my blood pressure." I stopped typing and looked up. I wondered what was wrong with the automated machine she used when I was away at school, but I stopped myself from asking. "I'm sorry," I stammered, guiltily. "I can do it now." I followed her into her room, where she sat down on the bed. I wiped off the layer of dust on the stethoscope and on the blood pressure cuff and cords. The routine did not seem as familiar to me as before. Had I forgotten how to take care of my own mother? She seemed older and wearier than I recalled. My father walked into the room and I hugged him good night. I squeezed his hand and noticed that it was thinner, the veins more distinct. His dark hair had turned the color of light pepper, his wrinkles deep. Looking at my parents, I realized sadly that they had grown much older in my absence. I hugged them again, as if to make up for all the days I was not there to see them. I had become so preoccupied with my personal goals that I had nearly forgotten the very people who gave me so much. I said good night to them with a light voice, trying to conceal my sadness.

As I turned off the lights and opened the door to leave, I detected something swinging on the doorknob of my mother's closet. I recognized the handwriting that read "Do not disturb" on one side. I flipped it over and saw a photograph of myself in third grade, surrounded by childish hand-drawn hearts and stars. It read: "Although we fight a lot and sometimes disagree, you have always been there for me. Happy Mother's Day to you! I'll be there for you always, too." I smiled at the thought of the eight-year-old writing that simple, silly rhyme. I turned around once more to see my parents peacefully sleeping, lit by the light coming from the hallway. I closed the door softly and walked through the dark hallway back to my room.

The decision to become a physician does not always happen in a single moment. For me it is an ongoing process of self-reflection and questioning, as well as gradual realizations of my impact and role in relationships with people around me. It is a search for the heart of one's motivations, experiences, and values, a search made in hope that they will continue to guide my way through the darkness.

N.B.: Marlynn Wei wrote this essay in the summer of 2000 while applying to medical schools. She is now a student at Yale University School of Medicine and Yale Law School.

A Pre-Med Major

Tackling the Pre-Med Decision

I spent the first two years of college doubting my choice of medicine and the required pre-med courses. Some of that uncertainty was a result of my own growth, and some grew out of ethical issues surrounding medical practice in the recent information-age explosion. Like everyone else, we pre-med students have watched the physician's role evolve and respond in various ways to a range of social and economic challenges. Clinicians have had to adapt to HMO and insurance guidelines; many doctors have become more specialized in their fields; and technological innovations have changed the way health care is delivered and experienced.

The increasingly complex role of the physician in today's society has created new issues for the pre-med student to consider. These issues led me to acknowledge my own doubts about a career in medicine as a physician and to struggle with such questions as "Is this career the best way I can serve my community? And, even more important, if I make this choice, do I make it for the right reasons?"

The last thing I want to do is enter the medical profession simply because it seems respectable, pleases my family, or answers my general desire to help people. Although the respect that physicians have traditionally received as professionals, as well as family suggestions for my career choice, have greatly influenced me, but I know that these motivations would not meet the needs of the patients for whom I'd care as a physician, nor my own needs. And while the gratification gained from helping patients is a powerful motivating force, there would be times, I know, when I would be expected to provide care without receiving that gratification. Respectability and personal gratification are necessary reasons, but during these first two years of college I have realized that they are not enough to motivate me to excel in courses or devote my career to a profession in medicine. So even though I was on a fast track to medicine, I came face to face with my own uncertainty about that track.

Surprisingly, that uncertainty has provided a positive aspect to what came to be my decision. Over my past two years in college I began to see a "pre-med mentality" develop in my classmates. An obsession with becoming the "perfect" medical school applicant seemed to evolve around me, and that focus prevented me from questioning whether the career itself was appropriate for me. This mentality portrayed activities such as community service, clinical experience, intense laboratory research, and indefatigable striving for grade-point averages as a laundry list to be completed, or as "resume builders," rather than as ways for students to recognize and strengthen their talents. I was, at times, vaguely aware that medical school might *not* be the right choice for me, but the pre-med mentality made it much easier to avoid real uncertainty by equating a medical degree with happiness. My real reasons for embarking on a medical career became buried in such piles of activities and accolades. I didn't yet realize that my decision to attend medical school should grow out of my academic and personal desires, goals, talents, and skills.

At the beginning of my first year in college, when asked why I wanted to be a doctor, I replied, "Because I want to help people." As that first year of college progressed, and as I began to choose coursework that would lead to a career, I realized that my vague desire to help was not a rich enough reason for me to pursue a career in medicine. There are, after all, many other careers that directly benefit individuals or society. I needed a deeper reason, no matter which career I chose. A desire to help could have motivated a decision to pursue any health-promoting career. Why was an M.D. the goal to which I clung? I had to have a better reason to enter medical school—or any professional school, for that matter. So, in my effort to better understand my uncertainty, I refined the question to: "*How* do I want to help people?"

Since my sophomore year this question has guided my exploration of other career possibilities. I began to investigate a gamut of health-promoting careers and attended several career-planning talks. These talks often addressed medical school as the goal or reward for a committed student and suggested that other health care professions were less prized. Why do we not give these graduate study programs and careers the same consideration we give to medicine, I wondered. Services cannot be provided to the individual unless the framework for care exists—and in our society, that framework rests on a wide range of health-related careers.

Aside from learning about the traditional roles of health care providers, I became aware of how medical knowledge was being used to create new types of therapy and technology, some of which created much discussion in my classes and in the news. I became aware that stem cell therapy, for example, calls on physicians' scientific prowess but also on their ethical and societal knowledge in the regulation of this new technology. These kinds of discussions led me to begin my own micro-investigation. Through it, I found that medicine, law, ethics, public health, business, and economics all affect health care and contribute to individual and community health. Lawyers can work toward adoption of regulations that will promote a safe environment and improve access to medical treatment for underserved populations. In that space between law and medicine, ethicists often resolve medical dilemmas or work out "ethical" use of new technologies. In epidemiology and public health and in business and economics, researchers and practitioners analyze the health needs of a community and then propose ways those needs may be addressed through allocation of resources and implementation of new programs, locally and internationally.

Through allowing myself to become aware of my uncertainty and explore it and many career options, I have learned two things: that apparently irrelevant and even seemingly disparate disciplines can have a real impact on health care; and, most important, that my talents and inclinations led me to explore social, political, legal, ethical, and economic aspects of medicine and how each can enhance individual health and health care in society.

I also came to realize that my passion to help people was at the core of my drive to study medicine. But this passion alone was not enough to clearly and completely explain my motivation. Through the exploration of my uncertainty I came to understand that medical school is the right choice for me, and I came to understand why. For me, it is through the practice of medicine I can best serve the physical and overall health needs of individuals and communities.

N.B.: Mike Mann graduated with a biology and Spanish double major from the University of Notre Dame in May 2002. He is pursuing a medical degree from the University of Texas School of Medicine at San Antonio. His quandary persists, however. In order to address ethics and justice in medicine he now considers also pursuing a master's degree in public policy.

JULIEJUNGKANG

A Science and Humanities Major
The Inspiration of Purpose

Unlike a job, a vocation suggests work that has deep purpose, meaning, and even happiness. These graces accrue from the career, not just the salary, and are what I seek in my life, especially as I strive toward a profession. However, I realized that I could attain these goals only by developing a genuine awareness of who I was and what I hoped to become. I came to realize that, for me, "the purpose of life is a life of purpose" (Robert Byrne).

The most valuable aspect of my early education was the study of the lives of great men and women. These were historically significant individuals, but reading about how they became significant inspired me to make my own contribution to the world. The scientists and physicians I most admired were role models for the way a person could pursue a valuable and meaningful career. The work of a healer appealed to me, and I believed that becoming a physician would lead to a life of service. But I was also inspired by such activists as Martin Luther King, Jr., and Susan B. Anthony, who courageously struggled on behalf of all of society; their lives served as evidence of the power of caring individuals to make a difference in the world through humanitarianism, activism, and optimism.

Armed with idealism and motivation, I approached my education with the intent of gaining knowledge in a variety of subjects and participating in activities that would facilitate friendships with people of diverse backgrounds and interests. My high school education gave me trust in myself and reinforced the idea that becoming a physician would reconcile my intellectual and social interests.

The boundless opportunities at college prompted me to explore different options through experimentation. When I applied to Yale University, I naively thought that I was a finished product—already aware of my interests, abilities, and aspirations. But the college environment compelled me to reevaluate my interests, rediscover my identity, and ultimately reconstruct my perception of the person I hoped to become.

Heeding the advice of my advisors, I took classes in diverse subjects in an attempt to acquire a wide knowledge of the liberal arts. I knew that medical school would provide ample exposure to scientific knowledge. To be honest, my quest for a broad education was probably more the result of uncertainty and the desire to explore all options before subjecting myself to the grimace-inducing "pre-med" experience. I soon realized that there was no inner impetus driving me specifically toward medicine. To the contrary, I was drawn to exploring my options so as to uncover hidden interests. That was the central pursuit of my college experience, and that questioning and exploratory period led to self-discovery and a sense of mission.

My English classes were mentally rousing and provided me with experience in analyzing and synthesizing information to find meanings and conclusions about broader issues. But I chose not to major in English because my enjoyment of literature was not paralleled by a passion for that subject. Rather, I sought to use aspects of English to gain insight and appreciation for other academic areas. Through practical lab courses I rediscovered my interest in science and the satisfaction that comes with understanding important principles and seeing their relevance to everyday life. I enjoyed learning fundamental scientific theories and applying such knowledge to problem solving. I was inspired by a growing feeling of accomplishment and usefulness as I gained practical and readily applicable knowledge. I was moved by the prospect of possessing the ability to help people by solving problems. Furthermore, the intellectually stimulating nature of science courses motivated me to pursue an understanding of science for its own sake. Although I loved the physical acts of lab research and seeing the changes that could be wrought, I came across a passage from Colin Wilson that synthesized this understanding of knowledge: "The mind has exactly the same power as the hands; not merely to grasp the world, but to change it."

Though my interest in science was based on this synthesized pursuit of knowledge, my attraction to the subject was not enough for me to pursue a career in that field. Education could give me confidence and perspective, but I could not see a life for myself devoted to the pursuit of knowledge without the practical use of that knowledge. For me, intellectual growth had to be supplemented by the act of doing something, of changing the world. With increased exposure to physicians I came to understand the reason I wanted to be a doctor: through medicine, one can help many individuals and thus make an impact in the lives of men and women, as well as on humanity. From youth, my conception of a good person was one who did good things; the doctor's active work of healing, treating, and curing was the consummation of my desire to use my interests and abilities to perform helpful deeds.

Once I knew that I wanted my hard work to be of use to people in need and had decided that medicine would be the culmination of my intellectual interests and innermost aspirations, I felt a sense of comfort and peace. With that foundation of security I felt confident enough to explore various other disciplines that I found simply interesting. My religious studies courses constantly challenged me to evaluate my beliefs and come up with moral conclusions. That brought me to a level of comfort with myself, and an awareness of my hopes for life.

Then I found a revolutionary discipline that once again forced me to reconsider my ideas and decisions. Bioethics was a field that immediately moved and inspired me. In this field my intellectual and emotional passions spoke to each other. I chose to pursue medicine because it was a humanistic application of scientific knowledge, but bioethical thought expanded my perspective so that I could see how good medicine depends on both science and moral responsibility. Ethical medical practice demands acknowledging the moral dimensions of helping and saving human lives without depreciating the centrality of scientific understanding to medical care. As I gained more knowledge of problems and issues I craved more exposure to the interface of science and ethics, not only for their relevance but because of the insight they gave me into my own views and ideas. As my exposure to bioethics increased, I felt the need to consider these pressing moral dilemmas and sought to be involved in discussion whereby possible solutions could be found. I had finally found inspiration and a calling for my professional life.

Through more experience with bioethics I found my great need for conscience, care, intellectual conversation, and action could work together toward the betterment of lives. The obvious need for large-scale ethical and legal reform pointed me toward law, a principal instrument of social reform. That new commitment to seeking solutions was my calling to pursue an MD/JD degree, allowing me to pursue my interests in helping people on an individual as well as on a larger scale.

When some people hear about my plans, they wonder at my willingness to subject myself to seven more years of dense reading and hard work before I enter what may be two of the most stressful occupations around. However, I have never felt more comfortable, secure, and optimistic about my professional life. Finally, after so much searching, I have found a vocation (and not a job) that inspires and challenges me. The conflict I had to resolve in order to find my way toward law *and* medicine was not academic in nature, though certain pre-med courses made me question my willingness to suffer the means to reach the end. Rather, my dilemma was one of learning about myself and finding inspiration so that I could find a profession that embodied my needs. My quest for the possibility of happiness and meaning in my career demanded that I search for understanding and, ultimately, do something with myself. As a result, I learned about and re-created myself. The perspective I have gained on education and life has allowed me to begin spinning my inspiration into action.

N.B.: Julie Jung Kang is applying to medical school and working in a research lab at Yale University School of Medicine.

Preparing for Medical School

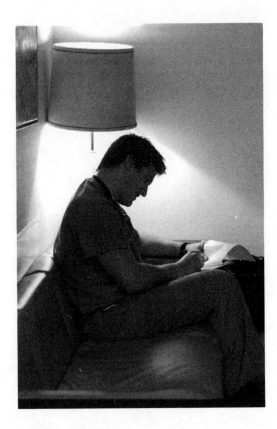

As you consider a career in medicine you are likely to wonder whether you will be able to get into a medical school. After all, everything you hear suggests that gaining admittance is next to impossible, that students need extraordinary grade-point averages, remarkable extracurricular experiences, and record-breaking MCAT scores just to be interviewed. At the more popular schools the ratio of applicants to available positions can be as high as 150 to 1. It all seems so depressing.

Yet all sorts of people actually do gain admission to medical school, and they follow all sorts of routes to get there. The ratio of applicants to acceptances at any one school is high because many students apply to more than twenty different schools. But the admission rate at U.S. medical schools should reassure you: overall, only two or three people apply for every one person accepted.

The first question, though, should be "Do I really want to be a doctor?" rather than "Can I get into a medical school?" And knowing whether one really wants to be a doctor may be more difficult to determine than it seems. The students writing in the previous section grapple with this question, as does Peter N. Herbert in the first essay in this section. Herbert discusses in detail the process of choosing medicine as a career. He indicates how much the process has changed over the past forty years, and he offers sound advice on how to prepare yourself for medical school.

Stanley H. Rosenbaum, Thomas L. Lentz, and James Jamieson are all experienced medical school administrators, and their businesslike essays offer practical suggestions for applying successfully to medical school.

From a wide range of perspectives, other authors offer more general advice about preparing for medical school. Vivek Murthy, writing as a third-year medical student, emphasizes the importance of using preparation time for self-understanding and self-improvement. Christopher P. Coppola, a surgical resident, advises taking time to understand and address your strengths and weaknesses. Stefan C. Weiss develops a year-by-year plan for making the college experience most productive. Richard Belitsky, who directs a training program in psychiatry, describes the broad scope of career options available in his field and indicates that before preparing to become a psychiatrist you must prepare to become a doctor. Steven Wolfson, an experienced cardiologist, writes eloquently and persuasively about how a liberal education can enrich your life as a physician. Gerard N. Burrow, a former dean of Yale University School of Medicine, indicates that the best preparation for a productive career in medicine comes from research-intensive, university-based medical schools that emphasize both the science and art of medicine.

A common theme that runs through these diverse essays: the central importance of being true to yourself in your preparations. Only an honest, inner-directed approach yields a productive experience. If getting into medical school becomes the only goal of your preparations—if you neglect your genuine interests—then you may have gained admission to a medical school, but you will have lost valuable opportunities and wasted precious time and resources.

PETERN**.HERBERT**

A Hospital Chief of Staff
The Medical School Decision

F
orty years ago, American culture, as well as the culture, theory, and practice of medicine, seemed simpler. Many young men and some women at least entertained the thought of attending medical school. Mastery of Latin was considered crucial for both understanding medical taxonomy and writing prescriptions for medications. The aptitude of undergraduates for studying medicine was judged by their mastery of arcane courses such as comparative vertebrate anatomy and organic chemistry, both largely irrelevant to medical practice. Medical school itself was viewed as a surreal ordeal, traversed with difficulty by even the best students. The body of knowledge in medical school, replete with anecdotes, half-truths, and falsehoods, supported more by tradition than by research, was in fact approachable and readily mastered. There was more content in the art as opposed to the science of medicine.

The apprenticeships (termed "internship" and "residency") were the primary vehicles for teaching the art of medicine. They were total immersion experiences. The stethoscope was one of the most powerful diagnostic tools. Most physicians were men and were held in very high regard in the community. Rightly or wrongly, physicians were not regularly challenged by the federal government, insurance companies, the legal profession, or their patients. Most of a physician's waking hours were devoted to the practice of medicine. Generally, practitioners were well compensated and had little life outside of medicine. Physicians virtually never complained, and their devotion to their profession certainly matched that of clerics and others committed to a religious life.

In contrast, medicine as a career today is clearly more objectively viewed and judged. Many young men and, now, many women still, at least briefly, consider entering the medical profession. Admission to medical school remains more competitive than admission to other graduate schools. Unsuccessful applicants to American medical schools can pursue other routes to their objective. These include many more positions in foreign and off-shore Caribbean medical schools where requirements for admission are more liberal and less restrictive. And medical school itself is not more difficult than other graduate schools. The theory of modern medicine is now deeply rooted in modern science, and the body of knowledge is so vast that no student can realistically hope to assimilate it. Also, the tools of modern medicine are as computer-based and as technologically advanced as those of any other discipline.

Postgraduate residency training ("internship," a term used to describe the first postgraduate year, is now outdated) remains the most challenging experience in the formation of a physician. Every-other-night call schedules have been replaced by every-three-to-four-night schedules, but these are nonetheless physically and emotionally stressful for all young physicians.

The community continues to regard physicians highly, and they remain better compensated than most other professionals. The compensation gap, however, has narrowed considerably. In addition, physicians are now held strictly accountable by all stakeholders—state and federal governments, insurance companies, lawyers, their patients, and one another. The level of proficiency expected of physicians creates intense pressure, which is daunting to many physicians.

Physicians increasingly want a "life" outside of medicine. They are less willing to sacrifice marriage, family, and leisure activity to their profession. Society has far fewer clerics and others committed to religion than forty years ago. Medicine likewise finds itself with far fewer physicians who desire total immersion in their professional life.

Alternatives to Medical School

There are many ways to make a living, and many professions now pay as well as the medical profession. The appealing aspects of the medical profession are also found in other professions. The committed biological scientist with a Ph.D. degree, for example, is in great demand in academia, pharmaceutical companies, and biotechnology corporations; availability of research funding has never been better. We need individuals who will continue creating bridges between basic and medical sciences; for some researchers, medical school education does provide that unique perspective and background. Nevertheless, successful laboratory-based physician-scientists must devote 80 percent of their time to laboratory research, and they compete head-to-head for research funding with investigators who have Ph.D. degrees and who are often better prepared for this work.

If the clinical aspects of medicine hold more attraction for you than its technical aspects, there are wonderful opportunities in affiliated health professions. Physician assistants/associates, midwives, and nurse practitioners enjoy almost all the rewards of clinical practice but experience far less aggravation from society's watchdogs. They also are less responsible for, and are, collectively at this point, less annoyed by the business side of medicine; they leave school with less debt than physicians; and they are often more successful in pursuing a life outside of medicine. Physician assistants, especially, have much more career flexibility than do physicians and can move from specialty to specialty with relative ease.

If a commitment to serve others and better our society is an overriding ideal, you should realize that opportunities other than medicine abound. These include government, teaching, many areas of law, a' the application of unique personal attributes to business, enginee' and other professions. Retaining one's idealism is, of course, th lenge, and this is as true in other careers as it is in medicin'

Women and Medical School

There were a half dozen women in my medi 1967, and they largely embraced the then prev?' manded total immersion in medicine. After gr?

cians found themselves paid less for comparable work, were slow to receive well-deserved academic promotions, were excluded from employment by their male counterparts, were subjected to a bewildering variety of harassments, and were tortured by conflicting priorities related to life choices. Because of their medical school experiences, many female physicians have avoided a number of medical specialties and subspecialties (such as trauma and general surgery, neurosurgery, orthopedic surgery), and they still have no parity in the governance of the medical profession. Women, however, are effecting a cultural change in medicine that was unthinkable forty years ago, and, it seems to me, they bring much needed civility and humanity to the profession. They define new career paths, set new standards, and satisfy an overwhelming need among women who want to be treated by female physicians. Women constitute roughly 50 percent of the population of medical students in the United States. They bring unique insights and skills to the field, they are slowly achieving leadership status, and they will create a profession that allows a life outside of medicine.

Preparation for Medical School
Take a Personal Inventory

Our personalities can evolve, but our capacity to "cope" in adverse circumstances is strongly conditioned by our genes and childhood environment. If you are easily frustrated, have a short fuse, find the thought of changing a loaded diaper distasteful, do not "suffer fools" well, are intolerant of certain ethnic or racial groups, or deal poorly with the frail elderly or with grief or death, then medicine may be a bad career choice. Physicians live under the microscope and are expected to be in control of themselves, even under the most trying circumstances.

Undergraduate Majors and Course Choices

It is a waste of college education to try to "get a leg up" on medical school. Most of us pass through college only once, so that is the time to fill in gaps in your knowledge and experience and pursue subjects that most interest you. Medical school admissions committees are amazingly heterogeneous and very open-minded in their consideration of candidates. Arts majors are as welcome as biophysics majors. Committee members will, however, look for evidence of the capacity to handle quantitative concepts. Mathematics and other science courses, particularly chemistry, should be taken. It is difficult to read current medical literature intelligently without knowledge of molecular biology and genetics, and some relevant course work in these subjects before medical school is very helpful. Opinions differ about whether courses focusing on human biology or psychology are helpful; medical school courses that deal with these areas do not require special preparation or a foundation gained at the undergraduate level.

Extracurricular Activities

These activities do capture the imagination of admissions committee members, perhaps to an inordinate degree. It is difficult, however, for committee members, presented with long lists of activities, to know whether involvement is deep or superficial. Participation in research as an undergraduate is particularly difficult to assess, since most undergraduates are insufficiently experienced to master the concepts and methodology of research. Still, pre-med advisors often push students toward laboratories even though students at this level will serve in a capacity somewhere between glassware washer and technician. If you claim research experience, be prepared to knowledgeably discuss what you actually accomplished.

Most impressive to admissions committee members are one or two areas of extracurricular interest, pursued throughout your undergraduate days, with more than one summer or semester of involvement. When choosing extracurricular activities, you should capitalize on your personal skills and attributes and further develop them. Then, when the time arrives for medical school interviews, it will be easy to showcase your activities.

The Application

Your transcript is your academic record, and it may or may not be without blemish. With near universal grade inflation, admissions committees tend to focus more on Cs and Ds than on As. Anticipate being asked about weak grades. I spent most of my medical school interviews explaining a D in Calculus III. To quote novelist Kurt Vonnegut, "So it goes."

Crafting the personal statement is the most difficult aspect of the application process. You will try to sell yourself without seeming self-aggrandizing. You may be tempted to portray yourself as the Second Coming of Albert Schweitzer, but saving the world from disease may be too lofty an ambition. Applicants tend to seize on a catalytic event—the death of a pet, relative, or childhood friend—but these are tough avenues to develop in a meaningful way. More credible are statements reflecting the lines of your decision-making, culminating in a choice of medicine as a career. If you understand how you reached this point, and can adequately communicate the process, admissions committees are more likely to recognize your statement as genuine. Accept some evaluation and editing of your statements by advisors, parents, and friends, but do not let your English literature professor create a publishable essay for you. You are, after all, an undergraduate and probably have not yet published your first collection of short stories.

Apply Now or Later?

The answer to this question must be individualized. Most college graduates have attained the statutory legal age, but most have minimal life experience beyond that of a student. Medicine is a very committed and narrow road that has few acceptable detours between matriculation in medical school and completion of residency or fellowship. Nothing is lost if you defer applying to medical school while you pursue some real life experience. This will permit you to gain a perspective that is unavailable to the college senior. It may change your mind or reinforce your resolve. It will undoubtedly contribute to your maturity and to your attractiveness to any admissions committee. This is true whether you are a ski instructor in Switzerland, a Peace Corps volunteer in Honduras, a Special Forces officer in Zaire, a high school teacher in the Bronx, or a sitcom producer in Los Angeles. Such interludes have provided material for the best personal statements I have read.

A Medical Career Today

It is common to hear of physicians who advise their children and anyone else who will listen to steer clear of the medical profession. Physicians have been buffeted by a major social revolution over the past decade, and many have emerged disillusioned and bitter. We have been buried in a mound of bureaucratic paperwork, have been pushed to see more and more patients in less and less time, have seen our income levels eroded, and have found our judgment questioned on all sides. We must accept some responsibility for this circumstance: we have not provided appropriate leadership or self-government, and there are those who have manipulated the medical enterprise. We have been too immersed in our traditional world to "take care of business."

Cultural turmoil notwithstanding, medicine remains to some the most rewarding profession imaginable. The intellectual content is unbelievably rich and spectacularly interesting. The variety of career options is unparalleled. The potential to contribute to the welfare of other individuals, to community, to the progress of humankind is simply exceptional. The privilege to participate as deeply in the lives of people when they are most vulnerable and needy is granted to no others. Witness the number of professionals who abandon careers in business, law, science, and communication to apply to medical school. To quote a line from *Peter and the Wolf,* "Sometimes it is necessary to go a long distance out of your way to come back a short distance correctly."

STANLEY H. ROSENBAUM

A Premedical Advisor

On Applying to Medical School

Medical schools in the United States generally require their students to have graduated from standard four-year undergraduate college programs. However, a few medical schools provide six- or seven-year programs that combine undergraduate and medical school education. In these programs, entry into the medical program is automatic for students who have done well in the initial years.

The process of applying, and being rewarded with an acceptance, to medical school in the United States is complex and often stressful. The two causes for this are the high academic standards that medical schools enforce and the fact that there are many more applicants than places.

Overall, medical schools accept approximately 40 percent of the students who apply. The actual success rate of students wishing to enter medical school is somewhat less than this because some undergraduate institutions will not support the application of students who, they believe, are weak candidates with little chance of success. Because many colleges, especially in the East, write an official letter from the undergraduate institution to the medical school, termed the "dean's letter," such lack of support can effectively block the application. Reasons for the decision to withhold support include the obvious judgment about a student's academic and other qualities, the comparative strength provided to the supporting letters granted to other students, and, for some, the improved "success rates" that many colleges view as part of their attractiveness in recruiting undergraduates. However, many schools, and all of the more selective colleges, will support all reasonable student applicants.

The conventional time for application to medical schools is at the end of the third year of undergraduate college. Most American medical schools use a uniform, standard application from the American Medical College Application Service (AMCAS), although about a dozen schools have their own individualized forms. The overall application includes an academic transcript, recommendation letters from the student's college plus several from individuals chosen by the student, a score on the Medical College Application Test (MCAT), and usually at least one essay written by the student. Recommendation letters may be solicited from teachers, advisors, or mentors of extracurricular activities. Wise students are careful to pick letter writers who are likely to hold them in high regard and who are sufficiently aware of the academic world to write suitable letters. A strong letter is always helpful, and a weak letter can be extremely damaging.

Medical schools begin interviewing students in the early autumn. There is generally a "rolling" admissions system wherein the first letters of acceptance are sent out in late autumn. As the admissions committee interviews additional candidates and as candidates accepted at other schools withdraw, more acceptances are offered. This process can continue until almost the summer before medical school matriculation. Prudent students get their applications in as early as possible because of the common belief that as open spots in the incoming class are filled, the admission criteria become more stringent.

In recent years, an increasing percentage of applicants to medical schools have applied later than the third year of undergraduate college. This is true for approximately half of current Yale College applicants. Also, a growing proportion of students may receive a medical school acceptance at the usual time but may wish to defer matriculation for a year after college. Most medical schools do not object to students applying after graduation from college, provided they can give a good accounting of their time and the reason for their late decision. However, not all schools will hold a place for a student who wishes to defer matriculation. Perhaps the greatest problem students have with late applications and deferred matriculation lies with their parents. A generation ago, most students did not pause between college and medical school because their parents viewed this delay as signifying a lack of seriousness. Parents need to be reassured (easily said!).

The academic requirements for admission to medical schools are generally straightforward. American schools intend to graduate practically all the students they admit. This differs from the policy of many foreign schools that admit large numbers but maintain high course standards and weed out students with lower grades. Hence, American schools want to be certain that all their admittees can do the course work. It is also fair to note that, given the superabundance of applicants, most schools wish to be meritocratic and accept the best they can get.

The required premedical course work varies a bit but always includes some math, English, chemistry, biology, and physics. Most schools claim to have no preference among student academic majors, many stressing the importance of a broadly educated individual. It is somewhat paradoxical that the science requirements are simultaneously inadequate for studying the high-technology and subtle foundations of modern medicine and excessive for the actual practice of much of clinical medicine. Many regard the organic chemistry requirement in particular as less a knowledge base and more a test model for how a student will perform when confronted with the subject material of medical school.

The student's grades, MCAT score, and letters of recommendation all contribute to the assessment of academic achievement and potential. Part of the "art" of writing a supportive dean's letter is explaining any transient academic dips and noting any academic achievements that are not obvious.

Any personal essay that is part of the application must be literate and coherent. These essays should reflect at least part of what is special about the student (remembering that the admission committee will be reading many hundreds of applications from academically similar students). All medical schools are very interested in the student's appropriateness for the practice of medicine. This means that students who claim (in their personal essay or interview) that they intend to be scientists must have demonstrated genuine interest with prior research experience and accomplishment. Similarly, for the majority of students who are heading toward clinical medicine, these schools are looking for some prior experience with social services and/or actual experience in a medical environment.

The personal interview with a member of the admissions committee often has great weight in the decision to accept or reject—the interviewer is attempting to judge sincerity, intellectual depth, and communications skills. Students who cannot explain why they want to be a physician or who cannot discuss what they have claimed in their essay to be their great abiding interest are not likely to have much success with their interviewer.

Any analysis of medical school admissions would be incomplete without mention of the social components of the acceptance process. Many medical schools are part of their state university systems. As such, they are state-funded and respond to state interests. Hence, many of these schools favor state residents, and some do not even consider out-of-state residents.

Most medical schools, especially the most academically selective, claim that given the outstanding academic and personal accomplishments of many of their applicants, they could fill up their classes multiple times over. Therefore, they may apply social criteria, often referred to as "diversity," to pick among the better applicants. "Diversity" has many meanings, ranging from geographical diversity (probably better to be from Montana than Manhattan) to unusual backgrounds (e.g., a rodeo-riding biochemist) to standard contemporary affirmative action criteria favoring underrepresented minorities. Overt, official discrimination against women and minorities virtually disappeared from American medical schools about a generation ago; subtle prejudices, however, remain within our society, although all medical schools are quite vocal in their official opposition to any unfair discrimination. In medicine, affirmative action programs are justified not only on the basis of fairness but also as a way for poorer, underrepresented communities to have their own members trained in medicine—the logic being that such doctors are more likely to return to their home communities to provide medical care. Nevertheless, some individuals feel discriminated against because they are not favored by the diversity criteria.

Financial issues also cannot be ignored in this process. A year in medical school typically costs more than the median American family's annual pretax income. Many students are obligated to go to their local, lower-cost, state schools. Almost all student aid packages require substantial borrowing before any scholarship money is granted, so that most students end up with large loans, sometimes reaching hundreds of thousands of dollars. This debt, especially when combined with prior loans from undergraduate education, can be so large that it becomes a factor in the student's eventual choice of type of medical practice (away from lower-paying research or community service and toward early entry into better-paying private practices). The size of the debt may even affect the student's choice of a medical specialty (toward more lucrative, procedure-oriented fields).

Given how strongly some desire to become physicians, it is not surprising that many of those students who do not gain acceptance to American medical schools persevere to attain their goal. They do further medically oriented schooling (hoping for better grades) or spend time in a research or clinical environment, and then reapply. Success in such circumstances is not uncommon, especially if the original failure was due to a poor choice of potential schools, a late application, or an inadequate record of appropriate experiences.

There are also other pathways to enter medicine. Some students will attend schools of osteopathy, which provide very similar didactic and clinical training, along with practice opportunities very close to the standard American M.D. degree. Others will go to medical schools outside the United States, particularly in Mexico or the Caribbean, or even to the few European schools that accept Americans. Unlike American medical schools, many of these foreign schools are run as for-profit institutions. Students at these schools can return home in various ways: some schools have clinical rotations in the United States; some are even incorporated stateside (although these schools are not officially "American" schools as recognized by the American Association of Medical Colleges). Nevertheless, most Americans trained abroad can receive graduate medical training within the United States, and eventually become fully licensed physicians practicing in this country.

Because applying to medical school involves multiple issues with some important yet subtle decisions, almost all colleges have professional, experienced advisors to help their students. These advisors, often very capable and knowledgeable, are key to a successful application, and the best source of further information.

THOMAS L. LENTZ

The Chairman of an Admissions Committee
Preparing for Medical School

P reparing for medical school is not as daunting as it first might seem, especially if you plan ahead and approach it systematically. You should take reasonable steps to prepare for medical school, but it is important that you do not let this process dominate your undergraduate career. Three major points in preparing for medical school are: become informed as to what the requirements are; determine whether you are sure you want to become a physician; and satisfy the premedical requirements and prepare to apply to medical school.

If you are considering a career in medicine, the first step is simply becoming informed about medical schools, premedical requirements, and applying to medical school. It is helpful if you can begin to do this before or early in your undergraduate years. Of course, it is never too late to start, as many people do not develop an interest in medicine until they finish college. The best way to begin is to consult the book *Medical School Admissions Requirements: United States and Canada, 2003–2004,* published annually by the Association of American Medical Colleges (AAMC). This book contains a wealth of information about premedical planning, applying to medical school, statistics, and financial aid, along with information for minority students. For every medical school in the United States and Canada, the book provides a description of the school, its programs, and its premedical requirements. You should become aware of premedical requirements so that you can begin to plan your undergraduate course schedule. For additional information, go to the web sites of individual schools. There are also web sites specifically designed for premedical students. Finally, you should go to the career counseling or premedical office of your school to discuss your plans and aspirations.

Once you have obtained this background information, you should take some steps to determine whether you are really motivated to pursue a career in medicine. Perhaps you are from a family of physicians and always thought that you too would become a physician. You may have a desire to help people and are considering medicine as a way to achieve that aspiration. Perhaps you are interested in scientific research and would like to investigate disease processes. Whatever your reasons for considering medicine, it is essential that you test this interest and learn as much about medicine as you can. Read about medicine in books, magazines, and newspapers, and become aware of issues, problems, and advances in medicine. Most important, though, gain some firsthand experience in medicine, especially in working with sick people. There are many ways you can do this. Undergraduate schools, medical schools, hospitals, clinics, hospices, nursing homes, and other organizations offer many paid or volunteer positions that undergraduates can participate in. It is up to you, however, to find one that appeals to you. If research is a part of your motivation toward medicine, you should perform research in a laboratory or clinical setting. It is important that you do not engage in these activities in a superficial manner, but that you explore them in depth. Many students even spend an extra year working in a medically related field. Through these experiences, you should be able to decide whether medicine is right for you or not.

Medical school admissions committees carefully examine the applicants' reasons for wanting to enter the field of medicine. What are your reasons for desiring a medical career? Whatever they are, you should be able to substantiate them with evidence and articulate them. For example, if you are interested in helping people, you should have extensive involvement in activities that involve working with people. These activities, besides telling you whether you are suited for medicine, demonstrate the depth and sincerity of your commitment to medicine. In addition, medical schools look carefully at personal qualities, especially the ability to interact effectively with people.

Finally, you should undertake the third step and actually begin to prepare for applying to medical school. It cannot be emphasized strongly enough, however, that the worst thing you can do is plan your entire undergraduate career with the sole goal of getting into medical school. Obviously, you should be aware of the requirements and make plans to satisfy them, but do not become obsessed or preoccupied with competition or grades or with what particular courses or activities might look best on your application. Instead, follow your own interests and work hard on what you like and enjoy. As a result, you will have a better undergraduate experience and will develop personally and intellectually. Also, because you are doing what you like, you will accomplish more and be a more attractive candidate for medical school.

With regard to undergraduate courses, students should acquire a broad liberal education that includes courses that provide the academic preparation necessary for the satisfactory completion of the medical school curriculum. Medical schools require that you take certain courses before applying. Most require a year of biology, general chemistry, organic chemistry, and physics. These courses extend a full year and include a laboratory. Taking these courses in summer school may be discouraged, depending on the medical school. The courses should be sufficiently rigorous to prepare you for the study of the basic sciences at a cellular and molecular level in medical school. Some schools have additional requirements such as calculus and writing. It is best if you can complete these premedical requirements by the end of the second year, or third year at the latest. In that way, you will have completed the basic science courses before you take the Medical College Admissions Test (MCAT) and apply to medical school. In addition, with those completed, you can devote the remainder of your time to your major, the advanced courses you are most interested in, honors courses, and independent study. In selecting your courses, keep in mind that a broad liberal arts education is fundamental to the making of a well-rounded physician.

Regarding your major, it is a fallacy that you have to major in the sciences to be accepted to medical school. It is true that most entrants have majored in science, but that is because most applicants have majored in science. Studies by the AAMC, however, have shown that humanities majors actually have a higher rate of acceptance. Remember that all you have to do is complete the basic premedical requirements in order to apply to medical school. You are then free to select whatever field of study most interests you. If you are inclined to study an area in the humanities, by all means pursue it. Your undergraduate years may be the last opportunity to pursue a nonscientific field in depth. On the other hand, if you enjoy the sciences most, major in a scientific field.

Besides gaining experience in a medically related field, it is helpful to become involved in other extracurricular activities such as campus governance, journalism, music, or athletics. Your outside accomplishments will distinguish you as an individual. Also, through these activities, you can demonstrate qualities medical schools value such as leadership, creativity, maturity, and independence. Be sure, though, to maintain a sensible balance between academics and outside activities.

Almost all medical schools require applicants to take the MCAT. This is a standardized test designed to assist admissions committees in predicting which applicants will perform adequately within the medical school curriculum. The four parts of the MCAT are verbal reasoning, physical sciences, writing sample, and biological sciences. The questions are designed to assess not only scientific concepts and principles but also problem-solving, critical thinking, and writing skills. The test is best taken in April of your junior year. If you wait until August, medical schools will not receive your scores until late fall, when the admissions process is well under way.

If you take the test in April and are not satisfied with your scores, you can retake the test in August. Because the MCAT is a part of the process, you should take reasonable steps to prepare for it. This can be done on one's own by reading the information sent to you about the test. Review basic material in the sciences, especially biology, chemistry, and physics. Sample questions will be included, and you should practice on these. Books with sample questions are also available. Practice answering writing sample questions. Simply being familiar with the type and format of the questions will help you. Also, a number of MCAT preparation courses are available. Some students prefer these because they are structured and because they have paid a fee, they are likely to adhere to the review schedule. If you have a history of not doing well on standardized tests, you should consider taking a preparation course.

You are now at the end of your junior year and ready to apply to medical school. Almost all medical schools participate in the American Medical College Application Service (AMCAS), and you can submit your application beginning June 1. You designate the schools to which you wish the AMCAS application to be sent. If you have carefully considered the schools you wish to apply to, ten to twelve should be sufficient. If you cannot gain entrance to one out of ten, it is not likely you will get into one out of twenty. Apply to a range of schools, from the least to the most selective. If you are from a state with a medical school, apply to it if it gives preference to state residents. It is also important to find the medical school that is right for you. Apply to schools you are interested in and suited for. They do not necessarily have to be those considered the most prestigious.

Remember that you can get a good medical education at any medical school in the country. If you are interested in primary care, for example, apply to schools that have strong programs in this area. Keep in mind, though, that your interests may change during medical school. After you submit the AMCAS application, schools will send you a supplemental application specific to that school. Some schools send a supplemental application to all candidates who have submitted an AMCAS application. Other schools screen the AMCAS applications and send the supplemental application only to selected applicants.

A few practical points in applying to medical school are important to mention here. Apply within the deadlines, and make sure your application is complete. Be sure you thoroughly describe yourself and your accomplishments in the application, but do not pad it with appendixes, excess letters of recommendation, or other items not requested. This information will dilute the effectiveness of the application and may not be read. Keep in contact with your premedical advisors, as they are in the best position to guide you. If you are not accepted on your first try, consider one of the following alternatives. Spend a year or two improving the weak aspects of your application. For example, if you did poorly in your courses during the first two years and your GPA is low, take additional courses to demonstrate the level you are working at now. You might also consider a related job, such as physician's assistant, nurse, or public health professional, where you can be of service to others and have a rewarding and worthwhile career.

JAMES**JAMIESON**

The Director of an M.D./Ph.D. Program

The Purpose of M.D./Ph.D. Programs

I t has become clear over the past couple of decades that fewer and fewer M.D.s are directing their careers toward academic medicine, in both the basic and clinical research areas. This is a cause of great national concern in the United States. Continued advances in medical care and especially in the understanding of the mechanisms of pathological processes are at considerable risk if physician-scientists become an "endangered species." Several mechanisms and programs are potentially in place to avoid this impending disaster, one of which is the M.D./Ph.D. program. This program started in 1964 with funding from the National Institutes of Health (NIH). It began with programs in three medical schools and has now grown to nearly forty such programs that are fully funded by the NIH. In addition, private sources support several programs.

The purpose of M.D./Ph.D. programs from the beginning was to train physician-scientists who would be equipped to apply basic and clinical research to problems of human disease. In most schools, M.D./Ph.D. students pursue Ph.D. programs in the traditional, basic life sciences (including cell biology, physiology, genetics, developmental biology, immunobiology, microbiology, molecular biophysics, molecular and biological chemistry, the neurosciences, and biomedical engineering).

Today, a growing number of students applying to M.D./Ph.D. programs are interested in nontraditional areas including epidemiology and public health, anthropology, psychology, the social sciences, medical policy and medical economics, philosophy (including medical ethics), and the history of medicine. In most institutions, cross-disciplinary programs are easily worked out in recognition of the diverse interests and career goals of this unusually well qualified group of students.

Course of Study

In most M.D./Ph.D. programs, medical/doctoral students pursue the first two years of medical school along with their physician colleagues. During this time, most institutions offer some graduate-level courses that students may take in anticipation of their graduate studies. In most places, some of the basic science courses in the medical school curriculum count toward graduate program requirements, but you should expect to take additional graduate courses as a Ph.D. student in order to be fully competent in your field of research. In the typical school, students between their first and second years will rotate briefly through selected graduate programs to determine the specific program that they will join.

In some programs, students are encouraged to have some minimal exposure to clinical medicine before they begin their research training so that they will be able to participate in clinical activities during their Ph.D. years. After joining a graduate program, usually at the end of their second year, M.D./Ph.D. students will typically spend four to five years on their Ph.D. work, including a year or more of graduate-level courses. Completion of the M.D./Ph.D. program requires an additional eighteen months or so of clinical clerkships prior to the next step of their education, which in most cases is the pursuit of a residency in a clinical area. In most programs, completion of the M.D. and Ph.D. degrees averages roughly seven and a half years. There are no shortcuts in the training period of these programs, but time is saved because some of the medical school courses count toward the Ph.D. requirements.

Application Procedure and Prerequisites

A prime consideration for admission to any M.D./Ph.D. program is the demonstration of a sincere interest in research. Most applicants begin research early in their undergraduate lives as freshmen and continue throughout college. Increasingly, students are taking a year after their bachelor's degree to carry out more research. The key here is consistency in research experience and the quality of that experience. Several brief, random experiences are not helpful, because we are looking for dedication and depth. Another important factor in the application is the letters of recommendation from people who know you well in the context of research.

Finally, we also look at the GPA and MCAT scores (most programs accept MCAT results for entry into the graduate portion of the program), and these are placed in the context of the overall research experience. Acceptance into an M.D./Ph.D. program of course also requires admission to the medical school. Some clinical experience is helpful but, in the experience of most programs, is not a determining factor in acceptance into the M.D./Ph.D. program within a given medical school. Medical school and M.D./Ph.D. program admissions committees always work closely together because we are looking for individuals who will also be competent clinicians. Applicants should consult the web sites that most M.D./Ph.D. programs have constructed. These will give comprehensive information on the application process and, more important, on the types of graduate programs offered. Applicants should be extremely well informed about the research opportunities at any place where they will interview. This will be one of the first questions asked at interviews to assess the seriousness of applicants. Be prepared! More important, you will make your decision about entering a M.D./Ph.D. program on the basis of the research opportunities available.

One URL that will link you to all M.D./Ph.D. programs in the United States is *http://info.med.yale.edu/mdphd/other/index.html*. An excellent source of information is the web site for the National Institutes of Health Medical Scientist Training Program: *http://www.nigms.nih.gov/funding/mstp.html*. The NIH supports approximately thirty-five M.D./Ph.D. programs nationally.

Sources of Support

As noted above, the NIH is a major supporter of students in M.D./Ph.D. programs, but many programs have additional private sources of funds that allow them to accept foreign national students who are not eligible for NIH support. You should inquire about a school's policy for admission before you apply if you are not a U.S. citizen or permanent resident. Most programs provide students with a livable stipend and tuition waiver for the duration of their training. No payback is now required for this NIH support.

Careers of M.D./Ph.D. Program Graduates

The NIH and several M.D./Ph.D. programs have tracked the careers of their graduates. About 75 percent have primary appointments in clinical departments in medical schools and academic medical centers, often accompanied by a secondary appointment in a basic science department. The remaining graduates have primary appointments in basic science departments in medical schools. About 2 percent of individuals are employed by biotech and pharmaceutical companies or by the government. Significantly, no matter where graduates of M.D./Ph.D. programs finally end up, most of them are actively pursuing basic or clinical research. They are publishing in top-rated scientific journals and are supported by peer-reviewed research grants. A detailed analysis by the National Institute of General Medical Studies that included most of the graduates from NIH-funded M.D./Ph.D. programs can be found on their web site at: *http://www.nigms.nih.gov/news/reports/mstpstudy/mstpstudy.html*. This analysis concludes that M.D./Ph.D. programs have indeed been successful in their mission of training combined degree students to become successful and competitive scientists and clinicians who are continuing to further the cause of the physician-scientist. In the early part of their careers, M.D./Ph.D. graduates devote 80 percent of their time to research and the remainder to clinical service, teaching, and administration. By mid- and late career, increasing numbers spend more time on clinical research (patient-based and outcomes research). This change reflects the fact that it is important early on in one's career to establish a labora-

tory and to obtain grant funding that will allow one to diversify interests in the future.

As I mentioned above, the M.D./Ph.D. combined degree programs are an important, but not an exclusive, training route for M.D.s
who want to pursue research. In my case, I became interested in science as a first-year medical student and worked summers in a basic
physiology lab at the University of British Columbia studying blood
pressure regulation. That first summer turned into a second and then
into an offer to take a year off between my first and second year to
do research and teach. This turned out to be a pivotal experience for
me because it made me realize that in order to carry out successful
research on an interesting problem, I would need more training. My
mentors were aware of this need and supported me. As a consequence,
I applied to the Ph.D. program at the Rockefeller, which I began after
finishing my M.D. (there were no joint degree programs in Canada
at that time and only a couple in the United States). The experience
of taking a year out of medical school to determine if research is for
you is again very popular with our medical students at Yale and often
will determine what area of clinical medicine or research they will follow after graduation. Most places have funds for medical students to
take a year off for research, and the Howard Hughes Medical Institute
supports medical students specifically for a research experience.

But what's the rush? Several of my most successful postdoctoral
fellows came to my lab after finishing their residency and fellowship
training, spent a few years as postdoctoral fellows, and continued on
to successful research careers in basic cell biology. This is a tough route
because debts and economic pressures are real after medical school
and residency, but the opportunities exist. Most labs are very happy
to take in seasoned M.D.s, who must have a true commitment to research if they are willing to take a cut in pay and prestige to become
researchers.

To attract another group of M.D.s into research, several institutions (Yale, UCLA, etc.) have begun programs that integrate residency
with a Ph.D. program, shaving a bit of time off formal class work by
recognizing the M.D. courses and training as part of the course requirements. Recognizing the "endangered species" up front, the NIH
has recently begun funding the "K" series of individual research grants,

which in effect support the salary of postresidency M.D.s at a reasonable level if they want to spend a few years working in a lab with minimal clinical responsibilities. This type of postresidency support at the salary level of a beginning faculty member will help rescue motivated physician-scientists who otherwise could not afford to consider research as a career option.

Probably the most important determining factors along your career pathway are serendipity and a supportive mentor who understands the needs and aspirations of medical students who want to do research. Find one of these mentors and your career options will be immeasurably clearer, and you will realize that you are not crazy to want to do clinical and basic research!

VIVEK**MURTHY**

A Conscious Evolution in Medical Education

For most of my life before medical school, medicine was an enigma. I grew up with a father who was a family practitioner, so medicine was by no means an unfamiliar art. But there was still an air of mystery that enshrouded the profession. How do doctors actually heal patients? How do they develop what seemed to be such close, loving relationships with their patients? Why does society hold doctors in such high regard? After beginning medical school, I began to understand that medicine is an occupation with incredible potential, rich experiences, and a complex, peculiar culture somewhat reminiscent of a secret society.

Most appealing to me are patients, a wonderful group of individuals who teach me not only about the body, but also about the emotional and spiritual dimensions of life. I also find myself surrounded by a stimulating group of peers of diverse persuasions and experiences. And, of course, there are the numerous traditions carried forward by generations of physicians that are frequently a source of interest and entertainment regardless of whether they mesh with my personal framework.

If I had to choose the most important realization I have come to in medical school, however, it would involve not so much an understanding of what was taking place around me so much as what was happening within me. I have come to believe that understanding who you are and who you are becoming through your experiences is the single most important part of medical training and practice. Medicine changes you. In subtle though profound ways, it affects how you think about people, health, and especially yourself. This change can be very positive. It can broaden your thinking, enrich your understanding of the human experience, and deepen your capacity to connect with the humanity in others. On the other hand, it can also generate cynicism, distance, loneliness, and an all too common myopia that allows medicine to consume one's life and distort one's values.

How one will change is difficult to predict, but change does take place. Over time, one thing has become clear to me: our ability to contribute meaningfully to the lives of others is rooted in our understanding of who we are and in our ability to care for ourselves on a physical, emotional, and spiritual level.

I would say that the best preparation one could make for medicine would be to develop a practice of caring for yourself and of understanding how you are changing over time. Before I came to medical school, I exercised, wrote in a journal, meditated, read for pleasure, and engaged in developing youth HIV/AIDS education programs in the United States and India. Each of these activities nourished me in important ways. They kept my body fit, exposed my mind to new and creative ideas outside medicine, and gave me a vehicle through which to reflect on my experiences and regularly reexamine my ideas and values. Perhaps the largest problem that physicians face is the fact that numerous demands and expectations often leave them little time for such renewing activities. Self-care, however, is one of the underpinnings of being a wholesome and successful physician. Without it, a physician's growth and ability to care for others are never fully manifest because he or she is always undernourished in some way.

Writing and reflection have helped me to be aware of my evolution. It is interesting, in particular, to follow the gradual change in my concept of "health" throughout medical training—keeping sight of this progression somehow makes it easier for me to identify with and understand patients' perceptions of their health. As an undergraduate, I initially tried to write in my journal every day. But writing soon became a chore. So I decided to write whenever I felt inspired to write or whenever a major development took place. Since then, writing has been an enjoyable opportunity to think about interesting people, ideas, and events that come into my life. Rereading many of these entries gives me a tangible glimpse of my evolution. It also reminds me of important values and ideals that I may lose sight of from time to time. Over time, my journal has chronicled the person I am becoming throughout this long journey.

Community involvement was another important part of preparing me for my medical training. Four years before entering medical school, my sister and I began a nonprofit organization dedicated to the creation of self-sustaining HIV/AIDS youth prevention programs in India and the United States. This proved to be a very humbling and enlightening experience. It allowed me to understand more tangibly what health means to people and what it is like to lose one's health. Working with people of diverse cultural, educational, and economic backgrounds was an important part of this learning process because it exposed me to a diversity in mindset and philosophies much like that which I would encounter in working with patients. These experiences prepared me to understand and more readily accept people with views and experiences quite different from my own. And although it is difficult to understand completely another's experience of illness, I find that I can come closer to doing so when I am able to ascribe more personal meaning to their illness. Any opportunity to work with people on issues of health can help one bring such personal meaning to how others experience illness.

Reading has become an important source of relaxation, learning, and humility for me. It reminds me gently but firmly that there is a rich world outside of medicine. It has also helped me to think about a question that every physician and future physician may benefit from pondering: "How can I best serve my patients?" Reflecting on the narratives of patients and physicians and using these thoughts to inform my own experiences with patients, I am beginning to understand the importance of equality, of being nonjudgmental, and of respecting the sacred dimensions of life. I am beginning to see that working toward "fixing" is quite different from working toward "healing." To heal is to make whole. By developing an attitude of service in my work, I find myself more able to focus on helping patients to restore their wholeness. Mother Teresa and later Dr. Rachel Remen said that we can serve only that to which we are profoundly connected, that which we are willing to touch. Reading has also helped me realize that service includes not only others but ourselves as well. When we serve others sincerely, we do much to nourish ourselves on a spiritual and emotional level.

The last idea I would like to mention concerns time. Medical training is undoubtedly a lengthy process. It is also a busy process that often leaves you feeling that there is no time for yourself, much less for extracurricular interests. But time that is invested in your personal growth is well spent. Taking time for yourself at any point during medical school and during each day of your training is an investment that you make in yourself. It allows you to give more of yourself intellectually, emotionally, and spiritually to your patients, peers, and loved ones. And it allows you to be enriched by them in the same ways. Without a doubt, this will make you a happier, fuller, and more contented physician.

CHRISTOPHER P. COPPOLA

A Surgical Resident

In Service to Nation and Medicine

The training of a physician includes mastery of scientific facts and knowledge, attainment of technical skills, and the spiritual and professional development commensurate with responsibility for a fellow human's well-being. Like many others, I chose medicine because I admired a strong role model. My father was a gynecologist whose kind and calming manner I constantly strive to imitate in my encounters with my patients. I learned early that the decision to become a doctor is the first step in a journey of experience and discovery that continues long after formal training ends.

Currently, most medical schools require a core of studies that comprises the minimum undergraduate background for medical school courses during the first two years. Almost all schools require a year each of biology, general chemistry, organic chemistry, and physics. About half require a course in English composition, and about a quarter also require calculus, humanities, and social science or psychology.

In addition to the required courses, I chose to study Spanish, including spending a semester in Spain, with an entirely liberal arts curriculum. French and German may have been valuable to physicians in the nineteenth and twentieth centuries because medical advances then were so often published in these languages. However, familiarity with Spanish has proved useful to me by enabling me to communicate easily with many of my patients.

You do not need to major in science to prepare for medical school; in fact, it is beneficial to choose a liberal arts major. Medical school is an experience so tightly focused on the sciences relating to the well and ill individual that it is better, I am convinced, to broaden your undergraduate experience. College is the best opportunity to develop the ability to think. For many, as it was for me, it is the first chance to live independently. It is a time of social discovery, and it should be a time of intellectual discovery. For these reasons, what matters is not the topics you study but rather the methods of research, inquiry, and synthesis of ideas that you learn. Patients appreciate a well-rounded doctor's ability to converse about a nonmedical topic.

I did not take the humanities pathway. Instead, I chose biochemistry as my major. I came to college interested in biology, but my first class disappointed me. It took place in a lecture hall filled with over 200 students and seemed to be a description of irrelevant taxonomy. Chemistry, on the other hand, struck me as a balanced and precise explanation of the world around me. The concept that all matter could be simplified to its basic building blocks was attractive. So, I chose the less popular biochemistry major and with the guidance of a mentor was able to complete a course of independent research.

Looking back, I am confident that I did not need to study a science to be properly prepared for medical school. Biochemistry was very demanding in that it left open only a few slots for electives, but I always preferred to take an extra course and explore a new field. I had a blast studying Italian, archaeology, and expository writing. I was lucky enough to arrange my courses to take that semester in Spain. The things I learned about interacting with people of another culture are much more valuable to me as a physician today than learning to balance chemical equations. I took my electives on the basis of "pass/ fail," and never worried about grades because I was taking them for the fun of it. In retrospect, I should have taken all my courses with this attitude because it was the exercise of stretching my mind around something new that was the true point of college. Although I wished I'd had a broader course of study in college, things worked out well, because when I arrived at medical school I was able to place out of the biochemistry class and take a seminar.

The goal of a medical education is the skillful care of others; however, there is a long road to be traveled through classrooms, libraries, and laboratories before you will ever see a patient. Therefore you should test your decision to become a doctor by seeking out experience in the medical profession before applying to medical school. Most hospitals have a great need for volunteers and have a volunteer or public relations office for recruitment and training. Volunteers answer calls, provide information, speak with patients' families, transport patients from place to place, or perform any number of other minor tasks. So, what do these mundane chores have to do with being a doctor? Being a doctor is mundane. Rare are the moments of snatching a person back from the brink of death. Much more common are the experiences of answering a question, holding a hand, or soothing a sore limb. Spending time in the company of the sick will test your commitment to doctoring. Working in a nursing home is a great way to use the tools everyone has: a warm smile and a helping hand. They often do more good than pills or procedures. Even caring for children in a school or day care center is a way to test your ability to interact with others who need care.

During college, I became an emergency medical technician. I drove the campus ambulance and responded to emergency calls. It was a great way to jump ahead to my goal of caring for people, and it taught me a lot about myself. I learned that, most of the time, the skills used to put people at ease so that they can describe their symptoms are much more important than the techniques of treatment. My time on the ambulance was also a good test of my resolve to become a doctor and provided me with some reassurance that I enjoyed taking care of patients.

I hadn't realized that training to be an EMT had changed my position in the college community. I was part of a coeducational fraternity, and we lived together sharing in one another's victories and trials. One night, one of my fraternity brothers fell from a balcony and fractured his facial bones. The cry rose up "Somebody get Chris," and I was awakened from a sound sleep to take care of him. My brothers looked to me with respect and trust and believed that I would know what to do. It was quite shocking to feel so useful and needed simply because I had the extracurricular experience as an EMT. It gave me confidence that my choice to become a doctor was the right one.

Once I had made the decision to become a physician, I had to face the fact that the cost of medical school tuition and living expenses is quite formidable. Some medical students finish school with very large debts. But don't worry, you will find a way to get through this obstacle if you believe in becoming a doctor. I am the oldest of five children, and my parents were very generous in paying for my under-graduate education, but I was on my own for medical school. In addi-tion to school loans, I considered paying for my tuition by delaying medical school and working, by competing for scholarships, and by going into military service. I chose a scholarship from the Air Force and made a commitment to four years of active duty in exchange for tuition, reimbursement for medical school fees and books, and a monthly stipend.

The choice to take a military scholarship was a difficult one, and I'm not sure I would do it again, mostly because I made the choice when I was single. Now that I am completing my training and must enter military service, I have the lives of my wife and two children to consider. The first thing to realize when choosing a military career is that the needs of the military come first, which means that at times your ability to choose where you will work and what you will do is sacrificed. I was first attracted to the scholarship for financial reasons, but that rationale warrants reevaluation. If you can earn a high salary the first few years after residency, you might be able to pay off a school loan in less than the four years of commitment to the military.

However, even without the financial motivation, I was attracted to the service. I had just spent time in Spain, where military or govern-ment service is mandatory for all citizens. I admired that policy and believed it was important for me to give in some way to my country. I was also attracted by the idea of a set job after residency without the worries of office staff, practice buy-in, malpractice insurance, or the other headaches that seem to detract from patient care. Also, I was excited by the possibility of working in a part of the country or the world that was new to me.

I have done well with the military scholarship, just as my colleagues with loans have done well. I have learned that the military has a complicated bureaucracy of paperwork and it is wise to double-check all orders and forms, always keeping copies for myself. There are official communications and publications for the doctors in the service, but I have learned everything important by word of mouth from the people who are a couple of years ahead of me in the program. I found that I have been able to get what I have wanted in terms of residency and fellowship, but it has required diligent work in contacting the people in charge of making the decisions and keeping current with any changes in administration. The military scholarship has been a good choice for me, but I would advise anyone considering it to talk to as many people as possible who have experienced the program. And, before committing four years of your life to the military, consider the reality that you could see active duty service during wartime. If the benefits of military service outweigh the drawbacks, I recommend seeking a military scholarship.

The brief thoughts I have offered provide only a starting point for your preparation for medical school. Each of you must find your own unique strengths and weaknesses and master them. It is these personal characteristics that a doctor must call upon to transform the dispassionate science that governs the workings of the body into the compassionate art that brings a patient back to health.

STEFAN C. WEISS

A Medical Resident
Preparing for Medical School— The Four-Year Plan

I t is easy to become overwhelmed when you begin thinking about what you need to do in the years before you apply to medical school. What major would be "best"? When should you enroll in the core science courses? Such questions are inevitable. Along the way, you will have many doubts: Can I sing with an a capella group, or row crew, or join a fraternity and still be a pre-med?

The great thing about college is that you *can* do it all, as long as you set your priorities and balance your responsibilities. The best piece of advice I can offer is never to let your desire to go to medical school interfere with, or dominate, your college experience. That is not to say that you should ignore your studies. Grades are important, but going to college should not merely be a four-year interlude between high school and medical school. The college experience is a process of enculturation. It is a time to discover who you are and what contributions you want to make both in medicine and in the world. College is a place to, as Robin Williams says in the movie *Dead Poet's Society,* "learn how to suck the marrow out of life."

In my opinion, though not all will agree, the best way to prepare for medical school is to remember that it is four years away. During the first year of college try to sample courses in various disciplines that interest you. Enroll in courses on art history, Shakespeare, or the history of the American South, while at the same time registering for courses in general chemistry and the level of calculus most appropriate for you. In this manner, you can check off two of your pre-med requirements while surveying the humanities landscape. Of course, also spend this first year meeting people in your college and finding the extracurricular activities you enjoy.

During your second year, while continuing to register for the required pre-med sciences, choose a major and begin to focus on developing an academic plan that will enable you to write a thesis on something that stirs your interest. Unlike what you probably encountered in your high school, a college or university offers vast resources. Your goal should be to find the one tiny area in which you can become an expert. This expertise does not necessarily have to be related to medicine or health. Studying the influence of Oliver Cromwell on the social development of seventeenth-century Dublin, for example, is as important as evaluating the similarities between the pellagra epidemic at the beginning of the twentieth century and the AIDS epidemic at the end of it, or researching the role of the crx gene and its regulation of phototransduction proteins.

The third year is the time to begin to assume leadership roles in the activities that interest you as well as to continue to refine your academic interests in seminars and tutorials. Most likely, you will have at least one premedical science left to take. It is often best to leave physics for the third year, which is what most students do. Your preparation for the Medical College Admissions Test (MCAT) should begin in the winter of junior year, and by the end of that year you should begin to develop a personal statement expressing why you want to attend medical school and how the past three years of college have contributed to your personal development. The personal statement is the document that allows you to paint a picture of yourself, one that integrates all your diverse experiences into a coherent message. Sell the value of your unique background by describing why you would be an asset to a class of a hundred medical students.

Senior year is the time to interview. Applications, both the universal application and the applications mailed by medical schools, should be completed by September. Letters of recommendation need to be collected as you progress through the college experience. They can usually be kept on file at your dean's office. The seminar professor with whom you studied social psychology sophomore year is better able to write a letter immediately following the class than after a year has passed. You might not use all the letters you collect, but at least they will be available at the end of junior year when you must create your file with the office of career services. The remainder of senior year is best enjoyed with the friends you have made during your four years of college. You probably will not be enjoying your favorite pizza wherever you attend medical school, so now is the time to do that.

The two aspects of creating the "perfect application" for medical school that most concern pre-meds are research and volunteer activities. Research is important. However, if you are a history major, spending a summer in a lab at the biology department using the pipette and running a few gels is unlikely to provide you with many valuable skills. During your undergraduate years your research should be in the field that you consider most interesting, because at this point the value is in the process. Developing a research question and creating an investigative plan are skills that transcend all disciplines. Dedicating many hours to research for your political science senior thesis, and following an unexpected path revealed by uncovering new documents is not much different from reevaluating a scientific hypothesis when a gel produces a novel gene product. Important to medical school admissions personnel is evidence that you have demonstrated the capacity to engage in research and that academics and research are important to you. Do not feel disadvantaged if you've studied existentialism rather than protein chemistry. Your time to engage in basic science will come soon enough.

Your approach to volunteering within the community should be similar. Ideally, the spirit of contributing to the welfare of society is something you bring to college, as most universities are situated in communities with many needs. In this environment, tutoring students at a local middle school, working in a home for the aged, and volunteering at a community soup kitchen are all important. A consistent experience within a particular social action organization is more meaningful than spending what many find to be the compulsory three hours a week in a hospital. It is true that volunteering in a hospital may help you determine whether medicine is indeed the right career path for you. But if you are looking for an outlet to contribute to the community, do not feel that nonmedical service is any less valuable. Again, the purpose of your personal statement is to explain to medical school admissions committees why what you did was important to you and how it will make you a better doctor for your patients. People who live only for molecular biophysics are not any better medical students or physicians than those who demonstrate a passion for theater.

In my case, the path to medical school was anything but direct. As a philosophy major, I took the minimum premedical science requirements. I spent two of my summers in research labs and one summer in Washington, D.C., working at the Department of Health and Human Services. During my junior year, I took a semester at Oxford reading metaphysical poetry and philosophy of mind.

After graduation, I deferred matriculating to medical school for a year to sample corporate life, taking a job with a major consulting firm. I found this to be a valuable way to learn how the private sector influences the delivery of health care. Even in medical school I was not satisfied to blindly enroll in the specified courses. I created a lecture series focused on the role of the humanities in medicine. I helped edit *MSJAMA*, the student section of the *Journal of the American Medical Association* (*JAMA*). I even considered taking time off to attend law school. During the summer between my first and second year I returned to Washington, where I lobbied on Capitol Hill for the Health Care Bill of Rights. As a third-year medical student, I went to the National Institutes of Health (NIH), where I spent the year as a fellow in the Department of Clinical Bioethics and concurrently received a master's degree in clinical research.

Now I will enter a dermatology residency. Along with my clinical training I plan to continue my work in health policy. I am interested in how a society makes decisions about the delivery of health care services, including the role of health outcomes and how we determine which outcomes are appropriate end points. I am also interested in the role of the human genome in health care delivery. This encompasses both ethical issues, such as privacy, cloning and ownership, and pharmacogenomics, the ability to target drugs specifically to individuals.

As reflected by both my interests and my journey through college and medical school, it is unlikely that I will make a career of being a community physician. Despite my nontraditional path, however, at each step along the way I have been well received by committees mythically regarded as looking for a specific mold.

Thus, the best advice I can offer as you begin college, the best four years of your life, is simply to make them the best four years of your life. Take advantage of the resources available to you, and do not become embroiled in the medical school admissions game. Use your summers to pursue interesting opportunities. You can often find a variety of exciting externships, and your institution's office of career services can be valuable in helping you locate experiences in policy and corporate work. Spend time conducting research for your senior thesis with the help of school fellowships designed for summer research experiences. The summer is also a good time to study in a foreign country. In short, the summer is a time to enrich your academic plan and color it with interesting experiences.

The truth is, if you are successful on the path you choose, whatever it may be, then you will be a solid candidate for any graduate school and you will gain entrance to the profession you seek.

RICHARD**BELITSKY**

A Psychiatrist
Becoming a Psychiatrist

You would expect a dentist to have nice teeth, an oncologist not to smoke, and a dermatologist to avoid direct sunlight. After all, they should have learned something from their professions. So, I suppose as a psychiatrist I should at least know why I became one. What was there about my background, my environment? What were the critical events and influences that led me to my career? I do spend a lot of time trying to understand why other people do things; so, fair enough, I'll take a stab at explaining why I chose this pursuit rather than some other. I must admit, though, that it feels funny to write about myself. For one thing, there is so much I don't know—a feeling I often have as a doctor. But, if I've learned one thing from all my years in medicine, it's that although not knowing may be your only true and reasonable excuse, it's never quite good or reasonable enough to remain there.

I really hadn't planned on becoming a doctor. You see, there are no doctors in my family, let alone psychiatrists. In fact, my early images of doctors all came from television. Doctors were young (Dr. Kildare), arrogant (Ben Casey), handsome (Joe Gannon), and kind (Marcus Welby). They all fought for, and sometimes with, their patients. And in the end, they were always right.

At the time I grew up, during the 60s and 70s, the stories of doctors and their patients seemed, like most of television, to be compelling drama but not real life. What seemed real, and important, was the Vietnam War, peace, the Beatles, long hair (mine came in the form of a ponytail that went halfway down my back), protest, and rebellion. I was concerned with, and confused about, the meaning and purpose of life—others' and mine. I became a philosophy major, somehow hoping that somebody had figured out the meaning of life and had written it down for people like me. Physical science didn't seem relevant to my pursuit—literature, psychology, sociology, history, and poetry did. So I studied humanities and never gave a career in medicine a thought.

Science, however, was a requirement for college graduation. So I signed up, begrudgingly and fearfully. I was surprised to find myself fascinated and enthused with what I was learning. I realized how little I knew about the empirical world, and I found myself studying things that were known rather than just thought or believed. It added a new perspective about life—one I didn't want to abandon.

I wasn't sure how I was going to combine enthusiasm for science with my study of the humanities. Then one day, during a discussion with a classmate who was pre-med, it came to me—medicine is both an art and a science. It deals with the ethical and the empirical, the mind and the body, the person as a social and physical being. It requires empathy and understanding as well as the application of scientific principles. Medicine is about making a difference by helping and serving others, and I thought it might offer me the chance to find the meaning and purpose in life I was seeking. I certainly didn't understand at the time that what had prepared me most for a life in medicine was not a particular course, some special knowledge or specific set of skills, but rather a thoughtful examination of life itself.

I was thrilled when I got into medical school. I wasn't at all sure that I would. There is always that fear that once you've decided what you want, you won't get it. And ringing in my ears, at least as I remember it, is the raspy voice of that organic chemistry professor who, on the first day, looked around at the class of about 500 and said: "Look to your left, look to your right. Only one of you will get into medical school." The guy on my left looked like Einstein, and the guy on my right looked like Galileo. What chance did I have?

Well, I don't know what happened to "Einstein" or "Galileo," but I did get into medical school. And it was every bit as amazing as

I had imagined. I never felt as young, arrogant, handsome, or kind as the doctors I remembered from television, but my medical school experiences matched the drama of TV step for step. I never knew it was possible to feel so excited, sad, afraid, overwhelmed, astounded, disappointed, nauseated, lightheaded, embarrassed, or tired. (I could actually recount a story for each of these adjectives, if only time permitted.) But mostly it was about the privilege of getting to know patients, hearing their stories, examining their bodies and their lives, and learning about how their illness had affected them. It was about sharing knowledge, providing treatment, and offering hope. For me, the experience of caring for patients during medical school was powerful, meaningful, and moving.

When it came time to choose a specialty, I was indeed torn. I loved caring for patients, and there are so many wonderful and satisfying ways to do it. Internal medicine is fascinating, surgery is a blast, and delivering a baby is off-the-charts exhilarating. But in the end it was the relationship with patients that prevailed, the wish to spend as much time with them as possible, to hear their stories in detail, to wonder along with them about their lives. And those earliest longings to combine science with the humanities, to think about the mental and the physical, the person and the illness all seemed to come together in the study and practice of psychiatry.

So, what do psychiatrists actually do? How do we spend our time? What is the day like? Psychiatry is a very broad field that allows physicians to choose among a variety of activities. What all psychiatrists have in common is an interest in mental illness—those conditions that affect the way people think, feel, and behave. This includes mood disorders such as depression and mania, psychotic disorders such as schizophrenia, anxiety disorders such as panic and phobias, and addiction disorders such as alcoholism and drug abuse. Some psychiatrists specialize in disorders of children such as autism, while others specialize in disorders of the elderly such as Alzheimer's disease. These various psychiatric illnesses can interfere with a person's ability to assess reality, communicate clearly, behave appropriately, and relate meaningfully. They can rob a person of their sense of self, their enjoyment of life, and their ability to function day-to-day.

Here's what psychiatrists in practice do. Like all doctors, we make diagnoses by taking a history, doing a physical exam, and applying information from diagnostic studies such as laboratory tests and imaging scans. We also do a specialized mental status examination to assess in detail such things as thinking, cognition, mood, and behavior. We see a wide range of patients and offer many different kinds of treatments. Suicidal patients might have to be admitted to and treated in a hospital to prevent self-harm. Psychotic patients might need antipsychotic medication to help them think more clearly. Drug-addicted patients might need a medical detoxification to prevent seizures and other withdrawal symptoms. And depressed patients might need not only antidepressant medications to help improve their mood but also psychotherapy to help them better understand and cope with their illness and life circumstances. But no matter what the clinical situation, psychiatry is always about the relationship with the patient, about effective communication, about listening patiently and carefully, and about trying to understand the patient's circumstances and experiences.

Of course, some psychiatrists spend their time doing basic science or clinical research. They want to understand what causes mental illnesses, figure out why some people have them, and develop the best possible treatments. These psychiatrists might be neuroscientists studying the structure and function of the brain or geneticists studying genes, chromosomes, and familial transmission. They might be pharmacologists studying the mechanisms of drug actions in order to develop new medications. Clinical researchers might be testing or comparing the efficacy of a variety of treatment interventions through medication and psychotherapy trials. Still others might be thinking, developing, and writing about theories of the mind in order to help us better understand psychological and social factors, the impact of life experiences, and the role of the environment in human development.

Finally, where do psychiatrists actually work? The same places all doctors work. In private offices, hospitals, clinics, emergency rooms, nursing homes, laboratories, and medical schools. We spend our time trying to understand how patients become the people they are, how they relate to others, and how they cope with life's stresses. We want to know how and why they developed a psychiatric illness and how we can be most helpful in their treatment and recovery. This is important, especially because in a single year more than fifty million adults and children experience a diagnosable mental illness, many of which are quite disabling. And there is good news. The stigma of mental illness appears to be lessening, and treatment success continues to improve. As a psychiatrist, I can now offer treatments to my patients with an efficacy equal to or exceeding those of many common medical illnesses.

How do you prepare to become a psychiatrist? First, you prepare to become a doctor, the best one you can be. That means learning as much as you can in college about life—history, literature, philosophy, music, drama, science—anything that enthralls you and widens your perspective. And it means involving yourself in activities that demonstrate your willingness to give of yourself to serve others. The premedical requirements needed for your application to medical school will ensure that you have an adequate foundation in the basic sciences, and that you have the capacity to understand, and learn, basic, and then increasingly complex, scientific facts and concepts.

Sure, you have to be a good student and get good grades. But you don't have to be the best student there ever was or be perfect at everything you do. Just show that you can study hard, learn effectively, and persevere when challenged. And remember that being smart is necessary, but not sufficient. Show that in your life and in your relationships with others you try to be a thoughtful, kind, and caring person.

With these skills and attributes you will enter medical school, and you will build on them as your preparation for becoming a doctor continues. Then, if you are curious about people, have a willingness to listen carefully and thoughtfully to the stories of others, have an interest in patients with psychiatric illness, and have a fascination with how the brain and mind work, you will be as prepared for a career in psychiatry as you ever need to be.

STEVEN**WOLFSON**

A Cardiologist
Character Counts

A career in medicine is a lot like life. It includes good and bad, joy and sorrow, friends and enemies, known and unknown, connection and isolation. Much of the profession depends on preparation and skill, and much is out of our control altogether. We must rely on ourselves alone, and we must leave much to God. We seek self-fulfillment through service to others. We are at once supremely proud to the point of arrogance and the most humble of laborers. At times, our power seems limitless, and then we face our limits.

Modern parlance defines us as "providers" of health care. But we also belong to a priesthood as bearers of a tradition, a body of knowledge, and power. We are authorized by society to levy pain, to do harm, to injure, so that those who trust us may have less pain, less injury, and more life.

Our training is narrow and focused, and removes us from the world. But we bring to our work all we have, and we must remain in the world to function. If we know history, we are better doctors. If we can hear music, we are better doctors. If we have studied philosophy, we can deal with life and death. If we are mature, we can support others. If we are wise, we can heal. If we are connected, loving family members, then we can lean on our family in bad times. We can leave them when the beeper rings, secure that we will be there for them as well.

During my interview for medical school, I was asked for my favorite reading at that time. I replied that the essays of Miguel de Montaigne entranced me. The rest of the interview was a joyous acknowledgment of shared interest. All three of the interviewers had read and appreciated this sixteenth-century philosopher whose travail with painful kidney stones formed the basis of his approach to life. He was once a patron saint of physicians, I learned.

The best preparation for medical school is to acquire the best education possible. The broader our knowledge of this world, the better we can understand our patients and the lives they lead. The more we bring to medicine, the more we can contribute. If we understand ourselves, we can understand others. If we are secure, others can rely on us. If we are able to call for help, we can hear others call. If we can cry, we can comfort. If we know languages, and can listen and communicate, we can care for patients.

Self-knowledge, though, is perhaps the most critical tool a physician can acquire. What level of fatigue limits your ability to function? When have you reached the limits of your knowledge and ability? Can you call for help? Do you know how to tell if a coworker is trustworthy? Can you delegate responsibility? Can you work in tandem with those in charge? Can you work with your peers? Are you generous and courteous to those whom you employ, or those over whom you have authority? Can you recognize, and deal with, failure? These skills are as crucial as the pages we have memorized and the tests we have passed. We have all known people who are "often wrong, but never in doubt." They are dangerous.

The best doctors I have known have been good people who are evolved as individuals and good citizens. One, an ophthalmologic surgeon, has had a sustained interest in government. He turned this interest into a commitment to organized medicine, and to the difficult and challenging effort of bringing the legitimate concerns of physicians to the attention of state and federal legislators. To many of our well-intentioned elected representatives, this surgeon is the dignified, informed, persuasive face and voice of medicine. Another, a general surgeon, was long known for his humanistic approach to his patients as well as for his superlative skill in the operating room. Friends of mine, entrusting their son to his care, remember most of all the picture of their terrified boy falling asleep on the shoulder of this kind surgeon as he carried the boy into the operating room. That the boy subsequently recovered fully was the most important factor, but that he was cared for and loved while doing so was memorable. This sensitive surgeon began writing about his work and his patients and eventually retired from surgery to pursue a distinguished career as a writer. One of the most respected internists in our community is justly famed for his attention to detail and for comprehensive care of his patients. He is also known for his encyclopedic knowledge of classical music. We shared in the care of one marvelous man upon whom the fates imposed a terrible burden of disease, pain, and disability. I learned along the way that my colleague spent hours at our patient's home playing computer games with this gallant man. A gynecologist in our town has published poetry dealing with the joys and sorrows he and his patients have shared, and uses this poetry to show his patients that others have walked the path life has set for them.

I am a cardiologist, but I majored in history in college. My major has served me well in dealing with the changes society has imposed on the practice of medicine. In dealing with individual patients, my medical texts have helped me, but so have the jokes I have learned, the illnesses my family and I have encountered, and the life I have led. Last week, a patient called with a serious problem: his phone service was about to be turned off for failure to pay a bill. This would seem an economic matter. He has had several heart attacks, the last punctuated by cardiac arrest. If this man had no access to a 911 service, it might well be, as well, a death sentence. Calls to our local phone company brought no response. But a call to the office of our state congressional representative resulted in restoration of his phone service before the end of the day.

My advice is to seek the broadest education possible before joining the medical profession. The more tools you bring with you, the better tool you will be. In an era when technology is driving the future of medicine, training in the sciences is crucial grounding, and knowledge of informatics and information systems is an enabling act. But alone these disciplines will not help you understand your patients or yourself. A narrow, overly focused approach can lead to frustration and a waste of good training. Failure to understand your patient will lead you to miss crucial information in taking a medical history. Inability to communicate with patients will cause them to make mistakes in taking medications. Or they will mistrust you, which will lead them to abandon your diagnostic program or therapeutic regimen.

And there will come a time when you may want to retire. The interests you have developed will ensure that you continue your connection to life. And this connection will enable you to continue to be of use as a colleague, advisor, and friend.

GERARDN.BURROW

A Former Medical School Dean
Learning in the Twenty-First Century

I f you are reading this book, you may be interested in becoming a physician or at least you're seriously considering the possibility. Having read articles about doctors giving up their medical practice in disgust and patients complaining about the medical care they receive, you may be experiencing legitimate concern about the turmoil surrounding managed care and the practice of medicine. Should you really want to spend a minimum of twelve years after high school preparing to enter a profession that is so unsettled? My short answer is: if you find it is right for you, then absolutely!

There has probably never been a more exciting time to become a physician. Advances in cellular and molecular biology, the sequencing of the human genome, the explosion in neuroscience, and the computer age are causing a revolution in clinical medicine. While the science that forms the basis of health care is exploding, however, the system that delivers health care in the United States is imploding. The scientific basis of medicine and the way that medicine is practiced will change dramatically over the next twenty-five years, and these changes will occur in a world very different from the one we know today. By 2025, the earth will contain a population of 8.5 billion people, compared to about 6.0 billion today, and 95 percent of the population increase will occur in developing countries. As a result, the global burden of disease will increase and have direct effects on the population of the United States.

How should you prepare yourself to practice medicine in a health care system that can't be envisioned on a scientific base that can't be imagined? Tomorrow's physician needs to be flexible and able to adapt to the profound changes that are occurring in medicine. What is needed is a "liberal arts" physician, one who has been educated in the best university tradition. Educating intellectually curious physicians who are able to respond to new challenges is what schools of medicine do well.

Seventy-five years ago, Dean Milton C. Winternitz instituted the "Yale system" of medical education, in which medical students were allowed tremendous freedom to learn without the pressure of constant examinations. With ready access to faculty help, students assumed responsibility for their medical education but were free to pursue medical interests beyond their immediate course work. This system of medical education, with minor modifications, has persisted to the present day. The lack of external pressure results in "happier" medical students who become deeply involved in areas of interest ranging from basic laboratory research to health policy. A required thesis is an integral part of the system that fosters these interests. The thesis requirement also enables students to learn to appraise the medical literature critically, a skill that greatly helps individuals who will enter clinical practice. The physician in practice must decide whether the latest advance published in a medical journal is truly going to be helpful to his or her patients.

As good as this system may be, medical education cannot remain static but must change to accommodate the new era. Today's students learn medicine essentially as they did seventy-five years ago when Winternitz instituted the Yale system of medical education. The amount of material to be mastered, however, has increased exponentially since then and is overwhelming. Lloyd H. Smith, a leading medical educator, commented in the Alan Gregg Memorial Lecture (*Journal of Medical Education,* 1985) that, "Our students should be freed of the stupefying effects of fact engorgement which threatens to convert them into floppy disks encoded for our present ignorance." Medical students need to acquire a core of basic information equivalent to the multiplication tables in elementary school. The medical faculty needs to provide a conceptual framework on which students can integrate the acquired facts. With the information technology available, students have instant access to enormous amounts of information. They need to learn how to formulate the critical question to reach a clinical decision and then access the necessary information. Rapid growth of information technology along with access to the Internet makes long-distance learning completely feasible. The world's best teachers in any given field are now able to deliver a lecture that medical students could access whenever convenient.

If you enter medical school in the near future, you will be reaching the peak of your medical practice in about twenty-five years. With this background of issues in medical education in mind, you'll need to consider what clinical medicine will be like in 2025. Once we understand what causes heart disease and cancer, specific treatments will become available for these two leading causes of death. Better understanding of the immune system should lead to prevention and treatment of immunity-related diseases like rheumatoid arthritis. Although faced with a challenging task, research scientists will develop vaccines against viruses like the one that causes AIDS.

With increased understanding of the genome, physicians will be able to predict whether their patients are likely to develop a disease for which there is no specific cure. Important ethical questions will arise. Who should be tested, and who should have access to the information? Physicians will play a role in these decisions, and medical students need to be prepared. One of the great medical advances of the past century has been the eradication in the general population of the virus small pox. This deadly virus exists now only in microbiology laboratories and is a threat only if terrorists use it as a weapon. We all expected that tuberculosis would likewise be eliminated, but inadequate public health practices have made it more virulent than ever. Although people predicted at one time that infectious diseases would be a scourge of the past, new and emerging infections appear to be with us for the foreseeable future.

An issue of major interest is whether "aging" can be arrested. Despite incredibly exciting medical advances, the human body will probably wear out rather than become immortal. Although there has been a significant change in life expectancy, there has been little change in individuals living much past 100, and the increase in life expectancy has been mostly due to a decrease in childhood mortality.

The fastest growing group in North America is over 85 years old. This group is increasing at a rate three times the population at large. Medical schools have taught that death is pathological and part of a disease process, thus implying that eradicating disease would eliminate death. How much health care is enough is one of the most significant questions to answer over the next twenty-five years. Technology is available that can delay death almost indefinitely without prolonging meaningful life. Dealing with this issue is and will be an important facet of medical education. Medical schools have the responsibility to educate physicians so that they will understand the difference between sustaining meaningful life and delaying death.

Solutions to the problems of aging will also have implications for the health care system at large. Rising costs in health care have made hospitalization an increasingly undesirable option unless the patient is simply too ill to be managed in an outpatient setting. With the aging of the population, hospitals are gradually becoming geriatric intensive care centers. Managed care as it is now constituted is not acceptable. Optimal medical care is cost-effective care, but what is being "managed" currently is cost, not care. Patients are unhappy; doctors are unhappy, and the payers are unhappy because costs are rising. There are more Americans without health insurance than ever before. The United States cannot continue to have one in every five citizens lacking access to health care except on an emergency basis. Americans must have access to health care other than through an emergency room. Health care companies are ridding themselves of managed care programs for Medicare patients while the population continues to age. Some form of universal health care appears inevitable, whether controlled by the government or by a consortium of insurance companies.

Solving these complex issues will require the participation of physicians who are leaders. What the leading medical schools do well is to prepare medical students to become future leaders, to develop into physicians of the highest quality who will be comfortable with the changes they will encounter. A number of years ago, Dean Vernon Lippard described the Yale medical school and its objectives in his speech entitled "The Yale School of Medicine in the Twentieth Century." Dean Lippard's words are equally applicable to the twenty-first century: "Our objective, however, remains perfectly clear—the maintenance and cultivation of a community of scholars who, at various levels of maturity are learning together. In such an atmosphere, good physicians will be educated, and the frontiers of science and medicine will be advanced for the benefit of all of mankind. This is an effort worthy of a great university."

I can't imagine a more rewarding and satisfying career, nor could there be a better time to enter the medical profession!

PART THREE

Training to Become a Doctor

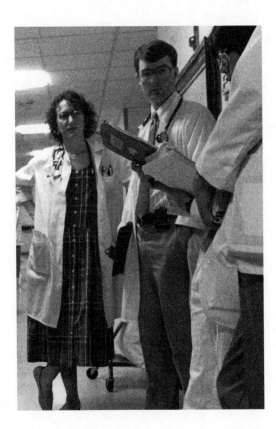

Medical School

If your preparations for applying to medical school have been diligent and coherent, you're likely to find yourself entering the completely new world that is medical school. Herbert Chase, Yale's deputy dean for education, discusses the directions medical school curricula will take during the twenty-first century. Although the fundamentals of medical training have barely changed in the past fifty to one hundred years, the complexities of the profession have increased so rapidly that the curriculum can no longer stand still. It is impossible to capture what this arena is like, but we can sample a few perspectives.

Julie Cantor, a first-year student who has just completed law school, writes about her early encounters with the preclinical sciences. D. A. Ross, in his second year and committed to obtaining an M.D./Ph.D. on his way to a research career, describes his interest in neuroscience and his desire to integrate this interest with his future role as a physician. A third-year student, Dena Rifkin, working on the wards for the first time, tells us how it feels to be directly involved in medical care. These students chose medicine for distinctly different reasons and decided on very different paths to get there. Yet all three convey the exhilarating nature of their medical school environment. For them, medical school has become a transforming event.

Teaching in medical school, particularly in the clinical years, differs greatly from the kind of teaching one finds on most college campuses. Peggy Bia and Frank Bia, a married pair of award-winning teachers, describe what it takes to teach medical students, and the rewards and frustrations of their efforts.

Nancy R. Angoff, Yale's associate dean of student affairs, residency programs, not only gives her view of today's medical students, but she also describes the unusual path she took to become a medical student and how she found her present position.

Residency and Graduate Study

A major problem with constructing a curriculum for medical students is that educators continue to assume that the goal of medical school is to produce independent physicians who can take complete care of patients. Although technically true, this assumption bears little relation to reality. Today's medical school graduates would find it virtually impossible to join a private practice, be appointed to the medical staff of a clinic, or independently care for patients in a hospital without considerable additional clinical training. A year of internship may be all that is required to obtain a license to practice medicine, but practically speaking such a license merely entitles a medical school graduate to perform limited duties under supervision in an approved medical center. Realistically, one must spend at least three years after medical school in clinical training to qualify as an independent practitioner.

To provide an idea of what this additional training involves, we have included essays by the director of residency training at Yale-New Haven Hospital, two residents, and two postdoctoral fellows. Rosemarie Fisher addresses the complex issue of whether residency should be regarded as a job or an educational experience. Fisher also considers a question that often worries medical students, residents, and attending physicians: do the rigors and long hours of residency training harden young physicians and make them less humane? Most physicians, of course, think of themselves as compassionate caregivers with an excellent bedside manner. Yet the public and patients alike believe that today's physicians are less empathic, and more impersonal, than their predecessors were. Moreover, medical students consistently attribute the bitter impersonal attitudes observed in residents to the wearying, stressful, and sleepless hours of work they must endure.

Essays by two current residents, though, reflect little or no bitterness about residency training. Although familiar with the hardships of their training, both Bobby Kapur and Mikhail Kosiborod express considerable enthusiasm for the skills and expertise they have developed and describe the empathy they feel for the patients they have encountered.

Many medical specialties require training beyond the usual three years of residency. This training is provided through fellowships funded by teaching hospitals for training that is primarily clinical, and by the National Institutes of Health or by private foundations for fellowships that primarily involve research training. If your goal is a career in academic medicine, research training and experience are mandatory. The nature of the training can involve patient-centered investigations such as those described by Julie Rothstein Rosenbaum, who looks forward to a career of teaching and research in the field of general internal medicine. In contrast, Jonathan A. Dranoff, who intends to specialize in gastroenterology, depicts what it is like to train to become a biomedical laboratory investigator. Training after medical school is long, arduous, and at times wearying, but most people who have been through it remember it fondly as a special time indeed.

HERBERT**CHASE**

An Overview of Medical School Education

The goal of a medical school is to create a rich learning environment where students can master the knowledge and develop the skills and attitudes of a caring and informed physician. The format and mechanisms used to achieve this goal differ among schools, as does their primary mission. Some schools are committed to training primary care physicians who will directly serve the community, whereas others foster development of scientific leadership.

No matter what the ultimate mission of a medical school may be, however, its students must become equally versed in the art and science of medicine. Before the current modern era of molecular medicine, the art prevailed; there was little to do for patients whose illnesses were not understood and for whom no reliable treatment existed. The pendulum has reversed in the modern era, where the explosion of molecular understanding and pharmacological and technological interventions often trivialize the art of caring for patients. Time and time again, however, we have learned from patients that they are healed by physicians who have mastered both the art and the science. A modern medical curriculum must include both.

A typical medical curriculum spans four years of training and is usually configured into a two-year preclinical and a two-year clinical curriculum. During the preclinical experience, students spend most of their time learning the language and basic principles of biology in health and disease. Although the actual format that provides the opportunity to master the body of modern medical information differs widely, the overall goal is the same.

The format by which the knowledge is mastered differs from one school to the next. At opposite ends of the spectrum are the traditional approach and the problem-based approach. The goal of both approaches is to enable the student to master a core curriculum. In the traditional approach faculties define and deliver the curriculum, whereas in a problem-based approach students construct the core curriculum on their own using clinical cases to guide their studies. Both approaches have many pros and cons. The traditional approach may be complete but is often overloaded, redundant, and at times irrelevant. The problem-based approach is always relevant but is usually incomplete. Despite the weaknesses of each approach, most authorities agree that they both get the job done.

Learning the art of medicine also formally begins during the preclinical years with activities that prepare students for their ultimate clinical role. During this time they learn the skills of clinical practice: interacting with and effectively communicating with patients, taking a history of a patient's illness, performing a competent physical examination, and communicating their findings to other physicians. They begin to develop the attitudes of physicians, such as their deep commitment to their patients, profession, and society.

During the clinical years, students are exposed to the activities and practices of the major specialties—internal medicine, surgery, pediatrics, obstetrics and gynecology, psychiatry, and neurology—as well as a number of surgical subspecialties such as neurosurgery and urology. During these so-called clerkships students attain the knowledge of the basic illnesses typical of that specialty. They also learn the skills necessary to become an effective and understanding caregiver.

During their time on each specialty, students finally assume the role of a physician-in-training and serve as an apprentice. The venues for clinical training should include both the hospital and doctors' offices. For most of the twentieth century the hospital was the major location of the apprenticeship, and it still is. There, students shadow the interns and residents from early morning into the evening, learning the procedures and mastering the skills that are required to provide care. Students also participate in "rounds," where the attending physician who is a member of the faculty meets with a "team" of interns, residents, and students to discuss the diagnosis and management of patients assigned to the team. Students also meet separately with faculty preceptors several times during the week to discuss aspects of their patients' care in greater depth than can be achieved during rounds. Students now spend anywhere from eight to twelve weeks in "outpatient settings," including doctors' private offices, where they see patients and are mentored closely by the faculty. Here the students see how medicine is really practiced in situations where a physician must not only focus on the patient's illness but also make sound decisions that are influenced by the patient's support network, home and employment situation, and financial circumstances.

An essential component of any typical four-year medical curriculum is the possibility of enrolling in clinical electives. Students choose from a panoply of activities and sometimes travel to far reaches of the world to observe medical care under different political, economic, and cultural influences. The elective experience has several purposes, not the least of which is to identify which specialty the student is interested in pursuing after graduation. An elective can solidify or dissolve a student's resolve to enter a particular specialty. Electives are also an opportunity to hone the doctoring skills only recently attained during the previous clerkship year. Electives can serve a practical purpose as well by allowing students to travel to other medical centers where they might want to go for their residency training. Students who subsequently apply to an institution where they are already well known are more likely, if their performance warrants it, to receive favorable consideration from the committee that selects students to become interns and residents.

Many schools have recently instituted various classroom activities for fourth-year students, the purpose of which is to revisit the basic sciences after a year and a half of clinical experience. The precise formats differ from school to school, but the overall goal is the same: to reinforce the dependence of clinical practice on knowledge of basic science. Students usually consider cases of patients with particular diseases and review an up-to-date summary of scientific breakthroughs that bear on the patients' diagnosis and management.

Certain thematic threads should weave their way through all years of the medical school program. These include medical decision making, a patient-centered approach, public health, professional responsibility, and the use of information technology.

Medical decision making is a theme that has only recently begun to be developed and implemented. The simultaneous revolutions in biomedical understanding, information technologies, and managed care have created the need to train physicians to be critical thinkers. Although physicians have throughout their history "thought critically," the complexity of the modern world has made no clinical decision simple. In fact, the flow of information through the Internet threatens to inundate the physician rather than clarify the path to be taken. A central task is identifying which information should become part of the base of knowledge that a medical student should learn.

The assessment and analysis of information, and its application to patient care, should be part of a medical decision-making curriculum. In the preclinical years such an activity as a seminar or journal club should provide students with an opportunity to master the skills of scientific reasoning and thus become proficient in assessing the quality of information. Having mastered scientific reasoning, students can enter the clinical years and learn clinical reasoning, which involves the appropriate application of accepted evidence. This is the first step in practicing evidence-based medicine, which allows physicians to use the best available evidence to guide their patients' therapies.

Another theme in a medical curriculum that should be reinforced throughout the four years is a patient-centered approach. The explosion of biomedical information, while providing explicit details of health and disease, runs the risk of pulling the patient apart so that an individual physician becomes comfortable with an ever-diminishing portion of the patient. Although deconstruction is a pedagogical strategy for teachers as well as a learning strategy for students, there must be a reconstruction of the patient before the student leaves medical school. This is best accomplished during interdepartmental clinical activities, such as a women's health clerkship or a geriatric clerkship where students can attend to all the needs of the patient, no matter what discipline is involved. The student will ideally feel comfortable caring for all the patients' needs, even though these needs may fall out of the range of the student's immediate expertise.

The health of the public is another crucial theme. Physicians must concern themselves with society at large and be attuned to issues of public health. Most medical schools have courses during the first two years in epidemiology and public health that examine the basic principles of the health and behavior of populations. Mastery of these principles is ultimately required to analyze and assess the clinical studies that guide evidence-based medicine. Also germane is exploration of the potential conflicts a physician faces when the rights of an individual patient place an entire population at risk.

Professional responsibility has become another subject that warrants continuous attention throughout medical school. The practice of medicine has always been influenced by ethical and legal considerations. Yet recent developments have increased the complexity of taking these issues into account when making medical decisions. Managed care and the development of expensive therapeutic interventions have made rationing of medical care in the United States a coldhearted reality. Conflicts of interests are far more widespread now that the pharmaceutical industry and academe have married in order to carry out clinical trials of new pharmacological agents. Physicians on the payroll of a drug company are unrealistically expected to be objective when caring for patients who are taking drugs that the company makes. With the rise of for-profit clinical trial organizations, the problem now involves community physicians in addition to those who staff academic institutions. Medical school curricula must create a forum for students to discuss these issues so that they will not only better serve their patients, but also become patient advocates.

Students need to use the tools of information technology throughout medical school. The explosion of medical knowledge and maturation of information technologies have made it mandatory for physicians to master the skill of obtaining information via electronic libraries. In the practice of medicine, it is said, you're only as good as what you know. The modern physician is able to access vast databases and useful searching programs to diagnose and treat patients. Skill at these activities does not usually come naturally, even for those who grew up on video games and Napster. A modern medical school must not only teach information technology but also ensure that the curriculum and its delivery are electronic whenever appropriate. Students spending time in a practitioner's office during a primary care experience should have access to an electronic portal linked to the school's curriculum.

A curriculum must never stand still! During the twentieth century medical students received their education from physicians who had acquired a similar, if not identical, education. The teaching faculty practiced medicine in a manner that was largely unchanged from that of the previous generation and one that the current students could expect to replicate when they went into practice. As the twenty-first century unfolds, however, students can expect to enter a world that is completely unfamiliar to their teachers: a postgenome, biotech, managed care, gene-chip, dot.com Internet era. Genetics, genomics, and proteomics will occupy increasingly important places in all aspects of the curriculum.

A medical curriculum, now more than ever before, must be continuously evolving. As the rate of discovery accelerates, so must the pace of curricular reform. Medical schools should go through "major curricular revisions" every five to ten years.

In conclusion, patients are best served when those who take care of them are informed, sensitive, caring, and objective physicians who are lifelong learners. Today's premedical students will be most apt to provide that care if they are enrolled in medical schools that give students the opportunity to master both the art and science of patient care.

JULIE**CANTOR**

Beginning Medical School

Time was, I could do science in my sleep. But by the time I slipped on my short white coat, months had passed since I had thought about metabolic cycles or biochemical pathways or anything remotely having to do with equations. Rather, I had spent my academic energy during the past three years studying, of all things, contracts, torts, and constitutional law. I came to medicine via an unlikely route: law school.

Before that, in what became a season of LSATs, MCATs, and personal statements, I had simultaneously applied to both professional schools. I was drawn to that place where law and medicine converge—a place where we ask if patients have a right to die, if parents can refuse to have their premature baby resuscitated, if physician training should be reformed.

Odd as my route may seem, nontraditional paths to medicine are not so unusual these days. Three lawyers took anatomy this year, and at least four law school students have nearly or completely finished their medical training. And no fewer than four medical students have approached me with questions about applying to law school. Rounding out the first-year class at the medical school are a handful of writers, a peace corps volunteer, a semiprofessional musician, more than a few scientists, and a nurse. Clearly, what admissions experts say about becoming a doctor is true: many paths may lead to medical school.

I am often asked which I liked more, medical school or law school. Perhaps predictably, I respond that they are completely different. A mundane observation: my medical school class is less than half the size of its law school equivalent. On a more theoretical level, the two thought processes operate within entirely different frameworks. Legal analysis teases out shades of gray. It employs arguments that persuade and rhetoric that inspires. Winners and losers may emerge, but rarely are there a right and a wrong. And the outcomes of court battles and policy decisions are not always fair or even just. Medicine is more absolute. Lab values are elevated, or not.

I suppose that this is one similarity between the two professions: the outcomes are not always fair. Cancer, for example, can strike even those with the healthiest lifestyles. But medical students don't spend time discussing the policy behind cancer. Although we do have discussions, they center on facts that can be found in a textbook or a journal or on a web site. Inventing ideas out of whole cloth will not get you far in deciphering a disease or performing a procedure. In terms of the body of knowledge we are learning, you either know it or you don't. In law, by contrast, the rules are rarely ends in themselves, and making things up along the way is not necessarily problematic. Still, both fields ask their students to apply their factual knowledge creatively, whether through astute diagnosis and gentle bedside manner or through clever writing and impressive oral argument.

Perhaps a legal education is more useful to everyday life than a medical one, but some medical schools do encourage an education that is general and broad. Quite a few physician-slash-something types—physician/writers, physician/scientists, and physician/journalists—have spoken to my class about their careers. There are more opportunities to incorporate doctoring into a broader life experience than one might think.

Entering medical school marks a process of acculturation. In medicine, as in other fields, there are rituals and dress codes, specific ways to present information, even an unfamiliar language that is crucial to master. Everything is new, and everyone is at least a little uncertain. During the first year of medical school, students thank patients profusely for speaking with us about their illnesses or letting us examine them. We have little to offer them by way of medical skill or acumen, so their generosity becomes our learning opportunity.

Most strikingly, the classroom-based preclinical years of medical school mirror the process of learning a new language. We may have been exposed to the "CBC, chem 7, type-and-cross" lingo of television shows like *ER*, but otherwise we live in a world of relatively new vocabulary. We are told to practice our newly learned words and phrases on each other, but to the trained ear, the din we create must sound like that of preschoolers just learning to talk. We can hardly speak in full sentences; the language just isn't there.

From what I can tell, learning the basic sciences can range from an enjoyable process to a painful one, depending on the school you attend and on your own abilities. Certainly the information is the same, but it can be conveyed very differently. Some schools have weekly quizzes, complete with grades. Others have only a handful of tests and a pass-fail system. The key is to choose a program that complements your learning style and ups your odds of having an enjoyable preclinical experience. The Yale University School of Medicine, like many schools, values a progressive, independent-minded education. In recognition of different learning styles, the school minimizes in-class time, gives computers a pivotal role in anatomy and other courses, and uses a stress-reducing "pass now or pass later" grading system: if you fail, you take the test again until you pass. The system fosters collaboration rather than competition. A world without class ranking is a pleasant place to be. Still, students accustomed to the use of the stick instead of the carrot could be lulled into complacency.

The particulars of the teaching philosophy aside, I have felt some confusion over the preclinical material. How much detail do I need to know? That is perhaps the classic question of the medical student. The problem is that the answer varies. Those who have gone before me, from medical school friends to well-established practicing physicians, tend to de-emphasize the importance of knowing the details. "Big pictures!" they bellow. They say that I don't need to learn x fact, and that y biochemical pathway will be repeated eleven times, so if I forget ten times, I'll still be fine. Even budding surgeons have told me that they learned anatomy during a clinical rotation, not on a cadaver.

Others say to learn as much as you can, as fast as you can. It's a bit disconcerting. Wanting to minimize risk, I try to follow the "it's better to learn as much as you can now" school. I don't have the benefit of hindsight yet.

I do, however, have the benefit of time. And that is something that those who are further along in their training lack. The preclinical years, compared with life on the wards, hemorrhage time so much that I have time to think, sleep, exercise, and even teach an undergraduate seminar on reproduction, bioethics, and the law. I am anticipating those long hours on clinical rotations with some measure of anxiety and uncertainty. And I hear that free time becomes largely a memory during internship and residency.

So far, medical school has been a fine balance between learning the foundational material (dusting off all that science) and trying on the beginnings of doctoring. For me, this experience has done quite a bit to demystify the body, its diseases, and medicine itself. I am learning how to listen to patients, how to examine them, how to take their medical history. It has been empowering to realize that mastering medicine is less magic than tenacity.

For those contemplating a career in medicine, or one that incorporates medical training, I'd have to say that, at least in the beginning, the preclinical years are not as arduous as the war stories suggest. The material is manageable, even interesting. For the uncertain, it may be helpful to realize that a medical school education is more widely applicable than one might think. Today more than ever, physicians have career options from writing to law to journalism and, of course, to research and clinical medicine. There is even the opportunity, cliched though it may seem, to be useful, even to have an immediate impact on someone's life. And that's something even we lawyers would like.

D.A.**ROSS**

Choosing the M.D./Ph.D. Program

I never wanted to be a doctor. In fact, when I was growing up, about the only thing that felt certain about my future was that I didn't want to be a doctor. My father and both my older brothers were physicians. Both my grandfathers were doctors, as were five aunts and uncles. In "a nice Jewish family" (insert Yiddish accent here), becoming a doctor seemed a matter of destiny. Teachers always assumed that I was a premedical student, and when I came home from college on break, my family always asked when I was planning to take the MCAT (Medical College Admission Test). But somehow, this high-level Judeo-deductive logic was lost on me. And in spite of (or perhaps because of) all this familial pressure, I remained actively against the idea of a career in medicine. Frankly, I could not fathom how working with sick people all day could be fun.

Yet as much as I was disinterested in medicine, I had an innate and profound fascination for the complexity and diversity of life. I found myself taking course after course in organismal biology, ranging from entomology to herpetology and ichthyology to ornithology. I loved staring into a glass case of beetles and marveling at extraordinarily subtle nuances that distinguished the different species. I loved dissecting families of amphibians and reptiles and teasing apart the structural differences that adapted them to their unique niches. But, more than anything else, I loved looking at diverse ecosystems and trying to understand and explore the "big" questions: What forces had shaped the evolution of a given system? How was it that one form of life happened to have been favored over a myriad of others?

The summer before my senior year in high school, as I started to consider seriously the possibility of a career in environmental biology, I accepted what sounded like the dream internship in field biology: I was going to be paid lots of money to go somewhere exotic and study the reproductive biology of mountain quail. To top it off, a large part of the summer would be spent raising my own flock of baby quail (which are, objectively speaking, completely adorable). But despite this seemingly ideal setup, the experience was a disappointment. Whereas I was initially drawn to environmental biology by the "big" questions, the project I worked on was beset by the smallest and most mundane details. I found myself spending eight hours a day weighing and measuring quail eggs, then holding each one in front of a light bulb and measuring the volume of the air sac. Much as I loved biology, there was nothing I loved about this research. And they made me kill cute baby quail. So as I left for college, I once again found myself with no sense of what I wanted to do with my life.

Conveniently, I found Yale to be the perfect place for an under-graduate with no career direction. With almost an infinite number of opportunities to learn, in both academic settings and extracurricular activities, it was an ideal venue for trying something new, improving on something old, or simply broadening my horizons. At the beginning of each semester I would flip through the course catalogue and select a list of ten or fifteen classes to "shop," planning on taking the five courses that I enjoyed the most. After narrowing the list down to seven or eight, I would invariably decide that they were all too good not to take, and with so little time before graduation it would be a shame to pass up any opportunity. Besides, with no thought of gradu-ate school in my future, why should I have any particular concern about grades? So what if I challenged myself with an extra course and got two Bs instead of one A?

In addition to a full course load, I also had the chance to begin studying music more seriously, after having treated it as a hobby for years. I started playing piano again, learned to play percussion and sousaphone in the marching band, and for the first time began taking voice lessons and singing in a small jazz ensemble. It was a wonderful time in my life, and music was taking on an integral role. With hindsight, it was inevitable that these two main interests of mine, science and music, would eventually intersect—the only question was how.

During my sophomore year, the director of my singing group was a woman with an extraordinary case of what I had heard referred to as "perfect pitch." Constantly, during rehearsals, she would turn to me with impossible instructions, asking me to hear things that I just couldn't hear ("Dave, you're a quarter step flat—can you come up to the B?" or "You need to be in major—not minor—sevenths with the sopranos"). Through all of these interactions I was continually struck by the fact that this person was fundamentally different from me. How was it that we could both listen to the same piece of music and yet have such radically different perceptions of what it was? How was it that she instinctively recognized a frequency that had no inherent meaning to me? At that point, I didn't even know what questions to ask, but I knew that I wanted to know more. So for the second time I headed off for a summer research internship. Knowing that I was unlikely to find something that directly matched my interest, I set out to find the next best thing.

I ended up at the Medical University of South Carolina studying how the brain processes language. My project was to design a paradigm for functional Magnetic Resonance Imaging (fMRI) that would allow us to locate language-processing regions in the brains of presurgical epilepsy patients. After learning that fMRI was a sort of magnetic magic trick that allowed researchers to visualize regions of heightened activity in the brain, I suddenly understood the allure of neurobiology. This was my epiphany. As much as consciousness and cognitive processing had always fascinated me, it had never occurred to me that they were immediately grounded in the circuitry of our brains. Now I found myself staring into a machine, a system of almost infinite complexity, and I became captivated by the idea of unraveling its inner mechanisms. Further, if functional MRI could be used to study how the brain processes language, surely it would be an equally viable tool for studying musical processing.

Meanwhile, as I became increasingly absorbed by the complexity of the brain's processing, I was also discovering that research doesn't necessarily take place in an isolated laboratory environment. In fact, the building that I worked in was a hospital, and the work that we did was almost entirely clinically motivated. Slowly, I came to realize that medicine wasn't always about the art of healing per se. Rather, it was also about the act of helping others, of reaching out to people in need and improving their quality of life, regardless of whether one could "cure" them. By the time I left South Carolina I was certain, for the first time, about what I wanted to do for the rest of my life. In the position of physician-researcher I saw the perfect synthesis of careers: the intellectual challenge of meaningful research and the opportunity to work with people and know that my work made a difference.

When I got back to Yale in the fall of my junior year, I redirected my studies and became absorbed in my new career path. As I started understanding neurobiology at the cellular level, everything shifted into focus. A year before, I had felt as though fields like biochemistry and molecular biology addressed biological minutia that undermined more interesting, broad-based fields of inquiry. Now I saw that they were essential tools for deciphering the complexity of organisms, and I understood that honing in on a single system opened more portals than I could have previously imagined.

At the same time, the interest that I gained in the classroom was immediately channeled back into research. After approaching the head of diagnostic radiology, I began working on a functional MRI study to determine simultaneously how the brain processes music and whether there are basic neurological differences between "normal" musicians and those with perfect pitch. Every day I went to lab and each day I enjoyed it more. By the time I graduated, we had completed three studies on musical processing in the brain. Rather than sating my appetite for answers, the work gave me an entirely new set of questions to ask. I was ready to begin working toward a Ph.D., to take these questions to a new level and explore new modalities for my inquiry.

In April of my junior year I took the MCAT, and that summer I began teaching for Kaplan (a test review service). Having personally been traumatized by the MCAT experience, I found it satisfying to help others through the test-taking process. At a deeper level, this was why I enjoyed teaching: rather than merely presenting material, it was about coaching, about establishing a personal relationship with students and reaching out to address their concerns. It was this personal dimension that made the job so fulfilling and the same factor that attracted me to medicine.

The medical school application process largely consumed my senior year of college. Regardless of one's qualifications, or how nonchalant one may be, applying to medical school is an extremely stressful endeavor. As someone accustomed to being in control of his life, I found it difficult to accept that I now had little control over my future. I have no idea how the average pre-med deals with this kind of pressure. Personally, I forced myself to adopt a sort of Zen approach: I had done the best I could—my MCAT was high, my GPA was relatively low—and there wasn't all that much that I could do to change things now. I accepted the process as a matchmaking ordeal, decided which schools would be good matches for me, and hoped that they would like me as well.

Since I had decided to apply to combined M.D./Ph.D. programs, most of my concerns about choosing a school revolved around the fact that I would be committing to be in one place for a long time (on average, it takes seven and a half years to complete both degrees). Location was important to me for overall quality of life (cross out Los Angeles, New York, and all of the South), and by this point in my life a noncompetitive environment was essential—I was going to medical school to learn, not to overburden myself with the stress of class rankings. Schools that had new, system-based, integrated curricula excited me, and finding a school with good opportunities for research in neuroscience was paramount. When the University of Rochester notified me of my acceptance early—in October instead of March—Yale was the only other school that I was still considering, and I pulled all other applications. I was excited about Rochester and would have been thrilled to attend. However, when I got into Yale several months later, it was impossible to turn down the cognitive neuroscience resources, as well as the opportunity to continue working in the same lab.

Contrary to popular mythology, my first year of medical school was not a nightmare. The basic science curriculum of the first year may be seen as a liberal arts education in human biology, and I loved delving into new material. Moreover, I discovered that a surprisingly large percentage of the material was information I had previously studied either as an undergraduate or in the course of my teaching—which left plenty of time to continue singing and to maintain an active social life.

I spent this past summer, following my first year in medical school, back in lab. I constantly feel like the movie character Shoeless Joe Jackson, as portrayed in *Field of Dreams,* wide eyed and in love, asking myself "Is this heaven?" It is impossible to describe the thrill of learning how to ask the "big" question and the intense satisfaction of developing the methods to answer it. With some regret I will return to medical school in September, setting aside for the moment the excitement of research. That is not to say that I don't look forward to continuing my medical education, but rather that I am highly motivated to begin work on my Ph.D. Eventually (if I ever graduate!), I hope to find a position in academic medicine where I can spend most of my time in research and continue helping others by practicing as a physician.

DENA**RIFKIN**

The First Clinical Year

I am neither a doctor nor a layperson. I can sometimes diagnose, occasionally treat, and rarely understand. Take a photograph of me now and you will see a person caught in the act of transformation: a girl trying on her mother's favorite dress or tromping around in high-heeled shoes three sizes too big. Though I don't always feel it, I am on the inside now, as I realize when I hear myself saying that someone has "syncoped" instead of "fainted" or had a "CVA" instead of a "stroke." But I'm still mostly an outsider, learning a new language and new rituals.

The third year in medical school is known in some places as the first clinical year, which means that for the first time in our book-bound lives my classmates and I will learn on the job instead of in the classroom. We spend the year caring for patients while moving from specialty to specialty: pediatrics, obstetrics, surgery, internal medicine, and psychiatry. It is a whirlwind tour through the hospital and its clinics, encompassing fields of medicine so different that I find it hard to believe that the basic training is the same for all.

I am glad to be on the wards, to have finished the often-dry basic-science part of medical education. I like the "hard" sciences—my undergraduate degree is in computer science—but I chose medicine so that I could work with people. And being on the wards means seeing people, sick people, every day.

Slowly I grow used to seeing sickness, to seeing faces as pale as the hospital pillows on which they rest. This is the first step in becoming a doctor, the statistical reality of working in a place where the illnesses and often the tragedy of life are concentrated. Cancer, car accidents, infection, congenital disease all become part of everyday life for me as I move through each ward of the hospital. This, I realize, is not "normal," in the everyday sense of normal I knew before clinical rotations began.

One thing you lose, immersed in the hospital for twelve months, is your sense of shock. I realized this the first time I saw someone die in the hospital. A woman we were caring for collapsed one morning just after we saw her on rounds. Of course, patients do not simply die in a hospital; instead, they "code," meaning that they stop breathing or their hearts stop beating and an alert is sounded. Emergency personnel come running, and vigorous resuscitation efforts ensue. I watched from the doorway as five or six doctors and that many nurses worked steadily for half an hour to restore a pulse. Finally the effort was called off, and we all drifted away from the woman, some staying to clean up needles and tubing from the floor. I felt sad but not surprised by this death, the first one I had ever seen, even though we had just told the woman she was healed and ready to go home. As we learned later, she had a massive, fatal blood clot in her lungs, killing her almost instantly. I ate breakfast just as I did each morning after rounds. After all, people die in the hospital, I thought. I am just one of the witnesses.

The clinical years of medical school are built around month-long "rotations" in different specialties; you may never be a psychiatrist or a pediatrician or a radiologist, but you catch a four-week glimpse of each of these lives during your clinical rotations. For one month of the year, I am a general surgeon. I enter into the ritual: the scrubbing followed by the gowning followed by the gloving. We move around the room with the sparseness and fluidity of a tribal dance, draping the patient with blue cloths, hovering over the table to assist the surgeon at his task. I spend hours staring into abdomens and pelvic cavities, at exposed kidneys and undulating bowels. Sometimes I meet the patient before surgery, sometimes after; sometimes I see the patient only in the operating room, open to the air. I am often bored, often uncomfortable, craning my neck to see or pulling steadily to retract the skin. Once we opened a patient's abdomen for a simple gallbladder removal and found cancer scattered like loose tea throughout. We closed her up again without touching anything, like children who have accidentally discovered something terrible in a forbidden closet. Another time we removed a colon tumor and the surgeon stretched her hand up to feel the liver. "Feel this," she said, taking my hand. I ran my fingers across the liver and felt a bump beneath my fingers. "Metastasis," said the surgeon, reading fates like Braille type beneath her touch.

I see people's lives saved by surgery. A woman came in delirious, vomiting. Her eyes had a strange glaze to them. The surgeon felt her abdomen once, twice. "Put your hand here," he said to me. I felt a tense something beneath my fingers. "Strangulated bowel," he said, and the next thing I knew we were in the operating room, looking at that same something with the overlying skin and muscle pulled away. The blood supply to a section of colon had been twisted off, and a foot or so of intestine was purple-black and swollen, about to rupture. We removed it, put the ends together, and sewed up the wound. The next morning I went to check on this woman who, without surgery, would not have lived through the night. We talked about her history research at Stanford, and I thought of her dark bowels, something only a few living people would ever see.

As I watch the bodies of other people fail them day by day, I begin to question my own. I do not yet have the practiced sense of distance or denial that older physicians seem to possess. I come home, go into the shower, and stare at my uninvaded abdomen, imagining its quiet dark organs performing effortlessly beneath the skin. I palpate for masses and tap out the shape of my liver. I caress the skin above my carotids, my thyroid, my sigmoid colon, and I revel in their internal balance, their unspoken loyalty. The next day, I know, I will return to the operating room and watch another unscarred abdomen yield up its secrets.

As a clinical student, I am assigned a few patients at a time to follow on a daily basis. I examine them, take a medical history, and talk to them about their dogs, their homes, and their families. This talk is probably the best thing I can offer now, although I can certainly look up their illnesses and bring journal articles about new treatments to the attention of the medical team, and I do. As I gain confidence and skill, I sometimes examine the patients and find things the residents did not have time to see—the greatest triumph available to a third-year student. One day, an elderly woman came to the emergency room with all the symptoms of a stroke: she could not respond to commands, and she did not speak or seem to hear our voices. I examined her, as the team tried to decide whether to treat her with an anticlotting agent, and I found soft yellow things blocking her ear canals. We removed what turned out to be her earplugs, and she turned in response to the sound of her name. It was my first cure.

There are so many simple cures, routine to the older doctors but miraculous to me. A child comes in with severe dehydration from diarrhea. A night of intravenous fluids and his once-sunken eyes are bright, his voice is strong, and he is playing happily in the hospital crib. A woman with pneumonia is given antibiotics and walks out the door in a few days. Even the vaccination clinic is amazing to me, a place where measles and mumps, diphtheria and rubella, are vanquished by a tiny needle stick.

Mostly, I am the person on the team with time to talk. I realize slowly that although I am often shy or afraid in the unfamiliar circumstances of the hospital, the patients are in far more need of comfort than I am. Sometimes the bedside table holds signs of a life outside this hospital: photographs, cards with uncertain purple lettering saying, "I LOVE YOU GRANDMA, COME HOME SOON." Sometimes patients have their own quilts or pajamas and the room fills with the hope of home. Sometimes they have nothing at all to distinguish them from each other except the location of their illness. We mix them up at morning rounds. Does Mr. Gerraro have the fever, or is it Mr. Frank? The residents cannot tell them apart. They call them by their diseased organs instead: "the liver in 5-A," "the pneumonia in 10-B," and so on.

They are all new to me, these illnesses, and I will remember these first patients I see. I have no regrets now about choosing medicine as a career, not with the daily excitement of seeing new things, the constant challenge of assessing problems I had encountered only in books and coming up with diagnoses. And ethical issues I had thought of in the abstract unexpectedly become urgent and practical. How will this patient obtain medication without insurance? What do we do if this fracture is from child abuse? Can an ex-wife make medical decisions for a comatose patient? How do we tell a patient that we accidentally damaged his bladder during the operation? Suddenly, the preclinical lessons concerning anatomy and physiology seem straightforward; there are no simple answers here.

Yet in a few years, repetition and sleepless nights will blur the patients for me. I watch the residents at work. They are there before I arrive at six in the morning, and when I leave at six or seven in the evening they are still there. Some of them seem rather hard. It's not a lack of caring but perhaps a lack of pity. They say bitter things about the patients, especially those who get sick at night. Any patient too demanding, too anxious, or too controlling of treatment is "difficult." I hear expressions like "circling the drain" used on rounds, in front of the patient, to describe what we think will be a slow but certain death. There are many such expressions, and many snickers exchanged. I know I am no better than they were when they started. I wonder what I will say when I am too tired to care.

PEGGY**BIA** and FRANK**BIA**

Teaching Medical Students

As we entered the medical profession and completed our training at the Yale University School of Medicine in the late 1970s, we were both wide-eyed and enthusiastic, filled with energy and a sense of calling. We had worked arduously, putting in many hours of studying and on-call training to get to our academic teaching positions, and we treasured the opportunity to serve in this way. At that time, the Yale faculty included several revered leaders in medicine whom we greatly admired, whose career paths we wanted to emulate, and whose high standards of medical practice we wanted to maintain.

During our first decade in academic medicine, as junior faculty members, we worked hard, but we also played hard. There were wonderful vacations on tropical islands as well as nights at the movies or at dinner parties with friends and colleagues. We also took several trips to work for a month or two at a time in developing countries. Those experiences taught us how to practice medicine in a challenging environment with limited resources. During those early years on the faculty we had much clinical responsibility, but we also tried to maintain active research pursuits. Eventually we gravitated toward roles with some clinical responsibilities but which allowed us to continue our research and to work closely with medical students, house officers (interns and residents), and fellows. One of us—Peggy—became a transplant nephrologist (a kidney specialist), and the other—Frank—specialized in general infectious diseases. Along with the many other jobs he performed to support his salary in academia, he remained most devoted to his first loves, tropical medicine and international health.

The phrase "supporting one's salary" bears explanation. In fact, within an academic institution the faculty are often accountable for finding the income to fund their salary. For this reason, an academic career often involves wearing many hats, with each job providing some salary support. A faculty member in a department of medicine, for example, might derive 25 percent salary support from a grant obtained from the American Diabetes Association to study some aspect of diabetes, in which case this function should take up about 25 percent of that physician's professional time. Other sources might include the income derived from seeing diabetic patients, directing a course for medical students in endocrinology, or administering a residency training program. This is a distinctly different situation from a private practice in which the income derived from providing patient care is used to run the office and to provide either an individual practitioner or a group with their income.

We have watched the landscape of medicine change around us, as people we admired moved on. We have become increasingly aware that the modus operandi in academic medicine, as in many other professions with long-standing traditions, is hierarchic and patriarchal. Changes result more often from power plays than from consensus. Some claim that the hierarchy of the medical profession is necessary so that those who are the most experienced control the difficult decision-making processes that involve the lives of patients. Yet a hierarchical system of authority, when carried to an extreme, makes it difficult for all members of a profession or a working group to contribute. Neither of us has a psychological style that readily accepts hierarchies, and we tend to react by trying to keep the playing field level whenever possible. On our daily rounds, we want a third-year medical student on a first clinical rotation to feel as comfortable offering suggestions as a senior resident.

Despite some disappointments, we chose to stay at Yale because of our great love for teaching. Some people might call it a gift; others might say it is a calling; still others might consider it an addiction. However one views it, there is no doubt that we have been seduced and fulfilled by the opportunity and privilege to teach the gifted students that come through the Yale School of Medicine.

Teaching medical students in their first two years of medical school can be very much like teaching college courses, which include seminars and even laboratories. But as each month of medical school passes, more of the teaching and learning experience becomes what has been referred to as a contact sport. Students must learn how to connect with patients, examine their bodies for signs of disease, and even deliver bad news. To learn these skills, one must work closely, often one-on-one, with experienced clinical faculty on the wards. By the time medical school comes to an end, teaching and learning at the bedside or in the clinic have come to supplant classroom learning, lectures, laboratory assignments, and seminars. In fields other than medicine, the typical graduate student aspiring to a Ph.D. degree begins to focus on the completion of a specific thesis project and the defense of that thesis before a faculty committee. The medical student moves in a different direction, working at the interface between science and patient care. Often the very students who did not excel in the classroom find themselves to be outstanding when interacting with patients on a daily basis. The opportunities we've had to teach at the bedside remain vibrant to this day, and they have sustained us through many hard times when other parts of our work lives have been less fulfilling. Largely for this reason we have remained strongly tied to the academic life. The ability to teach what we know, to model the high standards of practice, and to guide others toward priorities and goals that we feel are critically important—this is clearly a privilege.

We decided to have children later in life, after our careers were well established. The presence of children radically changed our sense of reality, especially for Peggy. No longer did the long hours at work seem as rewarding. The satisfaction of completing a project or a manuscript paled in comparison to the home life we were missing because of our commitments at work. We looked for opportunities to maintain our salary support without carrying the large clinical loads that kept us at work, especially on the weekends. We are tremendously grateful for the gifts that our children provide and view them not as sources of conflict between work and family but rather as opportunities to remind us of what is most important in life. Furthermore, we have discovered that many of the best skills of parenting are similar to the skills one must possess to be an understanding, compassionate physician. We have struggled with the time constraints imposed by full-time academic careers, family life, and changing job descriptions, and we still do not feel that we have achieved the correct balance. Life can be like a mobile hanging from the ceiling: when you move one element, the entire structure is affected.

In recent years, health care delivery has transformed itself into a business model in which the value of a physician is defined by the volume of patients seen, procedures performed, and money generated rather than by competence, compassion, and dedication to patient care. These changes in medicine have been devastating to clinicians like us whose lives could become dominated by paperwork, documentation, and a series of regulations created by administrators who know very little about the practice of medicine. Nevertheless, we continue to hope that a new life in medicine may evolve from the current chaos. This new life may be one where listening and compassion are appreciated as the essential components of clinical care. We also continue to hope for an evolution in our models for medical training—toward a model that recognizes teaching as a form of mentorship that must be respected and nurtured.

We find it helpful to be aware of the threads that connect each of us with our own predecessors in medicine. While we were students at Cornell Medical College in the turbulent late-1960s, we were fortunate to have been taught by one of the great figures in medical education, Benjamin H. Kean. He felt strongly that teaching medicine and doing it well was the most demanding of the performing arts. The response of his students proved him to have been successful, and many of us do what we do each day because of our connection to physicians like him.

Often we have asked ourselves whether, if we had to do it all over again, we would still enter the medical profession. Although each of us could have taken other paths, and although in recent years we have been disillusioned with many of the new values of academic medicine, we still believe that practicing medicine in an academic environment has been a fabulous opportunity. To be able to see patients, to serve, to teach what you do, and to receive a salary for doing so—it doesn't get any better.

To participate in this profession and in a medical school, it was necessary for us to master a body of scientific information and to learn how to apply it to the care of patients. Too often and too heavily emphasized, however, are the perceived certainty and security that the science provides. But we've learned from our patients that, as the poet Muriel Rukeyser writes, the universe, in all its breadth and depth, is not composed of atoms; it is made up of stories. This one is ours.

NANCY R. ANGOFF

Advising Medical Students

In September 1986, I walked across the metal seal in the floor of the library rotunda and heard the tap of my feet echoing up to the balcony. At the age of almost forty, I was on my way to the orientation for first-year Yale medical students, and I was in a state of disbelief that I had been admitted to Yale to learn the secrets of medicine.

My journey to the Yale University School of Medicine was an unusual one, a journey that for a long time I did not even know I was taking. I recall that when I was in the fifth grade and had completed a project on the human eye, I was fascinated with the human body, but it never occurred to me that I could become a doctor. As a girl growing up in the early 1960s, I was steered toward becoming a teacher, a dream my mother had had for herself. In college I met my future husband, Ron, and my roommate, Roslyn, both of whom intended to become physicians. I listened to them discuss the competitiveness of the pre-med program and chose instead the analysis of poetry and prose as an English major. My husband did become a physician, and I became a junior high school English teacher working to put him through medical school. During those years, I also got a master's degree in guidance and counseling, having no idea at the time that it would prepare me for becoming the associate dean for student affairs at Yale School of Medicine.

In July 1973 we arrived in New Haven, where Ron started his internship in pediatrics. One month later I gave birth to our first child, a daughter. A son followed three years later, at which point Ron had a fellowship in the psychological aspects of pediatrics. I was never satisfied with staying home, and I was a terrible housekeeper. I fantasized about becoming a doctor but felt I could not do it for a million reasons. Instead, I decided to get as close to medicine as I thought I could by learning about health care administration. Two years later I received a master's degree in public health from Yale and became the associate chair of the medical school's Human Investigation Committee. I had always been interested in medical ethics, and this position gave me an opportunity to learn more about informed consent in medicine and research and about the ethical principles that ground medical practice and medical decision making.

It was during a professional conference in Philadelphia that I had lunch with an attorney who asked me what I would do if I could do anything in the world. Without having to think for a second, I told her that I would be a doctor. She asked me why I didn't go into medicine. "I can't," I replied. "I'm too old, it costs too much money, I've got kids, and I've never taken a science course in my life." In response, she told me that I hadn't given her one real reason why I couldn't and that I wouldn't know that reason until I tried.

I went home that weekend and told my husband that I wanted to become a doctor. He looked at me and said, "I've always known that you wanted to be a doctor. You absolutely should do it." I spent the weekend crying, wondering if it was really possible for this fantasy to become a reality. The following Monday I called Tom Lentz, assistant dean of admissions at Yale School of Medicine, and asked him if I was too old to become a doctor. Without asking how old I was, he told me that the medical school could not discriminate based on age. But he also said that I would need to take full-year courses together with labs in biology, chemistry, organic chemistry, and physics. Furthermore, if I wanted to be considered by Yale School of Medicine, I would have to take these courses in a high-level postbaccalaureate program. He told me about a special program at Yale that allowed people to enroll in undergraduate courses without working toward a degree.

That summer I started biology at Yale. It took me three and a half years to complete the premedical requirements while I continued to work for the Human Investigation Committee. From the moment I started those courses, I was driven. The effort took on a life of its own, and I knew I was going in the right direction.

I was accepted at Yale University School of Medicine in June 1986, the week my husband turned forty. Forgoing the celebration I had planned for his birthday, we spent the day in the bank discussing how we, with our two young children and mortgage and car payments, would finance my education in medicine.

Perhaps because I was older, perhaps because it took me so long to get there, I recall my medical school days vividly, with great fondness and appreciation. That is not to say that they were without controversy. I also remember feeling disenfranchised as a student from time to time, as if I had somehow forsaken adulthood for a second adolescence. I slipped into the role of student as I slipped into my jeans and hoisted my backpack to my shoulder. A few other older students were in my class, but I never had any trouble getting along with my younger classmates.

Yale was the perfect medical school for a student like me. The Yale system emphasizes the maturity of its students. It is dedicated to the notion that at this point in one's education, one must pursue learning and knowledge for oneself, for the intrinsic rewards that come from knowing and for one's future patients. The object of the learning is no longer to garner the extrinsic rewards of grades or class rank. As a result, there are no formal grades in the first two years, nor is there ever a class rank. Tests are kept to a minimum, taken anonymously, and intended mainly for self-assessment. I found my classmates to be my greatest support system. Through their help, tutelage, and encouragement, I learned the science I had been so afraid of. The system de-emphasizes competition and values cooperation, camaraderie, and support. This is exactly the right environment for training future physicians in the art of caring.

I loved medical school and flourished especially during the clinical years. As I rotated through the third-year clerkships, I "tried on" each clinical specialty as if I would wear it forever. It was through internal medicine, however, that I found my sense of self as a physician. By a process of elimination that I now help medical students work through, I came to internal medicine because it allowed me to express myself as a physician in the ways that feel right. I know that I need patients with whom I can converse in partnership. During the pediatrics clerkship I found it too difficult to face the parents of sick children because I identified too strongly with their pain. In surgery, the environment of the operating room was too closed and sterile for me. But in internal medicine, I am the doctor that I had for so many years fantasized about. I am in a relationship with my patients. I need to possess the special knowledge that they come to me for, but I also need to know the special knowledge that they bring me, the stories of their lives that give shape and purpose to our shared commitment. I stayed at Yale for my three residency years in internal medicine, and during those years in the early 1990s I realized that it was through caring for people with HIV/AIDS that I could become the doctor I wanted to be.

Residency was hard and made all the demands that one hears about. I was tired much of the time. When I wasn't in the hospital, I was often nodding off. If I went for a ride in the car with my husband, I would fall asleep. If I sat long enough in a chair, I would fall asleep. My children were growing older. My daughter, who had been thirteen when I began medical school, applied to college during my internship. During those years, I knew there were things that I had to give up: I couldn't do everything. My family was most important, and my residency and dedication to my patients were a close second. At times, I was asked to switch these priorities. I have been blessed to have the undying and unquestioned support of my husband, Ron. He learned to cook, he carried a beeper so the children could reach him at any moment, and he took care of life's chores that would have competed for my time and energy. But my becoming a physician was truly a family endeavor in which my children, Carrie and Jeremy, also shared. They did their own laundry, cooked, and learned both family commitment and independence.

When I came out of the other side of the tunnel of residency, I divided my time between practicing general medicine, caring for patients with AIDS at Yale–New Haven Hospital, and teaching medical students. During medical school, I had watched Robert Gifford, my dean of students, and considered that being a dean of students was the only job, other than being a doctor, that I would like to do and could do well. It never occurred to me that this possibility would come about in my lifetime. But years later when I learned that Dean David A. Kessler was creating a search committee to find a new associate dean for student affairs, I knew I wanted to be considered. I was fortunate to be appointed to this position in 1998. As dean of students I take daily advantage of the lessons I learned as a medical student and resident and continue to learn as a practicing physician. Furthermore, my experiences as a junior high school teacher, a guidance counselor, and a mother of children now in their twenties have all prepared me for this role.

The students I meet are incredibly talented. Before they even get to medical school, they have done amazing things. They learn easily from books and the Internet, and they know how to study, how to take examinations, and how to function in the laboratory and classroom. They have been developing these skills all their lives.

But the four years of medical school are a time of tremendous searching and intensity. As students step from the preclinical to the clinical years, they meet some of their greatest challenges. Some who have been extremely successful as book learners may become insecure as they enter into intimate doctor-patient relationships. They open the door to a stranger's room and find themselves asking personal questions and laying their hands on the expectant body. They feel vulnerable because both they and others expect them to know things they may not know. They must decide how to deal with lack of information and uncertainty while at the same time they are seduced by the seeming ease with which others articulate their medical knowledge. For the first time in their lives, they meet people who are suffering or dying and who ask for their help. They may be confused by the tension between the technological promise of medicine and the truth that ultimately everyone must die.

The students I work with, though brilliant and talented, can be fragile whatever their age. The challenge for me is to encourage them to draw on and learn from their own vulnerability as a source of empathy when they are taking care of patients because, after all, their patients are also feeling vulnerable. At the same time, the students need to become highly skilled and knowledgeable. They must be able to apply to clinical decision making all that they have learned about people, about themselves, and about the practice of medicine.

In addition, throughout the years of medical school, students must make big decisions about their own lives. Their personal relationships may sometimes create stress or complicate their futures. Problems arise when they or their family members become ill, but even when two medical students fall in love, this happiest of relationships creates demands for compromise. Students must also decide about their future careers. Often they make more than one decision. They choose not only which medical specialty to enter but also whether to be involved mainly in research or in clinical practice. They may also decide to pursue additional training in business, law, or public health or, in some instances, to give up the practice of medicine altogether. Furthermore, as the financial demands on students have grown, their expected earnings have decreased.

I have the opportunity to watch the students as they grow and develop during medical school. They come in enthusiastic and open to all possibilities. I remember feeling that way myself not too long ago. I watch them mature and learn more about themselves. Some of that enthusiasm may be lost; some of it may be rechanneled. For each of them, as for me, the experience is a personal journey that requires care, support, and guidance.

It is my great pleasure as dean of students to be able to represent for students the practice of medicine and the satisfaction that one can derive from it. I love taking care of patients. For that reason, I continue to see patients in the AIDS clinic and on the inpatient AIDS service. Medical students spend time with me in the AIDS clinic throughout the year. I've also organized an elective course for first-year medical students in which they are paired with an AIDS doctor and an AIDS patient whom they follow for three and a half years. During this time they assume increasing responsibility for the care of that patient.

I'm available to hear about and help with the students' struggles and to support them in their journeys toward becoming a doctor. I also model for them the life of a woman doctor who derives great satisfaction from both caring for patients and caring for medical students.

ROSEMARIE**FISHER**

The Ups and Downs of Residency

Becoming a doctor! The undergraduate years seemed like a lot of work, but there was a lot of fun as well. Then came the decision to go to medical school, the elation of acceptance, the trying times in courses that never seemed to have much relevance to your chosen career, and the exciting and scary first contact with patients. How were you ever going to be able to do all that physicians did? Yet seeing patients made you feel like you were starting to reach your goal. Then there were the clinical rotations: medicine, surgery, obstetrics, pediatrics, psychiatry, neurology. How were you ever going to choose? And then the choice of field was made, the results of the "matching program" (determining where you would go for your residency) were in, and graduation was upon you. You were about to become a resident just like those people you had worked with as a student. Some of them you admired; some you didn't. All of them showed you that this part of training was different. It wasn't just books and seminars and tests, or being the one who watched as decisions were made with and for patients about their lives. The stresses might be greater than anything you had ever experienced. What was going to happen to you as a person during your residency? You had heard people talk about becoming hardened in order to protect themselves from others' pain and disappointments. You had seen some of these people change during your rotations on the wards. What was residency all about, and how were you going to get through it? Some people talk about "surviving" residency. I think that surviving residency is like surviving adolescence. I'm not sure which is harder, and I'm even less sure after having survived a third milestone: the adolescence of my children. I look back on all three "survivals" with a smile, though, for they have all brought great rewards.

As for residency, perhaps thinking that one becomes hardened during this process is part of the problem. Graduating medical students now enter residency with a sense that they are entering the "House of God" in Samuel Shem's novel of 1978. They begin residency with a preconceived idea (or plan) that they will be hardened and changed by this experience, that there is no other way. So is it surprising when some of these changes occur? I think not. I strongly believe that things are what you make of them—if you don't expect residency training to be like the House of God, it won't be—but people who think it's easy to become a doctor are kidding themselves. Maybe people harden during residency because this is the first time they're no longer solely a student but instead a mixed bag of trainee, employee, student, and physician. The resident is, after all, the person whom the patient counts on for real. As we continue to emphasize that residency is a training period, we need to stress that it is training for the profession. The behaviors and ethics that are learned during residency will be the basis for future behaviors. Sometimes it's tough to remember that.

Residency training has changed dramatically since "I was a resident"—a phrase I swore I'd never use except when defining a time period. Whereas some people believe that those were the good old days, that view is purely subjective. Still, I expected the same things from my residency training as do people becoming residents today. They expect to become experienced and more knowledgeable in their chosen field. There will always be clinical scenarios that do not fit the textbook descriptions, illnesses that do not follow predicted responses to therapies, and patients and colleagues who do not act as one might expect. Residents can expect to work hard, and there's just no way around that. A resident once suggested to me that residents should have paid time off (PTO), just like nurses and other employees. This would be nice, but most other employees can more than likely put their work in a basket on their desk and leave for a day without worrying. Nurses may be able to have someone else cover their jobs without making patients feel that no one is watching over their illness. But in my view, making sacrifices for the patients who entrust you with their lives is part of learning to become a physician in the twenty-first century. It will indeed be part of the rest of your life as a physician. One need only become a patient to understand the dependence of patients on their physicians. (Unfortunately, we as physicians are often some of the most demanding patients.) That's not to say that residency should be like boot camp; the sentiment "I did it, so you should" is no longer tolerated. That's what I think has changed the most. In my "good old (bad old) days," the every-other-night on-call system and the responsibility for twenty to twenty-five patients forced residents to learn certain aspects of medicine, but the experience could be brutal. It need not be so anymore, and I believe it is not. I repeat, however, that it will not be a picnic. But times after the training is completed will not be picnics, either. I think that new physicians are sometimes shocked, after they graduate from a training program and enter a practice or join a faculty, to realize that their new life may be even more trying than residency. I was once told that I was not a good role model because I worked too hard. This seemed to me a very sad statement. Neither residency nor medicine should be seen as a cushy job. Residency should be an enriching and rewarding process, and for most people it is. Talking to residents after their first year or after their total training is like talking to a new mother after the long and painful labor and delivery of her first child. Somehow it always seems like a different experience after the fact. The joy of knowing what you have completed and accomplished makes the pain of the process disappear, or at least diminish.

Hospitals and clinics have been accused of using residents as cheap labor instead of hiring more expensive health care personnel. Clearly, nurses, nurse practitioners, physician's assistants, and other health care professionals can do many of the tasks that the resident staff now does. The question is, what is the balance of the distribution of duties between the residents and the other health care professionals? Hospitals can clearly be run, and patients cared for, in nonteaching hospitals without residents. These are difficult economic times for teaching hospitals, and these are important times for striking a balance between educational and service activities for trainees. But what is the ideal balance between service and education? We continue to address this question in educational arenas, and as government funding for such house staff as residents decreases, we will see a change in staffing. I suspect that the change will be to decrease the number of house staff in teaching hospitals and to decrease their service responsibilities. Some activities have no educational value to the trainee and should be eliminated. These include secretarial work, transport of patients, and so on. Yet there is educational value to some seemingly mundane activities, such as drawing blood samples, placing an intravenous catheter, and so on. The benefit may be as simple as enabling the trainee to talk to the patient while performing these tasks so as to understand the patient's concerns, needs, and fears. Each activity needs to be examined individually to determine its educational value.

Dealing with people can be the best and worst part of clinical training. The reason that this training period is called residency is because the trainees originally took up residence in the hospital. The people around them became their family. Most residents were not married, and most residents were men. Things changed slowly. During my period of training, residents didn't live in the hospitals; more of us were married (although few had children), and more women were entering the field. We still were very much a family, though, and spent more time with our fellow residents than we did with our own families. This is one aspect of training that has changed over the years. Yes, residents still spend an awful lot of time with each other, and you will feel closer to your fellow residents than to almost anyone else. But there may not be the sort of strong "family" support that existed in the past. More residents now are married, have children, or have had other careers before entering medicine. After a day's work, they are more likely to want to leave the institution and not hang out with other residents. Is that good or bad? I don't know. Nevertheless, your peers will be more than friends to you. They will be your teachers and your managers. You will learn as much or more from them than from the attending physicians and professors who teach you. So, as you interview at various residencies, you must rate them not just on their academic standing and on how they fit into your planned career. You must also consider the personalities of your proposed residency family. You enter into a marriage, in a sense, when you enter into a residency. You do not want to look at the person next to you in bed one night and say, "What am I doing here?" In the same way, you don't want to find yourself looking at your colleagues in a busy emergency room and saying, "What am I doing here?"

Other groups and individuals will play major roles in the residency period: your patients, the other professional staff, and the attending physicians. You must learn to manage your time, your resources, and your temper. At times you will believe that no one else is working harder than you are, and that you will never work as hard as this again. You will believe that no one else is treated like you, and that no one else could feel more oppressed than you. Yet everyone around you has the same feelings. The nursing staff is rushed and hassled; the attending physicians are rushed and feel that the powers that be won't let them practice as they should; and the patients feel that they never have enough time with their physician.

Residency is a time to learn how to cope. And learning how to interact with people while maintaining your professionalism may be the hardest lesson. When you deal with a demanding attending physician or nurse, you may want to scream. Instead, figure out what upsets you most and determine ways to accommodate. Dealing with a patient with multiple illnesses related to self-abuse, who is abusive to you as well, will force you to expand the limits of your professionalism. Dealing with dying patients, both young and old, will challenge you. Many people feel that doctors should be able to confront death and dying without being too emotional. Yet this may be the first time that you are forced to face your own mortality. It will be difficult. I still sometimes cry with families when I deliver devastating news. Does that make me a weak doctor? I don't think so.

You may need help with all these issues. It is there for you from multiple sources: your peers, the chief resident, your program director, and the attending physicians. The hardest part will be to admit that you have to talk about these things. Don't avoid them.

After three to seven years, you come to the end of your initial residency. Initial residency, you say? Is more training ahead? Well, depending on the field you choose, you may enter the workforce and begin to practice medicine in the postgraduate phase of your career. Or you may decide to get more training, either spending a year as a chief resident or obtaining advanced training in a subspecialty in your field. You may choose sports medicine if you're an orthopedic surgeon, vascular surgery if you trained in general surgery, or gastroenterology (as I did) if you trained in general internal medicine. Subspecialty training, or fellowship, is focused training, both in clinical areas in the field, and in research. A lot of the same information I spoke of above carries through this period of training. The chief resident year deserves special attention, however.

In several fields, the chief residency is part of the final year of training and is split among several residents. This position carries administrative responsibility and involves counseling junior residents. By contrast, in such areas as internal medicine and pediatrics, the chief residency usually consists of an extra year after completion of the residency. The chief resident often walks a tightrope between being a friend to the junior residents, their teacher, and their connection to the administration. This can be a difficult year, and the position is an honor that a resident should accept only after careful consideration of the pros and cons. In the past, spending a year as chief resident was almost a guarantee of a position on the faculty or a practice opportunity in the community. Now that is not the case. Chief residency will, however, allow a resident to learn more skills, and furthermore, will boost managerial, teaching, and professional abilities.

So there it is. During your residency, you will grow at a steeper curve than you have ever grown before. You will grow intellectually and personally. You will love it, hate it, survive it, and prosper. And you will have met your goal of becoming a doctor! Congratulations.

BOBBY**KAPUR**

A Resident's Night in the ER

As I walk from the darkness outside into the emergency department glowing under fluorescent lights, the distinction between night and day becomes irrelevant. While most of the city sleeps, I will keep company with the injured and the ill, who also will be awake tonight. I head to a large board hanging on one of the walls, which is filled with lines of names, times, and symptoms scribbled with different-colored markers. This blur of information is our attempt to impose some order on the numbers of random people lying on stretchers throughout the department.

The incoming and outgoing residents assemble here for evening "sign out" rounds. For continuity of care, residents leaving the day shift hand over their sets of patients to residents beginning the night shift. This important exchange of information must convey all the pertinent details to the incoming physician, but time constraints dictate that it must be brief and yet convey all the pertinent details to the incoming physician. "Did he have a cardiac stress test in the past six months? Were his arteries clear? Did he get an aspirin? What are his latest lab values?" The two residents exchanging this information banter for a few moments in an attempt to make this transition seamless, and the process continues for each patient.

This evening I am assigned to the "major med" section of the department, where the most acute patients are triaged. After receiving the sign out, I walk to the bedsides and introduce myself to the patients. As I visit each one, I ask, "What's different today? What finally convinced you that you had to come to the emergency room?" Often, patients live with symptoms for days before walking (or being rolled) through our doors. A lack of an important piece of information can complicate a patient's course in the hospital. Being in the emergency department is stressful for any person, and the emotional uncertainties and anxieties make the physical discomfort worse. Will I have to stay overnight? Who will take care of the children or the pets? Can I get time off of work? Will my insurance cover this visit? People's thoughts are in disarray by the time I walk up to them. In addition to all these concerns, they now have to meet a new physician halfway through their stay. Another face, another personality to adjust to. "Hi, I'm Dr. Kapur." When I introduce myself, I always do two things: shake the patient's hand and smile. I hope with these two gestures to place even the most recalcitrant patient at some ease.

Human beings are very social, and we seek connection in even the simplest of interactions. With just the pressing of my palm into a patient's hand, I try gently to initiate a therapeutic rapport. The laying on of hands has begun. Medicine is half art and half science. The laboratory numbers and X rays can provide a portrait of the body's physical matrix: the calcium in the bones, the levels of hemoglobin in the blood, the amount of bile leaking from a gallbladder. But the person within the body does not want raw numbers and data; the person searches for meaning. As a physician, I have to interpret all this information for the patient, to convey the impact of the disease on the person's life.

Even though I have received a sign out from the previous resident, I meticulously review all the information about each patient. I read through old charts, look at lab data and X rays. I trust my colleague's oral history, but I use the presentation as an overview to prepare the direction of the patient's care. For the remainder of the night, the patient's well-being becomes my responsibility, and I must construct an immediate course of action for every patient. Do I continue the management program of the past few hours, or do I initiate a new direction of care? I look at the vital signs and assess the patient's response to the medications. I am searching for signs of change. Are you getting better or worse? Do you need to be admitted to the hospital, or can I send you home tonight? Information streams before me, and I must make quick decisions. I look at my watch and realize that it is still early in the evening.

One of the nurses comes up to me and says, in an excited voice, "Bed two's O₂ saturation is dropping, and her breathing has picked up." Bed two belongs to an elderly lady from a nursing home whose lungs are filling with fluid because her heart is having difficulty pumping blood from her lungs and into the rest of her body. I walk over and increase the oxygen flowing through the mask on her face, and I see drops of perspiration forming along her forehead. She is struggling to breathe. "Are you getting enough air?" She nods a slow "yes." She still can understand my words, which means she is still receiving enough oxygen to think and respond. I am searching for time. Because of her age and the possibility of complications, I am trying not to intubate her. The procedure contains some inherent risks, and I fear that once she goes on the ventilator she may never come off it.

In large auditoriums and small conference rooms, medical administrators and insurance executives and policy makers casually discuss such abstract terms as resource allocation and cost-benefit ratios, but in this starkly lit emergency department in the middle of the night all their dialogues and theoretical discussions seem distant, almost irrelevant. Am I going to use an economic formula to decide how to save this woman's life? No. Without hesitation, if she needs a ventilator, she will get one. I stare into her eyes, and she begins to appear drowsy. She is using every inch of muscle and tissue to breathe. The monitor indicates that the amount of oxygen in her blood is starting to fall, slowly at first and then more rapidly. I turn to the nurse, "Call respiratory, STAT!" My cauldron of time has evaporated, and I can no longer wait. As soon as the ventilator arrives, she will receive rapid doses of sedating and paralyzing medications, and I will then place a breathing tube into her mouth, through her vocal cords, and into her trachea.

About twenty minutes later, the triage nurse pulls me aside and asks, "Who can come out? I have a young woman who just overdosed on her lithium." The major med area has five beds, but if the area is full and a critically ill patient arrives, we place the least ill person in the hallway. After scanning all the patients quickly, I tell her, "The man in bed five came in with chest pain, but he's pain-free now and just waiting for a bed upstairs. Put him on a portable monitor, and he can go in the hallway." The paramedics wheel a lethargic woman with a slim build and disheveled brown hair into the emergency department. She is wearing a T-shirt, blue jeans, and a heart pendant hangs on a silver necklace. Her fingernails are short and clean. She wears no other jewelry. I scan her arms for signs of intravenous (IV) drug use and find none. I am searching for clues, for reasons why this woman would want to end her life. In an effort to understand this young person, I wonder: Is she a student? Does she live with her family or a boyfriend or alone? I smell a trace of alcohol on her breath and wonder what she chose for her potentially final drink. The paramedic begins his report, and I learn that she was found unresponsive next to a half-empty bottle of vodka and three empty pill containers: 100 milligram (mg) lithium tablets, 10 mg Paxil tablets, and 10 mg Klonopin tablets. The paramedic concludes, "I think she had a fight with her boyfriend."

As I order blood work, IV fluids, and drainage of her stomach, I find myself thinking about the proximity of our ages, about the emotional suffering that could overcome her will to live, and about the impact of her actions on her family and friends. To "manage" patients objectively, physicians must detach themselves somewhat from the patients they treat, but the boundary can be tenuous, especially when personal similarities begin to surface. During my residency, many people will educate me about the sciences of healing, but I am less likely to receive a specific lecture on the humanity of healing. No one will sit me down and teach me how to tell a young woman's mother that her daughter just attempted suicide and is critically ill in bed five. No one will tell me how to absorb an experience and not dream later of a patient's green eyes and disheveled brown hair lying against a stretcher.

Somehow I find a few minutes when my patients seem relatively stable, and I tell the attending physician I am going to go grab a bite to eat. I look at my watch: one-thirty in the morning. My shift is halfway through, and I quickly walk up to the second-floor resident lounge and find a sandwich and soft drink in the fridge and a small bag of potato chips and some chocolate chip cookies on a table. After a few bites of food, I pick up the phone and check my messages. An old friend from Houston and my brother in Manhattan have called, and

I wonder when I will be able to get back to them. Ironically, the rigors of residency require a person to have strong personal ties for support, but time constraints put strain on those very relationships. I have been gone about fifteen minutes, and I wonder how my patients are doing. I collect the remainder of my food: I will finish eating downstairs.

When I get back, the woman in bed three has been transported upstairs, and in her place is a middle-aged man. I walk over to the new patient. The nurse has just finished doing an electrocardiogram (ECG). I have not even said hello yet, but I need to make sure that nothing acute is occurring. At first glance the ECG reveals some subtle changes, but nothing indicates an acute heart attack. I will have time to talk with this gentleman. And I enjoy the art of taking a history in the emergency department. In most clinical settings, the resident can take time to let a patient's narrative unfold, and often the patient and resident have developed a rapport. But in the emergency department patients are usually strangers, and that situation presents unique challenges. I have to establish an immediate relationship at a time when patients are very anxious about their health. Most people who arrive at the emergency department at two in the morning do not have minor complaints. Because I am still treating four or five other acutely ill patients, I will have to focus the conversation to obtain the most amount of information in the least amount of time. Finally, I will have to persuade this new patient in bed three to have confidence in me. Most likely he would prefer to be seeing his own personal physician.

As usual, I shake his hand and, with a smile, introduce myself. Knowing that he arrived with a complaint of chest pain, I sort through possible risk factors he may have for heart attack: smoking, diabetes, high cholesterol, family history of heart disease, prior heart attacks. My intent is to determine how likely it is that his condition is serious. Even the healthiest-appearing person with the mildest complaints can be gravely ill.

"What brings you to the hospital at this time of the morning?" I ask.

"I actually never slept. I had a nagging tightness in my left chest and shoulder, and I couldn't get comfortable."

"Are you having the tightness now?"

"No."

"Have you ever felt something similar to this before?"

"Not really."

"Has anyone in your family ever had a heart attack? Your father or mother?"

"My father died of a heart attack."

"How old was he?"

He becomes very apprehensive, and his voice resonates with tension: "About the age I am now, in his mid-fifties."

With this one question, his hidden anxiety rises to the surface. His lips tighten, the creases in his forehead become more noticeable, and his right fist clenches. I have stumbled on the reason why this man, who currently is pain-free, would get out of bed, get dressed, and drive to the hospital in the middle of the night. He knows his risks, and he knows the legacy in his genes. I begin to wonder if he was with his father at the time of the heart attack. Did this same clenched right hand at one time hold his father's clenched hand?

After reviewing with him his risk factors for a heart attack, I tell him that he will need to stay in the hospital for at least six hours and have a series of blood tests to evaluate his heart. I reassure him that the ECG does not show an acute event, but the lab tests will confirm the findings. The creases in his forehead seem less noticeable.

Dunkin' Donuts opens at four in the morning. Around half past three, someone starts passing around an unused plastic specimen bag and a roll of small adhesive labels. We write our orders on labels—a separate label for each item, or you may not get both the coffee and the doughnut—and toss the money into the specimen bag. Often, by the time one of the emergency department's technicians arrives with a large cardboard box filled with our early morning nourishment, the patients are stable, and the staff congregates around the food, chatting for a few minutes. It is a ritual. Unlike the residents, whose shifts alternate between day and night, many of the hospital staff maintain a nocturnal schedule, and they all have different motivations for working these hours. Some prefer the higher salary, and others want to spend time with children during the day; still others have a second job. But they all share the Dunkin' Donuts ritual each morning. Like all rituals, it provides a moment of continuity and a sense of camaraderie amid all the chaos and uncertainty that seems to characterize the rest of the night.

After sign out rounds at half past seven, I put my trench coat over my white lab coat, grab my umbrella, and walk out into the autumn morning. Because I live a few blocks away from the hospital in an apartment adjacent to the medical complex, I have the opportunity to get some fresh air before going to bed. I try to notice some of the details along the way as a means of distancing my thoughts from the events of the night before. Have the leaves become more yellow today? What is the morning newspaper headline? Do I recognize any of the residents walking into the hospital? Why are they placing a podium and some chairs in the medical school courtyard? Finally, I walk through my apartment door and begin my own rituals. Even though it is almost eight in the morning, I need to prepare myself to sleep. The nighttime events of the past twelve hours unfold. Because my mind has been working at a rapid pace for many hours, I can't just come home and immediately fall asleep. So I read a few pages of something completely unrelated to medicine or watch a few minutes of the morning news. Eventually, the lure of sleep overcomes all other distractions, and I crawl into bed while the rest of the world begins pouring a second cup of coffee.

MIKHAIL**KOSIBOROD**

A Chief Resident Reminisces

I think that I first started contemplating the idea of becoming a doctor at a very young age. Without a doubt, I was influenced by my parents. When I was only about five years old, my father, a medical scientist and researcher, and my mother, a dentist, began taking me to work with them. To me, this arrangement had a lot of advantages, not least among them being stuffed with candy by their coworkers. And I am sure that watching my parents work influenced my perception of the medical profession. Even though their activities were quite different (my dad spent his day designing research projects, while my mom took care of toothaches), both my parents were tremendously respected by their patients and colleagues alike.

In Russia, where I was born and raised, doctors were very poorly compensated financially. Entering a medical profession would obligate one to an uncertain financial future and long hours of hard work. It was more of a calling than a job. Partly because of this deep commitment to their communities, doctors were regarded as highly moral professionals and were universally respected. As I grew up, I became more aware of my parents' positions as health care professionals in the community. Since they were my role models, by the time I finished high school I was sure that I would dedicate myself to the field of medicine.

Because the system of medical education in Russia is based on the European model, I entered medical school after graduating from high school at the age of seventeen. During the first two years of medical school, most of the coursework concentrated on basic anatomy and physiology. By the end of the second year I was ready and eager for exposure to more clinical areas of medicine. During that summer, however, my family was forced to leave Russia because of rising ethnic intolerance. My disappointment at having to interrupt my studies matched my frustration at leaving my friends behind. Knowing little English and even less about medical education in the United States, I headed into the unknown, with little hope of returning to medical school quickly.

The first few months after my arrival in the United States were emotionally and financially challenging. My whole life was turned upside down as I realized that I had to start my professional training all over again. Finally, having acquired enough language skills to ask for directions, I decided that it was time to get back into the swing of things. I walked to the nearest City College, filled out the application for the upcoming semester, and became a university student. That was the beginning of my odyssey toward becoming a doctor (frankly, the idea of choosing a different profession never crossed my mind), which culminated in my graduation from medical school about seven years later. On graduation day I was filled with exhilaration and pride. Yet I was also anxious about residency training. I would no longer be in the protected environment of medical school, and the knowledge and skills I had acquired there were about to be tested for real.

The beginning of residency was filled with long days of hard work, followed by long sleepless nights and emotional ups and downs. I saw some patients get better, whereas others were not as fortunate. Even though for many years I had had my mind set on joining the medical profession, I frequently wondered if medicine was really worth it. At those moments, one patient's story always reminded me why I was doing this job. During my rotation as a resident in the medical intensive care unit, a seriously ill patient had been admitted, suffering from a severe infection, kidney failure, and heart failure. Within a few hours, our team realized that his prognosis was very poor, a fact I communicated to his heartbroken wife. After several days of aggressive treatment, though, this patient made a remarkable recovery. Months later, walking on the street near the hospital, I bumped into him and barely recognized him, because he looked amazingly well. He told me about all the things he had done with his life since leaving the hospital, and how indebted he felt to us for giving him a "second birth."

Going through medical school in New York and then internal medicine training at Yale, I kept comparing the status and role of physicians in the United States and in my birthplace. Despite the different languages, customs, and cultures, the idea of being a physician is remarkably similar in both places. Medicine is not just a job, it is truly a lifetime commitment to put the interests of others ahead of your own. This profession requires many painful sacrifices on a personal level, and it is laden with grave responsibilities, but it also carries the incredible privilege of guiding patients through their most vital decisions, and constantly challenges the intellect.

Curiously, some of the most disturbing events in one's life can also guide one's most important decisions. During my last year of medical school, my father developed severe coronary artery disease and had to undergo several invasive procedures. These events brought me into contact with his cardiologist, who later became my role model as a teacher and physician. Our many interactions and his strong interest in my career choices were the most important reasons behind my decision to specialize in cardiology. This choice was further reinforced by my clinical experience on the cardiology service at Yale.

Thinking back to my medical school years, I find it remarkable how much the relationship with my mentor influenced my subsequent development as a physician. There is no question in my mind that it is of the utmost importance in this profession to have as a role model someone who exemplifies moral and professional integrity as well as intellectual achievement. The idea of first acquiring and then passing on knowledge and expertise, which is an integral part of academic medicine, is something that I had the honor of experiencing firsthand, during my service as one of the chief residents at Yale Medical School this year. This was certainly a period of tremendous personal growth, which, once again, reaffirmed my view of academic medicine as the embodiment of the best that the profession has to offer—compassionate care for patients as well as teaching and guidance. As I look forward to my subspecialty training, I sincerely hope that I will actively participate in both during my fellowship years and beyond.

JULIE ROTHSTEIN ROSENBAUM

The Inspiration of Medicine and Research

Somewhere it is probably written that you are not supposed to admit that television inspired you to go into medicine. As I think about my journey from childhood to medical school to residency to my current role as clinical research fellow, I consider how career choices are shaped. The potential influences toward medicine might include a person's pediatrician or parents, the pursuit of wealth or stature, or altruistic motives. But I have to confess that when I was a kid, I always used to watch *St. Elsewhere*. Something about Howie Mandel running around a hospital in his long white coat and baseball cap epitomized a combination of professionalism and irreverence that appealed to me. The situations that he and his colleagues faced were so diverse that no career could be as satisfying as medicine. All of this influence on my life occurred years before Mark Greene met Doug Ross on *ER*.

I followed this inspiration, and I have found that being a physician allows me to participate in other people's lives and experiences in a unique and gratifying way. I have learned how to help patients, but I have also learned the limits of what we can do for them. As a physician-researcher, I hope to be able to clarify these deficits and find ways to improve our abilities to serve our patients.

In spite of my interest in medicine, in college I found that many other things fascinated me. I took an engaging policy class about the hard choices in our society, focusing on such issues as abortion, euthanasia, and allocation of scarce resources. I found myself considering a career in law or policy.

Although many of these big problems remain unsolved, I decided that my way of addressing them would be through medical school. As a doctor, I can make a difference in the health care system by being deeply engaged in the questions of our time, whether they be constitutional issues regarding physician-assisted suicide or explorations of how best to serve patients while finding ways to control the costs to society. Instead of reading about these issues or arguing about them in court, a physician is directly involved.

I can remember the excitement of arriving on the wards to meet my first patients during medical school. I could not wait to start the conversation, examine their bodies, listen to the sounds of the heart and bowels, and try to fit this information into some pattern I had read about in my books. Sometimes the symptoms, signs, and tests all pointed in a clear, easily treatable direction. But I was very frustrated when the patients did not fit into the seemingly clear categories outlined in the chapters in my text. This patient has chest pain, but it is not classic angina. The pain occurs after he eats, but the symptoms do not sound like heartburn when he describes them. His electrocardiogram and blood tests contradict each other. How should we interpret all this information? We physicians know so much! So many books have been written and so many journal articles published; how could so much still be unknown?

I remember taking care of a patient who arrived at the hospital in the final stages of cancer. He had been deteriorating for months. He was having terrible pain in his bones and was seeking relief. We tried to give him additional medicine to ease the physical pain, but the patient said that he was tired of suffering, tired of being sick. The only way to control his pain was to give him so much strong medicine that he would be unconscious. Yet he was surrounded by loving family and wanted to be awake to spend his last hours with them.

I found myself thinking about the pathology of his cancer. I thought about the advances in diagnosis and treatment that had been achieved with science and technology. Much had been accomplished, but more-effective treatments still needed to be developed. And I was also faced with other dimensions. Could I ensure that the patient had understood our discussions and agreed with me about how we should treat his illness? What were this person's values, and how should we have incorporated them into the treatment decisions? How could we best allow this man to die with dignity? If this patient had lived in a place where physician-assisted suicide was legal, would our interaction have been different?

During training, you are thrilled to learn about medicine and how to work with and treat patients. As your skills and fund of knowledge increase, one of the most important facets of medical education is to learn the boundaries of what you know. Accepting and acknowledging the limits of our knowledge is an important aspect of what we do. By saying "I don't know" to a patient or colleague, we acknowledge that we are not omnipotent healers but physicians struggling with the interplay of several types of uncertainty. As Renee C. Fox outlines in her essay "Training for Uncertainty" (in *Essays in Medical Sociology: Journeys into the Field* [New York: Wiley, 1979], 19–51), one type arises from what we may not know because of our stage of training. Another type derives from what is not known more broadly in medicine as a whole. And the third type evolves when we cannot tell the difference between the first two.

By the end of medical training, many people develop a sense of their personal limits of knowledge as distinct from the limits of the field itself. Physicians eventually learn how to function and make decisions effectively in the face of this uncertainty. But sometimes one can be left wondering about the questions that are yet unresolved and might be answered with research.

At the end of residency, I decided that as much as I enjoyed the work of being a physician, I was also attracted to the other work that needed to be done to allow us to take better care of patients. There are many investigators hard at work to improve our understanding of the human body and its inner workings through molecular and enzymatic analysis. Many people are trying to find the next wonder drug to cure our ills. But other kinds of questions have yet to be answered.

Patient-centered research provides a framework for approaching some of these questions. Are there better ways to identify people with a particular disease so we can treat them as effectively as possible (and thereby reduce conundrums on the wards and clinics)? What are the best ways to set up studies to discover the most appropriate medication to treat someone's high blood pressure? How can we find morally and legally acceptable ways to help patients in the manner most fitting for them? This sort of research is an intellectual and logistical challenge completely distinct from medical practice.

There are many ways to learn how to do research. Some people choose to obtain a Ph.D. degree in biology or public health instead of going to medical school. Some people obtain a Ph.D. in addition to medical training. Another route is to pursue a fellowship after residency. By completing medical training first, a person has a wealth of skills and experiences to draw upon in generating relevant and interesting questions for research.

During my two-year research fellowship, I can return to the challenges of policy, legislation, and medical ethics in a more focused way. I will learn skills in epidemiology that will sharpen my ability to conceptualize these questions and to create the most appropriate research protocols to answer them. I will learn biostatistical techniques that will allow me to verify that the research is valid and statistically significant. I will also take courses in health care policy and management that will broaden my understanding of the context in which health care is provided, and of how the system might be changed.

With these skills in hand, I can examine the many questions that arose during my time in the hospital and in the clinic, and I can think about ways to answer them. I can consider how students are taught medical ethics and how conflicting forces in the hospital and beyond might counteract these attempts at education. I can examine the relation of physicians to pharmaceutical companies and how conflicts of interest might transform the physician-patient relationship. I also hope to evaluate ways of assuring that patients obtain the end-of-life care they desire.

Physicians with similar training are creating the evidence that contributes to the creation of national guidelines for cancer screening. Others, who are in leadership positions in the federal government, are trying to find the best ways to reduce errors in the health care system. Still others are teaching critical thinking and related techniques to medical students and residents.

Completion of a fellowship may allow a person to develop other skills besides research. Some fellowships provide specialized clinical training. To become a cardiologist, for example, one must go to medical school, complete residency in internal medicine, and then pursue a fellowship in cardiology. One can then pursue even more specific training to become a specialist in cardiac catheterization or electrophysiologic study. Similar tracks exist in each medical specialty.

For me, the fellowship will provide a breadth of experiences and potential avenues for my career, which might include academic medicine or health care policy. In whatever path I choose, I will continue to practice medicine. As a physician, I can enjoy the conversation, the interaction, and the relationship with patients. I can teach them about their health and the importance of medical care. But I also learn much from them about their lives and their values, and this information tells us much about how we should treat their illnesses. As a physician and researcher, I can work on both sides of the equation. I learn about the problems and complications from the front lines, so to speak, and I have the time and skills to work on finding some answers.

Some evenings I come home and think about all that I have done in one day. In a clinic session, I can enjoy an exchange with a patient, learning firsthand about her world, her family, and her experience with illness and life in general. Then I can return to my office and evaluate the results of a survey of patient attitudes that will guide ways to improve their care. Sometimes my role involves teaching medical students about many of the issues in policy and medical ethics that will affect their attempts to help patients. After a day like this, you might think that I would not want to watch any television program that has to do with medicine. But once a fan, always a fan. I turn the channel to *ER*.

JONATHANA.DRANOFF

Balancing Research and Medicine

For better or worse, today's academic physicians are strictly categorized on the basis of their day-to-day tasks. There are those who are primarily clinicians, those who are teachers, and those who are investigators in either clinical or basic science research. The advantage of these distinctions is that researchers are protected from such "mundane" concerns as patient care and administrative work, whereas the disadvantage of this approach is that it creates classes within the field of academic medicine. Whether positive or negative, this specialization means that prospective researchers must undergo extensive focused training.

Recently I completed my training in basic research. I learned quickly that basic research expertise was difficult to acquire (I do intend to acquire some before retiring), but I learned much more slowly that basic research training had as much to do with process as with content.

In almost all institutions, formal basic research training occurs during a young physician's fellowship, which in some institutions is called a postdoctoral fellowship. This period is meant to mirror the postdoctoral experiences of newly trained Ph.D. holders as they learn the skills necessary to become independent investigators. A postdoctoral fellowship generally takes place after the trainee's residency, and either before or after a clinical fellowship in the subspecialty of interest.

Thus, although research fellows are fairly young physicians, they are often fully trained in their specialties and subspecialties. They are, in essence, capable of practicing medicine, for which they have trained for the greater part of the preceding decade. Therefore, initial immersion in research training can be a culture shock.

For the years as a resident and then as a clinical fellow, one acquires expertise in medicine through a series of increasingly responsible regimented roles. By the time fellows have completed clinical training, they've often achieved mastery of the clinical field. Then the first day of research training begins. All of a sudden, a fellow is as much of a novice as a medical student. Although bearing the same responsibilities (and perhaps perceiving the same expectations) as postdoctorates with Ph.D.s, research fellows—even those previously trained in research—simply do not have the background for their new position. More important, learning the daily routines necessary to achieve their goals will take a great deal of time. Looking back, I believe that concrete training in the day-to-day activities of a new research fellow would have been quite helpful.

What are the daily tasks of a research fellow? They are relatively few: read extensively to acquire expertise in the area of interest, attend as many conferences as possible, and plan and perform experiments. Fellows have no (or few) responsibilities toward patients, patients' families, senior physicians, or other clinical fellows. For the first time since medical school, a fellow is free to make daily plans, to dress casually, to take meals when convenient, and even to sleep late or go home early. Personally, I found this freedom to be an enormous responsibility: my success or failure was determined almost entirely by my ability to use my time well. In my experience, research fellows respond in one of two ways. Either they stick to rigid schedules characteristic of their prior research training or they vary their schedules daily (I chose the second option). Both choices carry benefits and risks. The downsides of remaining on a rigid schedule are twofold: first, research does not progress on a rigid schedule, and second, many of these fellows end up suffering from burnout. The downside of adopting a relaxed schedule is that one could easily spend several years of research training achieving nothing concrete. In any case, a research fellow's success depends largely on the ability to adopt a style that maximizes reading, conferences, and experiments, but takes advantage of the flexibility inherent in the research training itself.

With the beginning of laboratory work, a fellow's social life changes markedly. A flexible schedule should allow the fellow to spend time with friends, spouses, or significant others, and in part it does. Yet the demands of experiments that take place at nontraditional work times (late evenings or weekends) can interfere with traditional social activities. Fellows with family obligations, especially those with children, find these constraints particularly problematic. As a single person, however, I sense that my married colleagues have an advantage. Coming home after an unsuccessful experiment at ten in the evening to a frozen dinner or some canned soup can be a lonely experience. I can imagine that seeing one's spouse and kids must immediately put lab work in perspective. And perspective is critical for the research fellow: most hard work pays dividends, but only after several unsuccessful attempts. For those without families, planning for social activities is easier as a fellow than as a resident; only once in a while will a fellow have to take a pass "for the sake of science." Generally, activities that are planned far in advance are easy to schedule, because research works on a week-to-week basis. Whether married or single, a fellow will find that research brings changes in social life, but the changes are not for the worse and may be for the better.

How does a research fellow decide what to study? First the fellow must choose a mentor. This critical decision is generally made many months before the fellow begins research training. Mentors vary widely, but successful ones share several characteristics. Most important, to be effective, mentors must be committed to training fellows and must understand that the fellows' interests and their own will occasionally diverge. Additionally, the mentor should study a topic of interest to the fellow, should be approachable (and even friendly), should be reasonable, and should be honest. Many fellows choose to train in the labs of the most famous or most senior investigator available. While this approach is often a safe one, it occasionally limits the abilities of fellows to excel. Younger mentors often study a cutting-edge topic, and they often understand a fellow's needs for advancement because they can easily recall what they needed in order to develop their own careers. In any case, the mentor-fellow relationship will be paramount in a fellow's life for years to come.

The research fellow will generally begin training by being assigned a structured project to complete. In my case, my mentor outlined the different areas of research taking place in the lab and invited me to select the area that most interested me. Then he and I (mostly he) decided on a logical set of experiments necessary to explore that area. It is hoped that by starting with a structured research project, a fellow will develop the techniques necessary to complete the project and, much more important, will learn to think scientifically. Scientific thinking is learned in several ways. First, fellows present proposals for experiments and findings at lab meetings in front of peers, their mentors, and other senior investigators. By defending their approach and answering difficult questions, fellows learn to think deeply about a topic and ideally to generate novel hypotheses likely to lead to further findings. Second, fellows will fail. Experimental medicine is a trial-and-error discipline. Often, well-planned experiments simply will not work. The fellow and mentor will need to design alternative experimental strategies to test the same hypotheses. Integrative thinking and reformulation of experimental approaches are the fundamental bases of scientific thinking, but they are not learned overnight. It is probably for this reason that fellows must invest three years or more in training to become independent investigators.

What kinds of experiments will fellows do during this time? (My mother asks me this question constantly.) The answer depends greatly on their areas of research and the approaches taken previously by their mentors. Approaches in wide use at this time include molecular biological techniques, microscopic imaging, animal physiology experiments, and an assortment of cell biological techniques. Although these techniques are complex and sophisticated, they are also becoming increasingly easy to perform. In fact, I have seen fellows with no lab experience become able to perform state-of-the-art experiments after just a few weeks' training. Much more important is the ability to interpret results; this skill is what distinguishes an investigator from a technician.

After a few months or so, a fellow will have generated sufficient data to form the rough outline of a manuscript. It is now time to submit an abstract. And submission of the first abstract can be thrilling. A fellow's months of toil are reduced to a few paragraphs, submitted to a scientific organization, and judged for their importance. A few months later, the fate of the abstract is revealed: usually the researcher is asked to develop it into either a poster or an oral presentation. An oral presentation is an especially exciting event for a young investigator. It is a chance to present one's data in a distilled, rehearsed form in front of many of the most famous investigators in one's field. I remember distinctly my first oral presentation. I was quite sure that I would fumble through it. By the time I reached the seventh or eighth of twelve slides and realized that I hadn't erred seriously, I hit a high I have not felt many times in my life. When the question-and-answer session started, I realized one of the forgotten truths in research: I knew more about my topic than anybody else, simply because I was the one performing the research. Presentation of my findings continues to be one of the best parts of my career as a researcher.

Parallel to presentation of one's findings is submission of manuscripts to scientific journals. After the research project appears complete enough to communicate a new scientific point or (in the scientific vernacular) to "tell a story," the fellow must dedicate time to reporting the research findings in manuscript form for future publication. Not only must the data be organized into publishable graphs, figures, and tables, but the manuscript itself must also include several features. These include a rational introduction, an accurate description of the research methods, and a discussion of the findings that puts them in the context of prior findings and clarifies the importance and novelty of the work. Then it is time to wait. Sit on one's hands. Wait a bit more. Eventually, a letter will arrive (generally via E-mail) explaining the disposition of the manuscript. Rarely will it be accepted without change (when this does happen, it's party time). Often it will be rejected outright. This is both frustrating and painful; it reflects some level of disapproval from on high. After a week of banging their heads against the wall, the fellow and mentor will usually resubmit the manuscript to a different (probably less prestigious) journal, and the two of them will cross their fingers. Perhaps the most common result of submitting a manuscript is a rejection with invitation to revise and resubmit. This is a good outcome! After reading and rereading the reviewers' comments, the fellow and mentor decide on a plan to address the critiques, and after several weeks or months of further experiments and rewriting, the manuscript is resubmitted. Manuscript submission is complicated and demoralizing, but incredibly rewarding when successful.

Once a fellow has shown promise by presenting and submitting work (generally taking more than a year), it is time to think about the future. To become an independent investigator and a full-time faculty member, a fellow will need to find funding that will support a research laboratory. Promise is terrific, but money talks. Institutional funds are limited, so a fellow planning to become independent will require as much personally acquired funding as possible. In fact, this money gives a fellow power; most grants require that a fellow's time be "protected" from clinical and other demands. Thus, the fellow must apply for a grant. After spending a year or more performing experiments, the fellow must again shift gears. Time must be devoted to assembling all relevant data and creating a hypothesis that will serve as the basis for a grant proposal. Grant proposals are difficult to formulate. Whereas twenty-five single-spaced pages may seem like a large amount of space to fill, complete communication of one's ideas can often take twice that space. Moreover, many of the smaller foundations limit grant applications to five to ten pages or less, thus forcing further distillation of the applicant's thoughts. For this and other reasons, the average grant requires at least three complete rewrites before submission. Grant writing, then, takes over as the primary goal of the fellowship. The fellow should continue to conduct experiments but will also spend a few hours each day reading journal articles and writing. When the time finally comes to submit a grant proposal, the waiting period for manuscript review, by comparison, seems like a fleeting moment. Grant review can take three months or, for a complete review, closer to six months. Depending on the funding source, only 10 to 50 percent of grants are funded, meaning that most applications are denied. Fortunately, funding organizations want applicants to receive funding (that is their raison d'être), so resubmissions are expected. Eventually, most fellows finally acquire funding, ideally with their self-esteem intact.

The rest of the research fellowship consists of more of the same: performing experiments, compiling and presenting abstracts, submitting manuscripts, and applying for funding. As you can imagine, this is a full-time job that requires frequent shifting of attention. The progress of research can be slow. Many weeks may go by before anything concrete happens. Frustration is common, stemming from both slow results and the rejection of manuscripts and grants that is inherent in the system. That said, my research fellowship was one of the best periods of my life. I realized that I had the power to control my destiny—at least in part. I could design and perform my own experiments. The words I submitted were my own (with great thanks to my mentor and other contributors). I could control the use of my funds. Moreover, I learned that science should not be intimidating; the chief aspect dividing senior scientists from me was time. And most important, I discovered that research is a process; the journey is the destination; and the joy of science is in the pursuit (rather than the acquisition) of new knowledge.

Professing Medicine

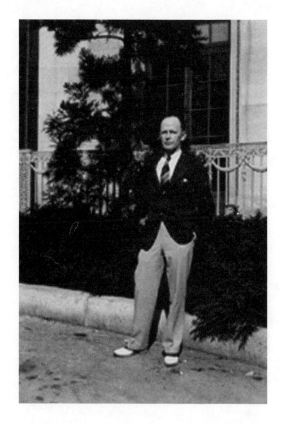

his book is all about the many varied ways that one can serve in the health professions. "Serve" says it all: to be a physician still means taking on an unselfish obligation to care for the sick. Ethicists question and struggle with the content of this idea, and it is sadly true that motives have grown mixed in these times. Medicine in the twentieth century provided the potential for very high incomes, and technology provided not only enormous benefit to sufferers of disease but huge rewards to doctors who performed procedures, and to academics who discovered—and patented—what they found.

In this section, a number of experts enlarge on the nature of the service of the medical profession. Some of these physicians are much older than you, but we ask you to remember that they were also young once; they too had passions like yours. Recall that human nature, along with medical training, changes very slowly, if at all.

The first quintet, Robert M. Donaldson, Jr., Albert R. Jonsen, Alan C. Mermann, Thomas Duffy, and Gerald Friedland, have a lot to say about what it has meant to them to be professionals while dealing with suffering fellow human beings. They describe and emphasize the profession's origins as an art, not a science. Donaldson, a physician-teacher, focuses on the personal qualities that a professional must acquire during training. Even though society rewards the physician for serving, true professionals always hold the patients' interest above their own. Jonsen, who trained first as a Jesuit and later through his academic training became a medical ethicist (now sometimes called bioethicist), agrees with that ideal. He stresses the primacy of the patient's freedom to decide, praising the good physician who holds high the patient's freedom to decide what to do— or not do—when facing disease and even death. Mermann, who first became a physician and then a minister, praises faith as the foundation of a medical career. His experiences and beliefs brought him to a chaplaincy for medical students. Duffy reminds us of the importance of the humanities in medicine, the recognition that narrative informs medical training almost as much as biology does. Friedland has always been fervid about social justice, and so, after a stint in the Peace Corps in Nigeria, it is not surprising that he has spent two decades working with patients ravaged by HIV/AIDS.

Ramin Ahmadi was born in Iran, where he suffered first-hand the abuse of human rights by the revolutionary regime. Not surprisingly, he turned to the borderless fields of medicine, as an educator in a community hospital in this country and as a physician working in wartorn areas abroad. You will not soon forget his descriptions of the anguish in East Timor ravaged by both war and terrorism.

Dyan Griffin, Laura R. Ment, Juanita Merchant, and John Blanton outline the major demographic changes of the past decades, especially the enhanced and larger role of women in the former male preserve, and the "rainbow"-like nature that, thankfully, now characterizes the medical profession. With her chief resident, Dyan Griffin, Laura Ment tells of the problems that women face, problems still quite different from those of men, especially in the never-quite-solved balance between family and professional life, and the slow progress of women toward academic equality and parity of salary. Merchant and Blanton each tell of the difficulties still encountered by black physicians in clinical and academic life. Finally, Vincent DeLuca and Howard Spiro comment on the many choices physicians must make throughout their professional lives as they warn about the tensions of a calling in which advances come so rapidly that physicians find their professional arrogance challenged by rapid obsolescence.

ROBERTM.DONALDSON,JR.

Medicine as a Profession

few months after completing my internship, I found myself in the U.S. Navy as the ship's doctor aboard an icebreaker. Hundreds of miles from the nearest hospital or other medical personnel, I took care of people with acute appendicitis, various infections, broken bones, lacerations, and other ailments. I even treated an Eskimo who had sustained life-threatening burns. The navy paid me for my services, and the Eskimo's family rewarded me with a fine pair of walrus tusks. At the time I did not doubt that I was a medical professional. After all, I had acquired the knowledge and skill that made me able to care for patients on my own, and I could earn a living as a doctor. Fifty years later, I realize that these limited attributes would hardly qualify me as a member of the profession today. In the first place, neither the navy nor society now gives so much responsibility to someone out of medical school for only one year. Moreover, being paid for technical competence might have fulfilled the requirements of the medical profession fifty years ago, but as we shall see, much more is required today.

One becomes a medical professional—that is, one takes on the values and attributes of a mature physician—gradually. The acculturation process, which begins in medical school, has changed very little over the years. The process influenced me most profoundly when I, as students still do today, dissected a cadaver during my first year in medical school. Although ostensibly meant to teach human anatomy, this gripping exercise really helped accustom me to the inevitable vulnerability of the human condition and thus protected me from feeling overwhelmed by it. My first two years in medical school also confronted me with a new language and a body of factual information more enormous than the human mind could possibly encompass. Most of the facts I struggled to memorize have now been proven wrong or irrelevant, but indelibly etched in my mind was the idea that lifelong study was necessary just to begin to understand something about medicine. Clinical training during the third and fourth years of medical school provided me with the opportunity to assume increasing responsibility for patients as a member of a health care team consisting of a hierarchy of residents and attending physicians. These early clinical years also showed me the line a medical professional must draw between being a team member objectively responding empathically to the patient's medical needs and being an individual so personally involved in a patient's troubles that objective judgment is lost. Added more recently to the acculturation process has been the "white coat ceremony," during which students make vows while donning a white coat before interviewing and examining patients for the first time. Today, the process of becoming a professional extends well into graduate (residency) training, a time when developing physicians become more independent and at the same time more and more dependent on each other. Given the magnitude of their responsibilities and the need to expand their knowledge base and skills, they increasingly recognize that, in an era of dramatic advances in biomedical science and technology, mutual dependency and a team approach are essential to medical care that is truly effective.

I was very fortunate to enter the medical profession when I did. During the past half century, American society has consistently and generously rewarded the profession's members with commanding authority, dignified social status, a comfortable income, and long-term security. Such was not always the case. Before the twentieth century, the American public had little use for physicians. In *The Social Transformation of American Medicine,* Paul Starr tells us how the medical profession rose from obscurity to become what he calls a "sovereign profession." Lacking transportation to doctors and hospitals, most eighteenth century Americans waited until they were seriously ill before seeking medical attention, and then they depended entirely on neighbors or members of their families to treat them at home. Doctors were relevant only to the comparatively few people who lived in cities. During the early and middle nineteenth century, urbanization and advances in transportation combined to expand the medical market by making physicians and hospitals more readily accessible. The medical profession, however, failed to take advantage of these gains because of internal conflicts and the rise of medical sects, such as botanical medicine, homeopathy, Christian Science, etc. These sects paralleled the development of religious sectarianism in early nineteenth century America and provided often-popular alternatives to mainstream medicine. In response, physicians united to form the American Medical Association in 1846, but for at least another half century the profession still lacked the internal cohesion and the external power to establish the primacy of mainstream medicine. Only in the late nineteenth and early twentieth centuries did physicians begin to consolidate the authority of their profession, but even then progress was slow. Over a period of decades in the twentieth century, accumulating scientific knowledge was only gradually transformed into authority and authority into market power. Entering the twenty-first century in concert with astonishing advances in biomedical science and technology, the American medical profession has now expanded its authority and market power enormously and finds itself a vital part, yet only a part, of a vast corporate health care industry.

What does it mean to be a professional as opposed to being an employee in a job? During the fifteenth century people used the word "profession" to describe the promise or vow one makes upon entering a religious order. Gradually the definition expanded to include other occupations to which one is dedicated and in which one "professes" to possess special skills. Members of the learned professions use their expertise to serve people with special needs. Thus doctors, lawyers, clergy, and teachers serve patients, clients, parishioners, and students, respectively. Professionals are generally paid on an individual basis according to the value society places on their services. Characteristic of a profession is its freedom to regulate itself primarily through professional societies. Members are held responsible for maintaining and expanding the body of knowledge their profession requires and for transmitting that knowledge to those entering the profession. Individuals are permitted to participate in the activities of a profession only after they have met standards that by and large are set by the profession itself. Participation may require licensure by the state, but the profession profoundly influences the licensing process. Generally, a profession has also reached a consensus concerning the code of ethics that governs its conduct. It is hoped that members of a profession will serve primarily the interests of others, sometimes at their own expense, whereas individuals involved in commercial occupations may seem to serve primarily themselves, sometimes at the expense of others.

The medical profession readily meets these criteria. But physicians are so powerful in relation to their sick and vulnerable patients that the medical profession has for centuries affirmed its special values and obligations. Unquestionably, physicians owe it to their patients to be competent, that is, to possess the knowledge and skill needed to provide high quality medical care. If they lack this knowledge and skill, physicians are obligated to transfer care of the patient to physicians who do possess the necessary competence. Other obligations include doing what is in the best interests of the patient, doing no harm, respecting the patient as a person, *accountability* or taking responsibility, *veracity* or truth telling, *fidelity* or promise keeping, and *confidentiality*. When individual doctor-patient relationships and continuity of care dominated medical practice, these values and obligations were readily apparent to patient and physician alike.

These obligations are not merely sold to the patient; nor do they represent philanthropy on the part of the physician. Nor is the patient merely purchasing a physician's services. Rather than a contractual relation, there develops between doctor and patient a central fiduciary arrangement, a moral interaction based on mutual trust. The doctor strives for the best possible outcome of the patient and the patient unreservedly endorses the physician's endeavors by making every effort to cooperate in the healing process. Both the doctor and the patient are freely giving to and receiving from one another. William F. May identifies this bond as a covenant and analyzes it in considerable detail in his book *The Physician's Covenant (2000)*. For many years, most physicians practiced medicine according to these tenets and received, in return, society's considerable investment in their professional careers.

In recent years, though, I've watched the medical profession come under siege. Most physicians put the entire blame on so-called managed care for what has happened, but I believe that this view is an oversimplification. I've seen dramatic advances in the technologies of medicine depersonalize medical care by emphasizing the treatment of the disease rather than the care of the people who are ill. Expanding specialization necessarily accompanies medical advances, but depersonalizes medical care further by interfering with continuity of patient care. After all, the involvement of many physicians in one patient's care tends to blunt the traditional doctor-patient relationship.

Biomedical advances have had other unintended consequences. These include the often-unrealistic expectations of patients and the public; the entrepreneurial, self-interested (and therefore unprofessional) activities of some physicians; and the astronomical increases in the costs of medical care. These costs in turn have led those who pay for health care to abandon the long-established fee-for-service system of payment, which provided physicians with incentives to perform procedures and services. To contain costs, payers have substituted a capitation-based, prepayment system that tends to reward doctors for avoiding or denying services. Large health care corporations are now employing more and more physicians who must deal with untenable financial incentives, conflicts of interest, virulent competition in the marketplace, and a disheartening deterioration in their patients' trust. The continuing growth of malpractice litigation undoubtedly contributes to the barrier between patients and their doctors as do the arrangements that managed care contracts impose on patients for selecting and retaining physicians.

Certifying boards and professional societies unquestionably deserve high marks for ensuring the technical competence of the medical profession, but I'm not alone in worrying about the profession's deficiencies. Critics emphasize that shortcomings were apparent long before managed care came on the scene. Particularly worrisome are examples of physicians acting in ways—such as charging for unnecessary or unproven procedures and treatments—that enhance their own financial position at the expense of patients. Over the decades, the medical profession, which has never policed itself adequately, has consistently failed to publicize and discipline all but the most egregious of such activities. I also find distressing the profession's desultory participation in relevant public affairs except when it comes to advocating positions that directly or indirectly favor its own special interests. Why doesn't the profession emulate at the national and local levels the selfless kind of advocacy conducted at the international level by organizations such as Physicians for Human Rights and Doctors Without Borders?

These days the medical profession is being urged to do better. For example, Wynia and colleagues argue persuasively in the *New England Journal of Medicine* (342: 1612–6, 2000) that the medical profession, in its interactions with the public, must actively and openly exemplify three core elements of professionalism—devotion, profession, and negotiation. Thus, the profession must consistently and unequivocally demonstrate its *devotion* to medical service, must publicly *profess* its long-held values and standards, and must *negotiate* with the public "the social priorities that balance medical values with other societal values." These challenges did not confront physicians who entered the profession when I did, and I wonder how we will respond. In fact, A. Relman, writing in the journal *Academic Medicine* (73: 1229–33, 1998), asserts that the medical profession can never respond adequately to the challenges of corporate medicine until we educate medical students and physicians-in-training about "the conflict between traditional professional values and the imperatives of the market." The students of today need to acquire a deep understanding of the many ethical, legal, and professional issues raised by the industrialization of medical care. Relman argues that without this knowledge and understanding, physicians will become "sophisticated technicians, future entrepreneurs, and managers" rather than members of a respected, learned profession.

Beyond understanding its role in the corporate world of medicine, the American medical profession must, at all costs, stand steadfastly by its traditional high standards and values. This means that physicians must continue to advocate the best possible outcomes for their individual patients, but they also need to recognize that unrestricted advocacy becomes untenable when it results in costs that prevent medical care from being equitably distributed. Above all, the medical profession, if it is still to be counted as a profession, must demand that its members unfailingly place their patients' interests above their own.

ALBERT R. JONSEN

A Physician's Character

When you began to consider applying to medical school, you sent for information about the schools you hoped would admit you. The materials that you received described the school's mission, history, and role in medical education and gave details about how to apply. In almost every one of these documents, you read that the school is dedicated to the production of physicians of competence and character. The idea of competence is relatively obvious: the courses and training provided by the school's professors will provide you with the knowledge and skills to practice medicine in a way that meets the highest standards. The idea of character is much less obvious. Even though the word "character" might not be used, the claim that the student will be formed into a physician with integrity, responsibility, fidelity, altruism, compassion, honesty, generosity, and a variety of other virtues is strongly suggested. Indeed, the school might announce that it expects you, as a candidate for admission, to have these virtues already. Medical schools, unlike most other institutions of higher learning (with perhaps the exception of divinity schools) claim to educate as much in ethics as in science.

When you were invited for an interview with the admissions committee, you probably encountered a battery of questions about ethics. You were queried about your dedication to the poor and the sick. Have you volunteered in a hospital, a clinic, a nursing home? Have you traveled to some deprived area to help the population? Many of you were able to answer yes, because you had been told by your admissions counselor that such service would demonstrate at least the inchoate virtues required of a physician. Some of you, of course, didn't need that advice because you felt drawn to such service. Whatever the motive, the admissions committee liked to hear that you had given of your time and talents unselfishly. An interviewer might then pose an ethical dilemma to test your skills at moral perception and analysis. Should a liver be transplanted in a convicted killer or rapist? Would you, as a physician, hasten the death of your suffering patient? You may have been warned of these questions and found a book on medical ethics to bone up on them. You might have been taken by surprise and relied on your instincts. Still, the interview seemed to confirm the published proclamation that medical education would be as much about ethics as about science.

Once you arrive at the place where you will spend the next four years in the absorbing and exhausting task of becoming a physician, you may notice that the ethics side of your education is not very conspicuous. Certainly, at orientation the same proclamations of dedication to the formation of character are repeated, perhaps quite eloquently, by the dean and senior professors. Also, you might see that an ethics course appears among the required courses of your first year. When you take the course, you find it quite interesting but you realize that anatomy and biochemistry and physiology make unremitting demands on your time and attention. Skipping an ethics class to study for an anatomy exam may seem imperative; an assigned article on euthanasia disappears under the demand to master the details of protein synthesis. The ethics course, come to think of it, dwells on the ethical dilemmas of practice, which are fascinating to discuss but very remote from the concerns of a first-year medical student. No one, in the ethics class or in any other class, is discussing the moral character of the physician, about which you heard so much before entering medical school. If anyone raises this issue, professors might confidently answer that the characteristic virtues of a physician were learned by experience, not by teaching, or if by teaching, it was in the subtle communication that flowed from the formed and experienced professor to the students as they observed the professor interacting with patients. A more thoughtful answer might allude to the difficulty, if not the impossibility, of defining and measuring moral character. Certainly, moral character should be encouraged but there seems no empirical data or method to teach it. It might gradually dawn on you (probably by the end of your first semester) that your medical education was thoroughly designed to convey to you the science and skills of medical practice; ethics was up to you.

Of course, ethics had always been up to you. Your parents might have conveyed by their behavior toward you and by instruction a certain moral tone to your early life and some notions about appropriate behavior. You may have emerged from your childhood with a strong sense of limits or with a deep feeling of freedom. Your teachers may have proposed certain ideals and imposed certain strictures. You may have encountered adults—a counselor, a pastor or rabbi, a coach—who exemplified some admirable feature and inspired emulation. Still, with all this moral ambiance, you made yourself. Sometimes quite consciously, sometimes instinctively, you selected elements of character for yourself. Working with some mysterious genetic resources, you shaped a conscious self with goals and values. By the time you entered medical school, you had made yourself into a person who could roughly be described in moral language (which we are not very eloquent about in our culture): you were generous or selfish, friendly or reclusive, thoughtful or thoughtless, calculated or casual, reliable or undependable. These descriptions are vague and oversimplified, yet they come easily to mind when we come to know others, or when, in moments of self-reflection (or criticism from our acquaintances), we learn something about ourselves.

Let me review the story of medical ethics to give you some perspective. As you become immersed in medicine—and ethics—you will learn that, over the past thirty years, medical ethics has indeed come into prominence. Beginning in the 1970s, public concern about advances in medical science and practice began to converge into a renewed interest in medical ethics and into a new academic field called "bioethics." The public learned about medical experimentation that put unwitting and unwilling persons, often patients, at risk for the sake of scientific knowledge. It learned that scientific discovery in the field of genetics and molecular biology was suggesting ways of treating diseases at their very cellular roots but also making possible the ambiguous "genetic engineering" that might shape human body and spirit to meet the specifications of scientists and others in power. The public was amazed by the feats of organ transplantation and life extension but worried by their implications for quality of life and fair distribution of medical resources. These broad concerns were focused into government and professional policies, and into educational programs in schools of medicine. Almost always, the topics of attention were the paradoxes posed when the human practices of caring for the sick encounter the rigid techniques of technology. Philosophical and theological ethics, which had a long tradition of analyzing such paradoxes in other fields of human endeavor, were invited into the world of scientific medicine. Unprecedented professors of medical ethics, with philosophical or theological training, were appointed to medical faculties. These professors produced books and articles, and a large literature appeared. Commissions and committees were appointed. Courts adjudicated certain cases, such as whether discontinuing life support constituted homicide; legislatures passed laws permitting persons to designate their desires at the time of death. Practicing doctors and medical students were expected to be familiar with the paradoxes and with means of analyzing them and resolving them when they appeared in clinical cases.

At the same time, the public became concerned that their doctors were becoming cold and distant. Technology was masking the personal face of concern. New economic and organizational structures for delivery of care placed obstacles between the patient and those caring for them. Physicians heard these complaints, and many medical organizations began to advocate greater attention to "humanism" in medicine, without being able to depict in any detail the dimensions of this desirable characteristic. Those who knew the history of medicine realized that even from the time of Hippocrates in the fourth century B.C.E., and even in traditions of medicine far from Western culture, a similar concern had surrounded the practice of medicine. In Hellenistic and Roman culture, in the Judeo-Christian tradition, in ancient Chinese and Indian medicine, exhortations to the practitioner to act kindly and compassionately, to treat patients gently and honestly, to refrain from exploiting the sick for the sake of personal gain or reputation, are heard again and again. Along with these exhortations, critics, often poets and playwrights, ridiculed stupid and vain doctors and vilified the greedy ones. The new call for humanism reiterated the ancient exhortations in the context of advanced technological and bureaucratic medicine.

What, then, do these noble proclamations about ethics and morality mean for the medical student? What does the practical negligence of ethical and moral education mean for the institutions of medical education and practice? As I have noted, you are likely to come to medicine as a young person with formed views, goals, and ideals, all of which are as diverse as the individuals who apply to medical school. Certainly, many students come from similar backgrounds and generally share the perspectives common to that background. Still, each person constitutes a unique being. Some of your classmates will be sincerely dedicated to the welfare of the sick and underprivileged. Others will be dedicated to self-promotion and self-aggrandizement. Some will be altruistic; others will be selfish and skilled at deception. Some will become the ethically good doctor that the tradition describes and the public seeks; others will successfully dissimulate until a crisis forces them to reveal their real values; still others will emerge as patently bad doctors, dishonest about their skills and unconcerned about their patients. Medicine is made up of all kinds.

Still, it is not enough to recognize the diversity of characters that come to medicine or the moral differences among practitioners. It is important to ask whether there is an ideal physician and whether the institutions of medical education and practice can contribute to the realization of that ideal. The vaguely described good physician of the past retains a great attraction for the public: patients always hope to find a doctor who is attentive to them, who will place their welfare above personal convenience and even above personal interests, who will add compassion to competence. However, a new demand is made upon the physician practicing in the cultural, economic, and institutional context of modern medicine. The physician of the past had a moral obligation to benefit the patient; the Hippocratic oath requires of those who take it, "I will act for the benefit of the sick and do them no harm or injustice." The benefit was not only the restoration of health brought about by medical skills; it was also the support of the patient's trust and confidence and hope. The physician of today must do this as well but has an additional duty: to respect and advance the autonomy of the patient, that is, the right and the power to make personal decisions about the course of one's life. The physician of the past was exhorted by Hippocrates to "treat the patient according to my ability and judgment." Today's physician must treat the patient according to his or her ability—but in accord with the patient's judgment. It is this duty that must be incorporated into the character of anyone who would practice medicine and that the experience of medical education in all its forms must foster.

There is a silly way to interpret this duty to respect autonomy: doctors must always serve the treatment that the patient desires, just as the ice cream vendor scoops the flavor the customer selects. Clearly, patients do not know what competent physicians know about diagnosis and treatment; seeking medical care is not shopping. And clearly, physicians must educate and explain when patients ask for something inappropriate or ineffective. Occasionally, physicians should withdraw from the care of a patient making inordinate demands. In other words, good physicians do not respect autonomy by granting every wish of every patient, nor do they even present all the options and let the patient decide without guidance.

Good physicians respect autonomy by recognizing that, in modern medicine, the effects of many of the most powerful technologies fall heavily on the patient. Treatment may alleviate and cure but may also damage human strength and capacity. Cancer chemotherapy, organ transplantation, psychopharmacology, and many other forms of treatment profoundly change the life of the person who accepts them in hope of cure. Extension of life is often at the cost of quality of life. The central issue for autonomy is whether the patient understands and desires to carry the burdens associated with hope of cure. One maxim of Hippocrates is often forgotten today: the work of the physician is to relieve pain, lessen the violence of disease, and to refrain from treating conditions that are beyond the powers of medicine. Many medical situations are beyond the powers of medicine, but physicians dissemble and patients hope against hope. In these complex situations, the good physician must have an exquisite sense and sensibility about the patient's freedom.

This is the essence of medical ethics. Learning about medical paradoxes should sharpen the sense and sensibility necessary for you to work constructively in complex situations, where knowledge, desire, emotions, and hope converge. Similarly, the exemplars of medical skill, the professors of clinical medicine and the clinicians whom you will encounter, must also become exemplars of medical virtue: sensitive to the autonomy of their patients and eager to show you the skill of making decisions within these complex worlds. No one comes into medicine with this virtue because the situation in which to exercise this virtue does not exist outside medicine and the other caring professions, such as the ministry, nursing, and social work. The physician takes on responsibility for the physical and psychological welfare of another human, often unknown to him or her, when that person is vulnerable in body and spirit. The ethics of such a situation are not part of life before medicine: even the best disposed of you, with the best intentions, will not have had the experience of one person placing health and life into your hands. Every human will encounter a physician, some much more frequently than others, and the awareness that physicians have the skills and the character to care for them must be universal. Everyone must accept that they can confidently put themselves in the care of a physician. The institutions of medical education and training must create the means to bring this aspect of medicine to the attention of students like you and create an atmosphere in which you can see how the difficult skill of respect for patients can be realized in practice. This is what medical ethics is about.

ALANC.MERMANN

Faithful Physician

Many of you may not yet have decided on medicine as a career. So as you consider it, I want to remind you that medicine is also a vocation. That is, in the true sense of that word, we are "called" to medicine as a profession. To be called is to receive a summons to a specific task, an invitation to a commitment that overrides ordinary obligations and duties. To be called, whether to a relationship, a profession, or any other position of responsibility for the welfare of others, carries with it the promise to serve others, and to offer guidance and instruction to those in need. Medicine is, traditionally, one of the three learned professions, theology and law being the other two. All three carry the same burdens of obligation and responsibility.

Another facet of medicine, as it is of law, is the attached and defining noun—practice—that offers a sobering reminder that the physician is always in the process of learning through experience. This is not to say that a doctor, even now, practices on patients to learn how to do some procedure or test! But it is a reminder to you as a potential physician that there is no final moment for a physician or surgeon when all is known and understood. Skills and knowledge must constantly be refined and expanded to include the latest information learned through ongoing study, professional conferences, and persistent clear-eyed evaluation of one's own experience.

But it is not enough to be intellectually up-to-date in the sciences, therapeutics, and technology. Most students admitted to medical school have impressive resumes that detail excellent grades, community service, laboratory experiments, and, frequently, mastery of a musical instrument! But this does not always ensure that the physician of the future will show all the characteristics of a good doctor. A major determinant of that good doctor will be the ability to be with and for patients as they proceed through their lives with the diseases and the disabilities that are part of the human venture.

One of the tasks for the students who hope to be physicians is to learn to be a companion—a sharer of bread—to persons traveling down the road of life, that journey that all we sojourners in a strange land, patients and doctors alike, will make. How do we learn to be with and for those in our care without breeching boundaries of the patient/doctor relationship, which can sometimes feel like friendship? That very breech can be destructive of the personal life of both doctor and patient, since this relationship is primarily fiduciary in nature, and therefore unequal.

How do we continue to do the work we are called to do when we are confronted with obvious evidence of our inadequacies and our failures? What will carry us through those difficult times confident that we are still true to our calling? These are questions that call to mind the importance of having a foundation that will support us in times of stress and help us understand who we are and what we do in the profession and in our private worlds. As has been noted, it is not wise to build your house on a bed of sand that rushing waters will wash away. We should all try to find a rock that will bear up under the stresses of living and working, pressures that can feel, at times, overwhelming. Searching for this stone foundation is often presented as our journey of faith.

A number of years ago I surveyed a number of doctors whose work, by definition, was highly stressful: cardiovascular surgery, neurosurgery, newborn intensive care, pediatric neurology and cardiology, oncology, *in vitro* fertilization, and others. My purpose was to learn *how* these doctors were able to continue their practices at times of severe stress. An outstanding finding was their ability to set feelings aside and focus on the intellectual and scientific aspects of their experiences. Expression of emotion, even to those closest to them—personally or professionally—was rare. There was a sharp focus on intellect, with only occasional and tangential references to religion or psychology as sources of support. I found it noteworthy that the moral and ethical components of their childhood exposures to religious faith were present, even though the formal commitments to religious practices were absent.

As a minister and a physician, I am reminded that the rock on which we build our lives is the god in which we profess—or confess—our faith. We all have a god in whom we place our final hope for understanding the reality of self and of world. There are no atheists: we all hold to some object in which we rest our final confidence for comprehending and interpreting our experiences, within and without. Be it the god of Abraham, Isaac, and Jacob, Muhammad, or our investment portfolio; be it the sensual and sexual delights of our bodies, or the revelations offered by the witness of the life of the Buddha or the moral philosophies of Kant or Hobbes; be it the final definition of the genetic structure of all living plants and animals or the interior reality of the presence of Jesus Christ as a present spirit—we all know a god, the final resting place of our faith.

For many of us, the search for a faith that will carry us through our day-to-day trials, disappointments, and failures is an ongoing struggle. Faith has never been an easily acquired prize. But it is a treasure to be sought so that we may respond to our calling with joy and the assurance that we are doing well what our profession demands of us. I think that many of us are hesitant to investigate the spiritual aspects of our lives since there are such extremes of expression visible. We see the spectrum that extends from Elmer Gantry to the purveyors of nostrums, and from magicians to massage therapists. But there is a life of the spirit that is attested to by generations of men and women who have sought it in many places, searching the depths of their hearts and minds for the strength to persevere in times of trouble and fear. There is also the praise and the honor that we express as we acknowledge our foundation in our faith in a creator and sustainer that carries us through the tests of living.

I have found that a readily available and competent resource for helping us in our search for faith is our patients. The questions posed by knowing the presence of pain, suffering, and the imminent death of others offer a source for dialogue about a personal foundation of faith that both empowers and supports in the times we all will know. The joys and the pleasures that are experienced in the birth of a baby, and the "rebirth" visible in the patient who has been granted a renewal of life by the skills of the physician and the surgeon are, again, sources for an enlivened faith. A common complaint of patients is the unavailability of the doctor to talk through with them their central concerns raised by disease. This retreat from opportunities for conversation with patients deprives the doctor of learning the riches of human experience that can then be offered to others and also applied to the spiritual growth of the physician. Although you may be uncertain of your own religious beliefs, as a physician your inquiry into and acknowledgement of the faith of your patients will be important.

In truth, I have found that the good physician must build on a foundation sufficient to bear the inevitable defeats we all shall know, while at the same time confirming the validity of our calling. As persons called to profess ourselves as doctors we are invited to join in that lifelong journey toward a faith that can sustain us and inform us in our work of caring for others, and we must build our house on a rock that will not fail.

THOMAS**DUFFY**

The Humanities
and Medicine

At the beginning of the twentieth century, the Carnegie Foundation hired educator Abraham Flexner to embark upon a demanding task: to evaluate the quality of American medical schools, which numbered one hundred fifty-five at that time. Many of these schools were of substandard quality with few faculty members and sparse to nonexistent laboratory facilities. The Flexner Report of 1910 resulted in the closing of many of these schools and an overall improvement in those remaining. As described by Kenneth Ludmerer in his book *Learning to Heal* (Basic Books, 1985, pp. 166–190), the standard of excellence Flexner employed in this undertaking was the model in place at Johns Hopkins Medical School, established in 1893. This standard was derived from a European tradition based on a biomedical model of disease. According to this model, disease was understood as an abnormality in biology; sickness was to be cured by identifying the physical disorder in the patient. Medical training was divided into the preclinical, bioscience years and the subsequent clinical medical years, a division that remains in place in most medical schools today. The desired end product of this training was a physician-scientist equipped to use the knowledge of science in the service of patient care. An additional role of the physician-scientist was the creation of new knowledge in medicine, an objective especially prized and rewarded in academic centers of medical excellence.

The subsequent decades of the twentieth century confirmed the wisdom and foresight of the Flexner Report, with its promotion of the biomedical model and its implications for training modern physicians. American medical schools have become preeminent in this realm, and their faculties have contributed to the extraordinary advances in medical science and technology. These advances, as one might expect, have resulted in such enthusiasm for the scientific dimensions of medicine that a significant imbalance has occurred in the scientist–physician dyad. The reign of technology has distanced the physician from the bedside, causing resentment among patients. Although physicians' ability to address disease has vastly improved, their skill in caring for patients has not. This imbalance has affected student selection for medical training, how students prepare for that training, the content of the medical curriculum, and the settings in which students and physicians live their lives in medicine. In their quest to fulfill science course requirements, many premedical students do not take advantage of a variety of college offerings, especially those in the humanities—English, philosophy, religion, history, and so on. Also, some students who are less sensitive or less attracted to the caring aspects of medicine have been selected for medical training. Because of this emphasis on the science of medicine, the art of medicine has suffered, along with patients, individual physicians, and the profession as a whole.

Many prescriptions have been written to right the imbalance that originated in the success of the biomedical model. Ironically, the source of that remedy is contained in the Flexner Report, whose purpose was to improve medical care in America. Abraham Flexner was firm in his conviction that a life in medicine required physicians to be educated for a learned profession. Physicians needed to be prepared to recognize and help resolve the social and moral problems of the communities in which their patients lived. The scientific foundation of medicine was to be improved and expanded, but it was not Flexner's intention that the art of caring for patients be sacrificed on the altar of science. An education in the humanities was the foundation for a rich life in medicine. Science is the basis of medical knowledge, but the practice of medicine requires artful skill.

Another corrective to the imbalance in medical training and practice was voiced long after the Flexner Report was released. In the mid-

1970s, George Engel, an internist and psychiatrist from Rochester, New York, correctly pointed out that the biomedical model—although it had been in place for over half a century and had determined the character of American medicine up to that time—had omitted several essential elements in the doctor–patient relationship. Engel's model, a bio-psycho-social model, recognized that the origins of illness are not entirely physical. It is most important, he pointed out, that in healing a patient the physician recognize the patient's social environment. Engel incorporated aspects that addressed the human element in patient encounters, and he cautioned that physicians need to have skills different from those garnered from a strict knowledge of anatomy and biochemistry. His work clarified the difference between disease, an objective phenomenon often reducible to a chemical or molecular understanding, and illness, the subjective experience of disease in a unique human being. The canvas of medicine was appropriately expanded and medical curricula have been altered to address the whole sweep of a person experiencing illness. Engel's commonsense model of illness did not make the physician any less scientific; in broadening the range of the physician's gaze, he demonstrated how the art and science of medicine are inextricably intertwined to the advantage of the patient. He described this model in an important paper entitled "The Need for a New Medical Model: A Challenge for Biomedicine," published in the journal *Science* in 1977 (vol. 196: 129–136).

Engel's bio-psycho-social model has received support from sources that emphasize the role of the humanities in medicine. The astonishing reach of medical technology in extending and creating life has taken society into arenas that border on science fiction. The ethical quandaries accompanying this broadening reach have, in turn, revived the field of philosophy by providing new and fascinating terrain for philosophic deliberation. The moral center of medicine in the doctor–patient relationship makes every patient a participant in a moral act. Questions of life and the definition of death introduce spiritual considerations that should be part of the conversation between doctors and their patients. The once inconceivable mapping of the human genome is now a reality, requiring a near comparable degree of wisdom in the judicious use of this new information. The cloning of the sheep called Dolly raises the specter of Frankenstein, and the potential of stem cells offers the possibility of a warehouse to replace worn-out body parts. The medical community is welcoming ethical and legal experts to help decide how and when to prudently and wisely open these Pandora's boxes. But the profession also recognizes that physicians must remain the primary decision-makers regarding how their discoveries will be put to use. Even greater involvement is necessary in the field of bio-ethics, where the medical aspects of any case are the responsibility of the physician and where command of this information is vital in any related ethical problems. If the physician relinquishes responsibility for these decisions, this shortens the reach of medicine and deprives the patient of an essential partner in exploring the ethical implications of medical technology. Training for a career in medicine requires expo-sure to ethical thinking in order to ensure that the ideals of the medical profession are upheld and supported.

Ethical problems arise frequently in medicine, but they are cer-tainly not part of every patient encounter. A different aspect of the humanities, though, is intrinsic to every first meeting between doctor and patient. When taking that initial medical history, every doctor must elicit and listen to the stories of patients' lives: who they are, where they are from, and what they will return to. The first doctor–patient encounter is the beginning of a relationship based on trust, and active listening enhances that trust. When a physician approaches a patient empathically—when she is willing and able to imagine what that patient is experiencing—she may come up with a question that might otherwise have gone unasked or she may have an emotional response that resonates with and comforts the patient. Possession of knowledge derived from literature brings a larger and richer frame of reference to the dialogue with patients, an advantage of special impor-tance in multicultural settings. An understanding of the particular cir-cumstances of a stranger's life may help the physician anticipate and prevent distortions in the doctor–patient relationship that differences in cultural backgrounds frequently create. Reading encourages empa-thy for those who live in worlds foreign to ours, and corrects stereo-types as ignorance gives way to knowledge.

In addition to listening, physicians can make the most of their encounters with patients by simply looking at them: looking can be a means of discovering the clue to the patient's diagnosis. One Renaissance physician developed a technique for authenticating the source of paintings; his technique capitalized upon "looking at the canvas for the minor detail." Painters' signatures are often in the details of their subjects' hands or the folds of their clothes and not usually in the more dramatic, obvious parts of their paintings. Similarly, illness has been described as announcing itself in a small parenthesis. The fictional character of Sherlock Holmes, who used observation to solve many crimes, was modeled upon a surgeon, Dr. John Bell. Physicians can be likened to detectives in the way they observe patients for clues to their illnesses. Thus, the encounter with a patient yields more relevant medical information when the physician not only listens to the details of a patient's story but also observes the patient closely as that story is told.

History, philosophy, ethics, literature, and art all are valuable to the practice of medicine because they expand the frame of reference a physician brings to the bedside and the consulting room. A grounding in the humanities helps the physician assume the caring stance that patients yearn for, and deserve, because of the vulnerable, frightened, and anxious state that illness imposes. An understanding of suffering equips the "complete" physician to better attend to the sufferer. The broader vision of the humanities, in cultivating this understanding, extends the physician's role especially in cases when the science of medicine has little left to offer. The converse situation is also true: the humanities may provide a perspective that helps the physician recognize and experience the joys that a life in medicine offers.

Another important aspect of the humanities is their ability to keep a creative spirit alive during the grueling and demanding periods of medical training and a life in medicine. The demands of that life may leave physicians with little time to entertain the ideas necessary for creative insight. Intellectual liveliness, present in nearly all people coming to medicine, is relegated to the back burner while heat, energy, and passion are applied to the all-consuming process of doctoring. Education in and appreciation of the humanities help improve the physician's performance by enlarging the scope of medical concern, addressing patients' spirits as well as their bodies.

The humanities have both applied and intrinsic value for the practice of medicine, a truth that is especially important in the face of the current romance and seduction that science brings to the practice of medicine. The symbol of the medical profession, the caduceus (staff) with two snakes intertwined, represents the two cultures of medicine. The snakes represent knowledge and wisdom in medicine, with knowledge derived from science and wisdom discovered in the arts. The snakes intersect at some points and diverge at other points: achieving knowledge in medicine is not the same task as achieving wisdom; each task yields different rewards, but both are essential in the daily practice of medicine. Art and science are joined in the service of patients, and the combination creates and sustains a healing sensibility in the profession.

GERALD**FRIEDLAND**

Medicine as a Calling

I came to medicine later than most. I was not a pre-medical student in college at Columbia. Rather, my interests were in sociology and history. I entered graduate school in sociology with the vague notion that this field would arm me with the skills and expertise to work toward social equity and justice. But I quickly learned that the discipline of sociology was concerned with methodology and social theory rather than with the more practical concrete issues that were calling me. I soon decided that the ethics, goals, and practice of medicine could satisfy my desire to be of use both to individuals in need and to society. Medicine, I thought, might be the vehicle that would provide the framework and skills to allow me to work productively toward social justice. Now, thirty-five years later, with some satisfaction, I can say that I was right.

My path in medicine has not been a straight line. It has been a journey of related but unpredictable career turns. The skills and expertise that are acquired in medicine—through difficult training—can provide myriad opportunities that vary over a lifetime. Good medicine is always interesting and always needed by societies and its members.

Having avoided the sciences in college, I crammed in physics, chemistry, organic chemistry, and zoology in postcollege classes and was accepted at New York University School of Medicine. I expected that the first years would be difficult for a liberal arts type like me, and they were. But I found biologic science both learnable and fascinating, and I reached the third year of medical school and experienced the thrill of clinical medicine at Bellevue Hospital in New York City. Poverty, race, and sad, self-destructive behavior had marginalized the patients at Bellevue, but they were very interesting, in great need, and grateful for the ministrations of even a lowly medical student. At the bedside, the manifestations of illness, both subtle and obvious, and the rhythms of disease slowly became apparent, as did the special and unique character of each patient. I knew that this was where I was at my best. But the demands were great and the support from colleagues and teachers inadequate, and my physical and emotional strains went unattended. I had come from a humble background and found it necessary to work through college and medical school to support myself. These difficulties made the rigor of medical school even more intense and at times dampened my enthusiasm for medicine. I learned then how important support and succor is for doctors as well as patients. The rewards in medicine completely outdistance the deficits, but the latter are real and problematic. We learn early in medicine to attend to the needs of others, yet we sometimes neglect ourselves in the process—an unhealthy paradox.

Early in my internship at Bellevue, I decided that it would be important for me to interrupt my formal training at the end of that year and apply my nascent skills in an even more exotic environment. I enlisted in the Peace Corps and the United States Public Health Service and spent two years in Nigeria. This was a life-changing experience for me—to work as a physician and to live in another culture was extraordinary. The powerful and defining relationship between disease and culture became apparent in revelation after revelation. The dearth of resources was an education in itself, requiring painful choices about what should be done and what could be left unattended. Do you develop programs to combat tuberculosis or malaria, since the funding available allows you to do only one? The sociologist in me was again aroused and I resolved to train further in infectious diseases and public health with the intention of returning to Africa to work in these disciplines.

Upon my return to the United States, I trained in Boston in infectious diseases and public health. It was the early seventies, the community health center movement was beginning, and the political and social climate in the country was exciting and compelling. I was, and remain, appalled that our extraordinarily wealthy society still cannot provide health care for all, and this disparity creates unfair benefits in health and burdens in disease. I remained for a decade in Boston and worked in both community health and infectious diseases. Before going to my next appointment, I took a six-month hiatus at the Ben Gurion University School of Medicine in the Negev desert in Israel, which had been recently established to integrate basic science, clinical care, and public health in medical education—an obvious but, at the time, still radical concept.

In the spring of 1981, I returned to work and teach at the Montefiore Medical Center and Albert Einstein College of Medicine in the Bronx. And soon after, in August of 1981, I saw my first three patients with *Pneumocystis carinii* pneumonia. They were desperately ill young men, and two of them were on respirators. A similar bizarre illness had just been reported in California among gay men. But our patients were different—they were intravenous drug users, with wives, girl-friends, and children. With this bizarre illness, the current chapter of my career began. I can remember a mixture of feelings at the time. I had had a dispassionate clinical interest in this most unusual cluster of cases. But the terror and pain of those young men and their families also brought on a great deal of personal distress. And I felt a profound sense of disbelief and dread as I realized something new and frightening was occurring. After working with infectious diseases for almost fifteen years in Boston, Africa, and the Middle East, I thought I had seen everything. But this disease was different. During the first year of what we now know as the acquired immunodeficiency syndrome (AIDS), an additional fourteen patients were diagnosed and treated at Montefiore Hospital for the disease—still without a name—that they all shared. During the second year, the number doubled and, each year thereafter, doubled again.

Albert Camus wrote in his novel *The Plague:* "The word 'plague' had just been uttered for the first time . . . everybody knows that pestilences have a way of recurring in the world; yet somehow we find it hard to believe in ones that crash down on our heads from a blue sky. There have been as many plagues as wars in history; yet always plagues and wars take people equally by surprise." So, too, was it with the present day plague of human immunodeficiency virus (HIV) disease and its most severe manifestation, AIDS. In one of those early years, I wrote about a patient of mine:

I had seen J. the evening before and knew he was soon to die. Years of cocaine abuse and careless sex had brought him to the edge. AIDS had been particularly cruel to him . . . and he was an impossibly angry man, demanding of everyone with such urgency and insistence that his family and the doctors and nurses caring for him often found it difficult to be compassionate. But he elicited a grudging respect as well. He accepted neither his disease nor its resultant disabilities. When he was no longer able to drive his taxi, he had his father drive it for him while he sat in the front seat going through the motions of his business. Rarely keeping his appointments, he usually showed up instead only when he was sick and then always expected immediate care. Each diagnostic test and therapeutic maneuver that was offered he met first with sneering refusal; yet eventually he would reluctantly agree. I knew that he was grateful for our efforts, but he hated his dependency and loss of control, and J. made it clear to us he was not going to extend his life with intubation or a respirator. Never ceasing to fight his disease, and us, he would nevertheless refuse those measures. And J. lived longer than any of us expected. Shortly before he died, a nurse called me on the phone and told me he was asking for me. She thought I should come as quickly as I could. I momentarily worried about not meeting my organized schedule for the day but went off to J.'s room. There he sat, still alive, upright in a chair beside his bed, bloated and breathing fitfully, an oxygen mask over his mouth and an intravenous line in one arm. His parents were hovering nearby in a corner of the room, and the nurse who had called me was sitting at his side. He grasped her hand tightly, holding onto her as his life ebbed, his courage having moved her to stay with him through the night. As I stepped into the room, he lifted his swollen eyelids, stared directly into my eyes, and slowly nodded.

J. was but one of so very many. In those years, my colleagues and I cared for hundreds of young men and women with this new disease. We established a comprehensive program to address the myriad needs of dying young men and women and launched several major studies, which helped define the epidemiology and established that HIV was transmitted heterosexually and among intravenous drug users via sharing contaminated needles and syringes. And, that HIV was not transmitted via close household contact.

In 1991, I moved to New Haven to direct the AIDS program at Yale University School of Medicine. Not unlike the Bronx, New Haven has been beset with poverty and drug abuse and, as a consequence, with AIDS. It has been one of the fifteen cities in the United States in which AIDS became the leading cause of death among both men and women between the ages of 25 and 44. Developing an AIDS Program at Yale has involved providing clinical care services, teaching, and research in which we have worked to develop new therapies to combat HIV replication and disease. By 1995, over 500,000 young men and women and children in the United States alone had died of AIDS. But, beginning in 1996, the tide of inexorable death and dying had been turned, and dramatic advances have reduced the rates of morbidity and mortality in a spectacular manner, unknown for any other disease in our lifetime.

Working as a physician in the AIDS epidemic has been difficult and painful, but also satisfying and meaningful beyond my expectations as a student embarking on a medical career thirty-five years ago. I have been fortunate indeed. In many ways, HIV/AIDS has crystallized my dual interests in medicine and in sociology by providing a precious and deeply personal contact with patients and an opportunity to participate in events in human history of immense social, cultural, and political consequence.

HIV/AIDS has illuminated the power of science but also its limitations. In the past twenty years, over thirty-five million adults and children have been infected with HIV worldwide and over fifteen million have already died. Ninety percent of those with HIV live in the developing world, where few have access to the therapies that have resulted in such a dramatic turnaround in our country. I am now planning to return to Africa, where I hope to find ways to extend the benefits of anti-retroviral therapy to that area of the world where the epidemic has had its greatest impact and where those afflicted have the fewest resources. I believe this to be a moral responsibility of the developed world and one with which I hope to conclude my personal journey in medicine.

RAMIN**AHMADI**

International Health and Human Rights

I t is the end of the twentieth century, and I am walking among the ruins of what used to be a vibrant downtown. This desolate place is the capital of the newly independent East Timor. It is two months since the Indonesian-backed militia rampaged the streets to punish the locals for exercising their right to self-determination by voting for independence from Indonesia. Four weeks of a vindictive military attack has defaced everything I see.

I am a doctor, and understand as a doctor all that I see. The Dili laid before me is on a gurney—its charm and vibrance damaged beyond recognition. In disbelief, I stare at the deformed skeleton of the buildings. These structures are gutted. Their flesh lacerated. The skin of their walls defaced and their skulls—rooftops—half exposed. The damaged columns are the city's broken bones, burned ribs, and clavicles; black smoke–filled fossae and fractured femurs of door frames are testimony to a catastrophe that followed a frenzy. One of the students working with me, Gina, murmurs with awe, "What a passion for destruction." Every building, every home, without exception, is burnt.

Gina, the other students, and I make up a small group of international guests brought to this site by East Timor's independence leader, Jose Ramos Horta, the 1996 Nobel laureate. Jose is making his historic return home after twenty-five years in exile, and we are accompanying him. What should have been a joyous homecoming is, instead, a return to a country ravaged by hatred, the inhabitants greatly in need of what little medical attention we can give them. In the eastern corner of the island known as Lospalos, we visit the only hospital in town. Dilapidated beds with occasional IV tubes penetrating the wasting bodies of abandoned East Timorese painfully remind us of the nation's deprivation. East Timor has sustained a massive trauma and hovers on that edge between life and death. Jose asks me to assess the condition of this hospital. He senses how desperate things are but wants an expert's view. I hesitate. Overwhelmed by the scene, I search my memory of my decade-long North American training in clinical medicine for words of wisdom, but feel embarrassingly inadequate. What is, after all, clinical medicine without diagnostic tools and pharmacy?

I see a two-year-old boy dying of starvation curled up motionless—with swollen belly and wasting extremities—and hooked to an empty IV bag. All of my training can render only a soul-wrenching tenderness. I approach his bedside, hold his little hand, but cannot help any more than that. No one can. He is alone in a world in which his little body is the very document of this world's terrifying inhumanity. Overcrowded facilities, the bullet hole–riddled walls, poor hygiene, filthy needles, broken tubes, dirty water, and a hospital out of basic medications—a slow and melancholic decay are all around us and I cannot tell Jose what I, a North American physician, truly see. I cannot tell him, nor can I tell the people who attempt to care for his people, that modern medicine in a place of such distorted humanity and such violated basic dignity seems a cruel and irrelevant joke. I cannot tell Jose that the massive human rights abuses of forced displacement render health workers speechless.

At home in my daily life, I am a physician living in the United States, specializing in internal medicine and employed by a community hospital in Connecticut. I came to this country in 1982, after living through the Iranian Revolution where, as a young boy, I saw my friends killed, and many others I knew suffer. From these experiences, an interest in human rights developed and has informed all of who I am. For all my adult life (I am now thirty-seven), I have worked for human rights. As a physician, I have striven to aid those caught in the crossfire of oppression and human rights. And as a human rights activist, I created the Center for Health and Human Rights at Griffin Hospital in Connecticut. Through a coordinated effort with other nongovernmental organizations (NGOs), I and other members of the Center work with leaders of these war-torn countries, as I did with East Timor's independence leader, Jose, to bring medicine where it is needed.

But I struggle with what to make of my Western clinical medicine training when confronted with these humanitarian emergencies in which I have a tendency to find myself. Can the physicians who are committed to the practice of health and human rights make a difference in humanitarian emergencies, or are they just a Band-Aid, a temporary relief agent whose time runs out with the money of the funding organization? And what lessons can we bring back home, to the advanced industrial world, that world in which the emergency is silent and pains of social injustice are hidden. We in the industrial world do not see the insidious harm of the violations to basic human rights. Our lives are so very different from their daily experiences.

In February of 2000, I visit another country and search again for answers to these tragic questions. This is Nazran, Ingushetia, and I am a member of a delegation of three from the Physicians for Human Rights, which intends to document the violation of human rights in Chechnya. The war in Grozney is ongoing when we arrive. Our mission is to conduct a survey of the refugee population—to gain an epidemiological understanding—and, not least, to report individual cases of human rights violations. A large population of refugees crosses the border daily. The agonizing shadow of war, fear, persecution, and homelessness is palpable even to a stranger like me. For weeks, the Chechens have continuously returned home only to leave for the border again under the heavy fire of bombs and artillery. We conduct the survey among a randomly selected group of refugees. We train young Chechen refugees to help us gather the data and then enter it into a database. In two weeks, we interview more than eleven hundred refugee families. I start interviewing the victims of torture and collect evidence of trauma through physical examination. Now my public health skills and knowledge help me analyze the survey results, while my clinical medicine training enables me to document the individual cases of torture.

In a modest refugee home, I talk to a mother who has lost her son in the war. From what I'm told, her twenty-year-old daughter, an exceptional student of mathematics at the University of Grozney, is experiencing post-traumatic stress syndrome. It has been weeks since she talked or walked. She lies in her bed, flaccid. She stares at everyone without a word. Her mother wants to know if I can treat her, cure somehow this mysterious disease that has debilitated her bright girl. I do not tell the mother that it has been a long time since we physicians cured anything and that our discoveries and research now focus on the management of chronic conditions. I sit across from her daughter and try to begin a conversation. She gives me a bewildered look and a smile. In her eyes I see my own reflection: a creature that knows and sees but is paralyzed, incapable of bringing about change. I observe with a scientist's precision, take notes diligently, and try my best to translate human suffering into collectible and measurable data. But is this all that modern medicine and public health can offer in the face of the atrocities of war? All I prescribe is "watchful waiting," like many other instances when the diagnosis is uncertain and treatment unclear.

In Chechnya, the war has taken its toll. The math student never uttered even a word to me. I had no miracle for her in my backpack. Before our delegation left Chechnya, I asked the young refugee volunteers who worked for us what they expected us to accomplish when we return to the United States. To my surprise, they had no illusions. They knew all too well that Russia, the superpower, would not budge under the international community's scrutiny, nor would it respond to the pleas of her own citizens. But the students had one request, as one of them passionately expressed it, "Don't let the world forget us. Tell them our story. Tell them what is happening to us."

We promise to do just that. And do. My colleagues and I, as members of Physicians for Human Rights, make a lengthy report based on our findings. The report makes its way to the United Nations High Commissioner for Human Rights, Mary Robinson. Through small efforts such as these and many others by the international human rights organizations, we hope the world puts more pressure on Russia to stop its war in Chechnya as well as the massive violations of human rights in the region. These dark wartime streets barely hide the destruction of the massive waves of violence. New mass graves are bound to be discovered in Chechnya. And more physicians will try to document the tragedy and bring justice to the victims. Will they succeed? I have learned to be content with small gains. A small clinic, a few reports of human rights violations, and a few more human rights projects for my trainees here in Connecticut. Will other physicians at our hospital at home decide to do the same? Perhaps.

I do know that a new generation of physicians committed to human rights and justice will arrive at a similar scene. They will be younger, more energetic, and innovative. The greedy competition of health NGOs abroad and HMOs at home will not weaken their determination and courage to fight the injustice. And those young physicians, who have given themselves to the experience, will return home with a different perspective on life, death, disease, human rights and wrongs.

Back in Connecticut at my own hospital, I see our interns with white coat pockets bulging with the small books and cue cards of clinical pearls and words of wisdom. I often wonder what I would write on such a card for those interested in applying their clinical medicine and public health skills to alleviate the suffering of war-torn communities. Perhaps such a card will have to remind us of observations—both theoretical and practical—some of which have been made by the practitioners who have trodden the path before me. Perhaps I would write that health and human rights are inseparable. Or that clinical medicine and public health practice are complementary, that unless you define the health problems in human rights terms your solutions will not affect the human rights condition and, without that, modern clinical medicine loses its relevance. And that the health and human rights field is young, there is much work to be done, so have manageable expectations, and be happy with small gains—the difficult and confusing circumstances of humanitarian crises pose a daunting challenge to the health and human rights practice. But, indeed, I would write: never lose your idealism; never forget why you were drawn to the cause—the terrain of health and human rights practice, human rights–centered care, and liberation medicine will be the fertile ground where clinical medicine and public health training merge and bear potential to heal.

DYAN**GRIFFIN** and **LAURA**R.**MENT**

Women in Medicine

The time is now—when Dean Rosemary Pierrel looked out at her freshman class at Brown University and said, "You can do anything you want to do. You can be anything you want to be. Be doctors. Be lawyers. The time is now," it was the fall of 1966. Against the background of the Vietnam War, Women's Liberation, and the advent of the birth control pill, she predicted that women would assume increasing representation in medicine during the next several decades.

Since then, women applicants to medical schools have steadily increased. Thus, although women accounted for only 9 percent of all new entrants to medical school in 1970, the number of women entering medical schools significantly increased in the next ten years. By 1980, women were gaining ground when they represented both 28 percent of all applicants and 28 percent of all new entrants to medical school. The increases remained steady until 1990, when 40 percent of all applicants to medical schools in the United States were women. During the past ten years this growth has slowed somewhat. The reasons for a slowing of medical school applications are not yet clear, but certainly more women are applying to graduate school in the biologic sciences—who needs an M.D. degree if molecular biology is your one true love? Also, more women are entering all areas of science as more women graduate students are now choosing the traditionally male-dominated fields of physics, engineering, and chemistry. Finally, although some medical schools such as Yale have routinely reported entering classes composed of 50 percent or more women during the past ten years, only recently have the national data reached 44 percent women entrants. Last year, women represented the majority of entrants at twenty-one of the one hundred twenty-five medical schools nationally.

Women want competitive graduate training positions, too. Parallel to the increases in women entering medical school, women have taken the opportunity to enter residency-training programs in increasing numbers. In 1980, women represented only twenty-two percent of all residents; by 1998, women represented thirty-six percent of all residents. Since women represented forty percent of all new medical school entrants in 1993 and forty-one percent of all new interns in 1997, these data suggest that the great majority of women graduates are entering residency-training programs.

Women are more likely to enter the "care-giving professions," and many surveys have shown that the traditional reasons for choosing specialties such as salary and prestige are of less concern to women than to men. Thus, recent data from the American Association of Medical Colleges (AAMC) (published in *Academic Medicine Statistics*, 1998–1999) demonstrate that women are most likely to enter internal medicine training programs, followed by pediatrics, family practice, obstetrics/gynecology, and psychiatry. Furthermore, considerably more women than men are entering both pediatrics and obstetrics/gynecology training programs nationally. Nonetheless, women still want to enter the finest training programs in this country, and the AAMC consistently shows that when training program match results are evaluated, women are just as likely as men to be awarded training at their first-choice institution.

Surgery, however, remains a largely male subspecialty, and less than 5 percent of women selected surgical residencies in the year 2000. The reasons for this are complex: certainly lifestyle choices, the prospect of many long years of training, and the persistent feelings of male camaraderie associated with surgical residencies all play a role. Lastly, the only specialties in which the proportion of woman residents has not increased over the past decade are emergency medicine, neurosurgery, otolaryngology, and radiology.

Despite these advances, women residents still feel the problems.

One of us, D. G. (chief resident in pediatrics at Yale–New Haven Hospital), expresses the difficulties experienced by women residents as follows:

> As an undergraduate student majoring in biology, I knew I wanted to enter a health care profession. I longed to go to medical school and saw myself working in academic medicine. But I was torn, because I knew I also wanted a family, and I believed it would be very difficult to succeed at both. Yet, when I looked at my college classmates, I discovered that a significant number of women were applying for admission to medical schools. This realization empowered me, and I told myself that if they can do it, I certainly can, too! So I followed my heart, and, seven years later, succeeded in becoming the chief resident of a prestigious pediatric program.
>
> Although I have never questioned my decision to pursue my dream, at times I have struggled with how to strike a balance between my professional and family responsibilities. Working eighty to one hundred hours a week has forced me to postpone starting a family. This is my personal decision. At the same time, I have been impressed with, and often marveled at, other residents and faculty members who have somehow succeeded at being dedicated pediatricians as well as devoted parents. However, as I look at the faculty, there continues to be an obvious discrepancy in the number of women who have attained positions as associate and full professors. Similarly, the number of women who work as surgeons, in surgical subspecialties and in critical care medicine, is far less than the number of men who work in those areas.
>
> I am encouraged, however, by the fact that women in medicine are continuing to make tremendous strides toward entering academic medicine and subspecialty fields. Many of my colleagues are constant reminders of how far we have come and how far we will go. Almost half of the graduating women from my class entered fellowships in various subspecialties. In order to ensure our continued progress, we must persist in our effort to support one another, and emphasize the necessity of equal opportunity and the importance of family values.

Career choices for women in medicine are numerous and varied. Women in medicine today are likely to find the same career choices that are available to their male classmates. While family responsibilities and the perception of gender bias may in the past have motivated some women to seek part-time employment in community clinics or private practice groups, most young women today feel that the choice is their own. Women are also more likely than men to be paid for employment that is less than full-time at some point in their careers. Nevertheless, a recent report in the *New England Journal of Medicine* (342:399–405, 2000) showed that during the past fifteen years women are more likely than their male peers to enter academic positions. This represents a major change from two generations ago! An informal survey of students and residents at our own institution suggested that both men and women were motivated not only by lifestyle concerns and family and/or financial responsibilities, but also by the mentors they had found during medical school and graduate training.

Academic medicine remains a challenge. As women began to enter medicine in increasing numbers, a major rallying point for women students and faculty became the paucity of women in academic medicine. During the 1970s and early 1980s, women represented a small minority of faculty members in medical schools nationally. The numbers of women who had achieved tenure were low, and in many schools women represented far less than 10 percent of senior faculty members. Women medical students subconsciously and not so subconsciously asked, "Where are the women role models for us to follow?"—and the few women who were on the faculty spent enormous amounts of time trying to fill the gap!

Recognizing that women represented half of all of the scientific community's brainpower, medical schools across the country began addressing the issues of women in medicine in the mid-1990s. Offices for Women in Medicine and committees dealing with the problems of women in medicine were established in many schools, and advisory programs for junior women faculty members became widely available. Furthermore, much has been made of the individual mentor—that professional who oversees a junior faculty member's academic progress, assists with research plans, and introduces the junior person to senior colleagues over lunch at meetings across the country or at breakfast on Saturday mornings in the hospital dining room. Not only were there were no "old-boy networks" for women—but women didn't seem to know how to make such things work. Indeed, most women who worked Saturdays and nights locked their doors and frantically tried to catch up. Recently, however, schools have taken a different approach. "Role models" don't have to be idols who are the classic triple threat (teaching, research, and clinical care). A recent study at Johns Hopkins School of Medicine showed that mentoring programs for women—whether provided by female or male mentors—help women climb the promotion ladder at the same pace as men.

These strategies have definitely benefited women, and last year women represented 27 percent of all faculty members at medical schools in the United States. Pediatric departments had the most women faculty member (41 percent), and orthopedic departments had the least (10 percent). In addition, rightly or wrongly, advancement in academic medicine remains largely dependent on research productivity—and a recent survey at our institution demonstrated that women faculty members were just as likely as their male peers to be awarded funding from the prestigious National Institutes of Health. The dollar amount of funding is important also, and women faculty members had just as many research dollars per person as the men had.

It's not a perfect world, and the problems of women in medicine are not unique to those in academic medicine, although perhaps the problems have been more clearly defined in this group of women. Furthermore, the problem of numbers tends to be most prominent in the upper ranks of faculty in academic medicine and medical schools, while the solutions must move upward with the continuous flow of women graduates. Nonnemaker has studied a group of women and men who graduated from medical schools between 1979 and 1993 and reported the results in the *New England Journal of Medicine* (342:399–405, 2000). Females were significantly more likely than males to seek a career in academic medicine, but women were significantly less likely than men to be promoted to the associate professor and full professor ranks. In this study, as the number of women graduates from medical school increased year by year, the number of women faculty members also increased—but the women remained at the lower ranks. If one looks only at the rank of professor—the ultimate achievement for most medical school faculty—9.3 percent of women were professors in 1989, and only 10 percent held the rank of professor in 1999. At this rate, it will take another twenty-five years for 15 percent of women faculty members to become professors. This is frustrating for many junior faculty members, who note that nationally over 30 percent of all males in academic medicine are professors. Furthermore, only 6 percent of all department chairpersons are women, and less than 5 percent of all deans are women.

Why are women leaving academic medicine? And why are they not promoted at the same rate as men? There are no easy answers to these questions, but the women themselves cite lower pay scales, inadequate mentoring programs, and the lack of access to leadership positions as barriers. Finally, as Catherine DeAngelis, the editor of the prestigious *Journal of the American Medical Association*, has said: women—and only women—can bear children, and as physicians they remain in large measure the primary caregivers for their children.

These problems are not unique to women in academic medicine; women physicians everywhere worry about lower pay scales, perceived gender bias in leadership positions, and the family responsibilities that encroach on their working hours. Also, it is no big surprise that when women juggle jobs, no one wins. The workplace loses brainpower, and the women themselves lose the self-esteem of a job well-done.

What are the solutions? There are no easy answers to the problems that women entering medical school today may face, but there is strength in the increasing numbers of women who choose to do so. Further, there is increasing recognition by universities that women are half of the world's brainpower and that it would be a big mistake to lose this valuable resource. Today, most medical schools appreciate that women are different from men, and that the choices they make and the problems they face are very different from those their male colleagues encounter.

Over 25 percent of medical schools nationally now have offices and/or committees for women in medicine, and these programs have worked well to ensure that women receive not only equal pay and space, but also the mentoring programs that appear to be so effective. Further, there is no longer shame in part-time employment and maternity leave, and the traditional tenure clock has been lengthened for all faculty who choose to work part-time for any reason. More students are spending five years or more in medical school, with time off for research or personal reasons. Child care is more widely available than ever before, and female students, residents, and physicians routinely access maternity leaves. Finally, medical school deans recognize that all students may need confidential mechanisms to air their problems, and, even as this is written, many schools are establishing committees to address the harassment of students.

At the end of the day, there are no idols. There are women out there—in the community, in academic medicine, in industry—all of whom so enjoy their lives that the movement is slowly but surely moving onward. Looking back, Rosemary Pierrel got it right; eight of those two hundred women in the class of 1970 became physicians— but in the class just five years later, forty-five of two hundred are physicians today.

We both are women in medicine who have benefited from the contributions of other women. Most recently, Merle Waxman, Giovanna Spinella, Kathleen Haslam, and Marjorene Ainley provided us with data and information on women graduates and programs for women, and contributed to our understanding of the experience of women in medicine presented here for you.

JUANITA**MERCHANT**

Embracing Diversity, Overcoming Adversity

I like to think of my life as affirmative action in action—or how to make the most of every opportunity!

I begin my workday with the sound of "Mummy, bottle." My nineteen-month-old daughter, Olivia, usually wants her bottle between 7 and 7:30 every morning, warmed to her specifications. She will throw it back at me if it's too hot. I need an extra hour to dress her for day care, and myself for work. To save time, I bathe her at night. In the morning, while she's downing her bottle of milk, I quickly take a shower and dress. An important tip for working mothers: dress yourself first, then dress the baby.

I became a single mother when I adopted my daughter on her first day in this world. At that time, I was already over forty. My mother and I had always been close, and part of my idea of success included becoming a mother in addition to having a professional life. My mother was a teacher and had blended her innate teaching abilities in the classroom with mothering skills at home, raising me and my brother—and raising us well, as I like to tell her. I had thought seriously about following her career path and pursuing my interest in math by becoming a math teacher. And I always thought I would marry another professional and raise my children in a more traditional family. I especially wanted to raise a daughter. But life does not always proceed as expected. By the time I got my career (medicine as it turned out, not math) headed in the direction of "success," I was divorced, childless, and over forty. Determined nevertheless to satisfy my maternal instincts, I elected to adopt a newborn. Olivia was born in Detroit on September 2, 1999, the baby of a fifteen-year-old African American mother whom I never met, and since the day of her birth Olivia and I have found our various ways of being a family.

Early in my career, and as a new faculty member doing my own experiments, I used to arrive at work between 7:30 and 8:00 A.M. Now that I'm a mother, however, I usually don't make it to work until sometime between 9 and 9:30. My days as a tenured faculty member in a clinical department consist of a mixture of teaching, clinical service, and basic research. In addition, my administrative duties have increased to include department search committees, faculty senate, graduate student thesis committees, service on study sections at the National Institutes of Health, and travel to give talks and to chair sessions at various national and international meetings.

There is never a dull moment in academia. Each day is filled with new challenges, so it's difficult to describe an average day. Some days I'm busy resolving personnel disputes in the lab, writing manuscripts, reviewing grants, attending research seminars, and reviewing data. On other days, I have a mixture of clinical service, such as endoscopy or "rounding," and meetings with visiting faculty or various university committees. My evenings are filled with household duties that include cooking dinner and feeding Olivia, play, bedtime stories, bath, then "nite-nite."

Twenty years ago, I never would have believed that I was capable of such a busy and complex life. I'm sure that students reading my daily schedule may believe the same thing about themselves. So how did I go from growing up on the streets of Los Angeles to joining the medical school faculty at the University of Michigan? Three important themes permeate my professional development. First, mentors at key decision points in my educational development directed me along the paths to the current position that I now hold. Second, each training period prepared me for the next challenge, which, on the surface, may have appeared beyond my grasp, even intimidating, but forced me to move beyond my comfort zone and grow. Third, I tried to make the most of every opportunity that was presented to me.

I grew up the oldest daughter of a self-employed electrician from

Tuskegee, Alabama, who did not complete high school, and a school-teacher who completed her college degree at a traditionally black college in Oklahoma. My younger brother is an electrical engineer for Motorola and has two sons. My father was an alcoholic and deserted us when I was in the fourth grade. At that point, I remember vowing to myself to finish my education at all costs. I was determined not to end up poor, depressed, and destitute like my father. Grades one through twelve were spent in the Los Angeles public school system. I was a straight-A student from seventh through twelfth grade and discovered along the way that I loved math and science. In retrospect, though, I regret not being an avid reader. I think it would have made it much easier for me to handle the volumes of medical literature and scientific writing that I must now do.

I engaged in typical extracurricular activities to increase my chances of getting into a good college—I participated in bowling, skating, and badminton, and I volunteered as a candy striper in a local hospital. I am not aware of anyone in my immediate or remote family who is in medicine or science, and the only indications of my aptitude for science in grade school was my request for a chemistry set and my work as a candy striper. I was pretty much the typical kid growing up in the sixties, listening to Motown music and picking up the latest dance steps. By the time I reached high school, busing inner city students in Los Angeles was in vogue, and I found myself at an integrated high school on the west side of Los Angeles. I was still able to maintain my grade point average and take honors and advanced placement courses despite an extended day riding the bus to school. Occasionally, Mom would pick me up from school if she didn't have a faculty meeting, or I would catch a ride home with my girlfriend.

Despite my 4.0 grade-point average and honors courses, I had low average PSAT and SAT scores. Nevertheless, I was accepted at Stanford, Yale, UCLA, and several other colleges that offered scholarships. Those of us from the inner city attending major colleges and universities assumed that affirmative action was the reason we were admitted. Still, I was determined to make the most of a great opportunity and the scholarship money to boot. I elected to attend Stanford to get out of Los Angeles but not be completely separated from family as I would have been had I moved East. But the East Coast intrigued me, and I decided that I would consider eastern schools if I decided to attend graduate school.

I loved Stanford. I managed to do well my first quarter with the exception of getting a D on my first exam in freshman chemistry (so don't despair!). I still ended up, after studying hard, with an A-minus in the class. Freshman calculus diminished my interest in math and my desire to become a high school math teacher. I declared myself a biology major and enrolled in the typical pre-med curriculum. By the end of sophomore year, I was told that I needed a "research experience" in order to improve my chances of getting into medical school. So I responded to an ad to do summer research in the biology department at Stanford. This was a very significant decision since it was my first exposure to bench research and was ultimately the reason I love engaging in basic research today. In addition, Renu Heller, the research associate, for whom I worked, strongly encouraged me to pursue both M.D. and Ph.D. degrees. I think she thought that I, as an African-American woman, would need the extra clout and credibility that an M.D. would bring to someone trying to become successful in academics. She and her husband had received their Ph.D. degrees from Yale, and she encouraged me to pursue a joint degree program (M.D./Ph.D.) there. So I did.

I was accepted into a joint degree program at Washington University, but elected to take an M.D. offer at Yale. I later applied and was accepted into Yale's M.D./Ph.D. program while a second-year medical student. I was wait-listed initially at Harvard, and received admission letters from the other medical schools to which I applied in New York, Pennsylvania, and California. I finished at Stanford with a 3.6 average, honors in my major, and top MCAT scores (a relief after my SAT experience!). I headed East to Yale, much to the delight of Renu.

What are my views about affirmative action, and do I think it helped to propel my career? Certainly during the early 1970s, when I was applying to colleges and eventually to medical school, affirmative action was a positive buzzword. Given my grade-point average in college prep and advanced placement courses, it was an easy gamble for most schools to make. In the current climate, the decision to admit me might be more controversial given my SAT scores. I think that now there are two important issues to consider regarding affirmative action programs. First, is it advancing the careers of minorities into areas where they have long been excluded? Second, have we done enough? We have had enough experience over three decades to answer these questions. The data clearly demonstrate that we are increasing the number of qualified minorities in high-paying, professional positions. However, from the academic point of view, we still have made barely a dent in increasing the number of faculty in higher education, and this is equally true in the upper echelons of other professions.

In the end, was I helped by affirmative action? Yes. Was a more qualified majority individual excluded? I hope not. And I used the opportunity given me to the fullest extent. What one must ask (and, ultimately, admissions committees must decide) are: what are the best indicators of who will succeed in the work environment? And, should we accept everyone who looks perfect on paper according to one set of criteria? Unfortunately, we all know that life is not necessarily fair.

After completing the second year of medical school at Yale, I joined the M.D./Ph.D. program and completed my Ph.D. in cell biology over the next seven years. During that time, I met several gastrointestinal (GI) fellows who were doing research fellowships in the lab next door to mine, one of whom, Fred Gorelick, continues to give me good advice on career directions. Years ago, as a graduate student, he gave me pointers on how to say no to the myriad assignments requested of medical school faculty, an important lesson. I earned high marks in both the basic and clinical sciences and received the nod from the chair of medicine to do my residency at Massachusetts General Hospital in Boston.

By the time I completed three years of an internal medicine residency, I realized I missed doing bench research. Thus, I deliberately searched for a postdoctoral position rather than a clinical fellowship. It was during my three years as a nonclinical postdoctoral fellow that I reestablished myself in the lab and developed the project on the gastrin promoter (on how expression of the gastrin gene is regulated) that I have successfully continued in my own lab even today. Moreover, it was during this period that I met several key mentors who subsequently shaped my current career in academia. Although I am an African American woman, I have not believed it necessary to choose only other African American women for mentors—and would have found them few and far between if I had!

My postdoctoral mentor, Dr. Stephen Brand, a tough physician-scientist from Perth, Australia, guided me in how to think about research, set up a lab, and write grants and manuscripts. While presenting my postdoctoral research at our national GI Society (American Gastroenterological Association) meetings I met and was recruited by another of my mentors, Dr. Tadataka Yamada. He tracked my career after I left Boston to complete a clinical year of gastroenterology fellowship at UCLA, then made me a faculty offer that I couldn't refuse. I have been at the University of Michigan since 1991. By the time I arrived at Michigan to begin my tenure as faculty, Dr. Yamada had become chair of medicine. In 1993, he submitted my name to the Michigan Howard Hughes Medical Institute committee and from there my name was entered into the national competition for a Howard Hughes investigator appointment. I was officially appointed in 1994.

I detail the course of my rise from a student in an inner-city grade school to that of a faculty member at a major university to illustrate the indispensable role a mentor can play in a student's life. The important thing to remember is that a good mentor is invested in your life until "death do you part." However, unlike spouses, you should have multiple mentors that remain influential periodically throughout your life. And, of course, it's not just the mentoring, it's the action you take with every mentor and every opportunity. It's how you put the mentor's advice to use at each opportunity that ultimately enables you to make the most of every opportunity.

JOHN**BLANTON**

Civil Rights, Civil Medicine

The decision to become a physician can be one of the most agonizing and anxiety-producing decisions you can make. It implies a commitment to years of difficult formal education and training, a lifetime of continuous education and service to others, more than rarely putting yourself and your family aside while caring for complete strangers. In addition, the cost of the education of the future physician can leave the new medical school graduate in debt more than one hundred thousand dollars. You probably have friends contemplating careers in investment banking and anticipating large starting salaries immediately after college. Students who read the news are aware of the controversies surrounding paying for health care. You may have heard physicians grumbling about the endless intrusions of managed care companies into their daily practices. Unhappy physicians may even have counseled you against entering medicine. For some students, it may be hard to remain focused on the rewarding side of a career in medicine when the difficulties loom so large.

For the minority student, the application decision is even more complicated. Simply contemplating a career in medicine requires enormous energy and faith. Many are still likely to have attended poor schools in poor neighborhoods, which have subtly taught them that they have no academic or professional future beyond high school. Moreover, minority students are likely to be the first in their family to go to college. Even now as a minority student, you are likely to have had no physician role models to emulate. You are also more likely to view the expense of a rigorous formal education beyond high school as being completely impossible to manage. You may worry that your SAT scores aren't as high as some of your majority peers and that you may not even get into college. If you have received any college counseling in high school, you may have been steered toward community colleges or lesser-known colleges rather than to prestigious Ivy League schools. You probably wonder how you will ever function in the highly competitive, seemingly all-white world of higher education, medical school, and medical practice. If you are like I was as an adolescent and young adult, the decision to become a doctor is daunting indeed.

For me, the decision to study medicine was made during college in the sixties. I had always liked science and had contemplated a career in physics or engineering. Or perhaps, I thought, I would become an astronaut. Then the civil rights struggle became very public and very violent. I became amazed by the power of nonviolence. I grew up in Buffalo, New York, in a family that placed great value on education. The civil rights movement provided the idea of serving others. At first I tried to tell myself that I could serve others through physics, but that just didn't ring true. On some level, I knew I wanted to be more actively involved with other people. Then my family moved to Cincinnati, Ohio, and I found that we were living just a few houses away from our new doctor, a black doctor. Visits to his office introduced me to a new world. His waiting room was always full of patients— black patients. He always stayed late until the last one had been seen. In those fee-for-service days before managed care, I watched him tear up bills of patients whom he knew had no money to pay. Taking care of them was more important than being paid. He began taking me with him on hospital rounds and on house calls. I had a role model. I was able to watch and learn from a black physician who was actually doing "doctor things" and doing them well. Volunteering in the local hospital served to support my new career interest. At first, I worked in the chemistry lab, learning to do analyses on blood, urine, and spinal fluid—tests that were important in the management of patients. The more I learned, the more my interest grew. The more I worked in the lab, the more doctors I met who would explain what was wrong with their patients and how their illnesses affected the tests that I was doing.

I had found a career that combined science with caring for others. And I was excited. I was excited, that is, until I began to examine the application process, medical school itself, and the training that followed. Then I became intimidated. Could I actually do it? Could I compete with thousands of other students for a place in a first-year class? I worked harder in my college courses than I had ever worked before. One biology professor kept my spirits up while another told me that he thought I had no business applying to medical school.

Medical school interviews were another new experience. I didn't know anyone who had been through the interview process. I only had books about the application process and had heard all of the myths about interviews, which seemed to be designed to terrify the applicant. Determination and support from my family, my doctor, and that biology professor got me through. On the evening news I saw law enforcement officers beating black people in the streets, unleashing ferocious dogs on them, and spraying them with fire hoses. I had visited my grandparents in Mississippi and had seen State Police officers enforcing curfews on black people. I realized that these people displayed more courage in facing the beatings, the dogs, the fire hoses than I would ever need to apply to medical school.

The first medical schools that I investigated were those in the Midwest near my home in Cincinnati, and my college, Purdue University, in West Lafayette, Indiana. None of them carried a prestigious name; applying to such schools seemed out of the question. I then read about the system of medical education at Yale and became excited again. It was completely unique among medical schools and seemed like it had been created just for me. I had realized long before that some schools would reject me, and that was the worst that Yale could do to me. I applied, was accepted, and off to Yale I went.

The experiences of minority applicants are different now from those of applicants of the 1960s. Today's medical schools understand the value of a diversified student body. They appreciate the diversity of their patients and the society in which they exist. There is the sense that admitting a student body that reflects the makeup of the medical school's patient population is a legitimate goal of a medical school's admissions committee. The richness of a diverse medical school class is stimulating in a number of ways. Most students are repeatedly enriched by the experiences of their classmates whose lives have been different from their own. Most medical school faculty members have lived and practiced among peers very much like themselves. Working with students of different races reinforces the reality that our world is composed of a wonderful mixture of peoples.

What advice would I offer a minority high school or college student contemplating a career in medicine? First, be sure you're willing to work very hard, serving others, for the rest of your working life. Practicing medicine is truly a privilege. Patients will admit you into the most private parts of their lives in ways that no others are allowed to enter. We must always be cognizant of this privilege and respect it. You must be able to work with the demands of managed care systems while always maintaining your allegiance to your patients and remain committed to what is best for them. They will always be counting on you. You must never let them down. Ask yourself if you're able to defer your own needs until those of others have been met. You'll enter a world in which there will be times when everyone else will seem to want something of you and you won't be able to find time for yourself or for those you love. Ask yourself if you're able to sit with the pain of others. Being able to sit with someone else's pain means not shrinking away from your patient's agony. Ask yourself if you can comfort the dying patient and the patient's family. Ask yourself if you're able to help people grieve the loss of a loved one. Ask yourself if you're willing to endure a prolonged period of rigorous training long after your best friends are working at high salaries, driving expensive cars, and living in fine homes. Ask yourself if you're ready to endure the looks from patients and instructors who wonder if you, the minority medical student, intern, or resident, are really able to care for them. Ask yourself if you're ready to remain modest after you've made a difficult diagnosis or saved a patient's life. Ask yourself if you're ready to tell your community that you've decided not to open a clinic in the old neighborhood like you promised, but plan to go into research instead. Chances are they'll still be very proud of you. Ask yourself if you can master the science and technology and also sit at the bedside and hold the patient's hand. Ask yourself if you're ready to enter what I believe to be the most honorable profession on the planet.

Deciding to apply to medical school is an awesome decision. It is more awesome for the student of color. Find yourself a supportive teacher whom you trust and who will offer you encouragement and guidance. It won't matter what subject he or she teaches. Just arrange to talk to that person about your dreams. Volunteer in your local hospital. Get a feel for the hospital environment. Try to picture yourself in the physician roles that you see. In college, work hard. Get the best grades you can. Don't try to guess which courses will impress medical schools. Major in whatever interests you the most, and also take the relatively small number of courses that are required by the medical schools.

Now just a word about career choice within medicine. Physicians can do considerable good for individual patients every day. Caring for groups or classes of patients is more difficult but equally important. As a pediatrician, I have the opportunity to care for the child in front of me in the examining room as well as all the children in the entire country. At this time of unprecedented national prosperity, a projected 5.6 trillion dollar federal budget surplus, and hundreds of billions of tobacco settlement monies, there are still many important medical problems facing American children. Every forty-four seconds, a baby is born into poverty. Every minute, a baby is born without health insurance. Nearly eleven million American children currently have no health insurance. Most of them live in families with working parents. Every eleven minutes, a child is neglected or abused. Every two hours and twenty minutes, a gun kills a child or youth.

I believe pediatricians are in a wonderful position to help remedy all of these ills by aligning ourselves with some of the wonderful child advocacy groups that work so hard to lobby for the good of children. This work might consist of letter writing. We have a body of knowledge that we can share with elected officials that will help them vote for legislation that will benefit children. Sometimes testifying before legislative committees is beneficial. Sometimes visiting our elected representatives and speaking directly with them or their staff members can help aid children. This part of our work is essential because children have no power in our legislatures. They can't vote. They can't send contributions to their elected officials. In general, they simply aren't represented. We must be their advocates.

I have been a member of the admissions committee of the Yale University School of Medicine for a number of years. The vast majority of our applicants have excellent grades at the best colleges and universities in the country, and excellent scores on the MCAT. At every applicant interview I ask myself two questions: What has this person done that actually demonstrates an interest in helping people? and, Can I picture this person as a compassionate, empathic physician at the patient's bedside? Unless I can give a strong affirmative answer to both questions, the applicant stands little chance of receiving a favorable decision from me. If you can overcome the barriers to becoming a physician, and you really want a lifelong career helping medicine, then there is no alternative for you.

VINCENT**DELUCA**

Transitions in Medical Life

TAY AWAY FROM MEDICINE! Is that the advice you have been getting? Do you hear that doctors are unhappy and can't wait to retire? And that doctors are tired of being confronted with an array of new hassles in recent years from HMOs that exert more control over the way physicians practice medicine? Often, nonphysician clerks use diagnostic codes to dispute a physician's decision to order tests for patients. Physicians may be forbidden to order appropriate tests and medications because of these HMO rulings and, subsequently, run the risk of being threatened with malpractice for providing poor medical care! Physicians are stressed by all the new bureaucracy: so many forms to fill out, so many phone calls debating with the insurance companies about the appropriateness of their medical management, so many hassles they never had before managed care. Physicians have increased the volume of patients they see in order to make up for reduced payments for patient care. Pulled in all directions, they find less time for family and recreation.

Well, if you are seriously considering going into medicine, you should understand that such problems do not provide the true image you should have of medicine. I will describe two features that, for me, still form the core of medical practice, despite the very real problems of modern medicine. The first is the meaningful *physician-patient relationship*, which is fundamental to medical care and should never change. The second is the climate of medicine, always changing with new methods of delivering medical care, the ever-growing technology of medicine, and new pharmacology.

I will address this second characteristic first. Physicians, insurers, and government legislators are currently struggling with the question of how best to deliver good medical care. That has meant that, during the past twenty years, physicians have had many distracting and discouraging experiences. Yet the basic goals, ideals, and purposes of physicians remain unchanged. When I began my medical practice forty-five years ago, the medical climate was quite different. Physicians were totally independent, and certainly we were not accountable to insurance companies, or even to patients. Only a few patients carried medical insurance, and most patients paid for their medical care out of their own pockets. That care was inexpensive by today's standards.

Accountability, the degree to which physicians were responsible to patients and society for the manner in which they practiced medicine, was a personal matter mandated by reviewing bodies. No physician was sued, and malpractice insurance costs were a pittance. Peer review, the evaluation of a physician's medical practice by other physicians, was very limited if it existed at all. Managed care, with its control of medical practice for the primary purpose of limiting costs, had not yet been created. Patients did not question their doctors and rarely considered seeking a second opinion. Patient education, the teaching of patients about their disease and how they could be responsible for many of their medical needs, was a novelty. Government and medical societies followed a hands-off policy. Physicians were islands unto themselves. Was this mightier-than-thou attitude of many physicians a good one? Fortunately, most physicians, I believe, were highly ethical and moral, as I believe they are today, and firmly adhered to the principle of *primum non nocere*—first do no harm.

Today, the field of medicine is much more inclusive and offers young physicians much that is new and exciting. In medical education, you can find opportunities to teach medical students and physicians in training. In medical research, possibilities abound in studies in clinical work and in basic science. Then there is medical administration, in which a physician manages a hospital department. I have been fortunate to enjoy all of these opportunities in my career, and you can read about these and other opportunities elsewhere in this book.

Yes, the climate of medicine will continue to change, and physicians will always have to adapt to the ever-evolving social order. Current problems in the delivery of health care are a necessary part of this evolution by which the practice of medicine will continue to improve, for both patients and doctors. Physicians will become more accountable for what they do, more aware of patients' rights and of the importance of being cost-efficient so that our limited medical resources will be available to all. Our patients will take greater charge of their own care as they become more educated about health and illnesses.

But the current changes in climate have not affected the goals and aspirations with which most doctors enter medicine, and hopefully they never will. Medicine today is more collegial than it was in the past. Physicians work more closely as a team, seek other opinions more often, and are more aware of their limitations when confronted with difficult medical decisions. Physicians freely exchange ideas at medical meetings and enjoy each other's company at social gatherings. We gossip more readily about the trials and tribulations we encounter concerning patient problems, medical politics, and pressures placed on us by hospital and HMO regulations. We are a vigorous and gregarious group of individuals with the same interests, aspirations, and purposes, and we can now offer patients so much more because of medical advances.

Yet our main concern is the welfare of our patients, and I turn now to the more important core of medical practice, which is the physician-patient relationship: within the medical profession there are many rewards and satisfactions for physicians practicing medicine, but the greatest is that of helping the sick. Like many of my colleagues in practice, I have been fortunate to experience that joy many times each day for many years.

William Osler, a role model for all physicians as well as a great writer and medical philosopher, expressed a century ago the values of medicine that remain true today: humanities—that is, honesty, truth, accuracy, and thoroughness; charity and fraternity; the importance of medical education, books, libraries, and medical societies; and physicians' devotion to duty, high ideals, and exemplary character. Osler cites the words of Bartlett: "Ever since the first dawn of civilization and learning they have been the true and constant friends of the suffering sons and daughter of men. Through their minister and disciples, they have cheered the desponding; they have dispelled or diminished the gloom of the sick-chamber; they have plucked from the pillow of pain its thorns . . . in the circle of human duties, I do not know of any 'calling,' higher and nobler than those of the physician. His daily round of labour is crowded with beneficence, and his nightly sleep is broken, that others may have better rest. His whole life is blessed ministry of consolation and hope."

Yes, that sounds a bit flowery. But, in fact, physicians' responsibilities and duty to their patient have not changed. Bartlett is describing the art of medicine, namely, a meaningful physician-patient relationship, as opposed to the science of medicine. I have not seen its importance diminish in my forty-five years of medical practice, and neither will you.

Why is this physician-patient relationship so important in any field of medicine? Human beings have feelings that cannot be separated from their illnesses. Current advances in medicine will dramatically help physicians carry out the mission of "stamping out disease and saving lives." However, the fundamental mission of physicians, the creation of the physician-patient relationship, must always be part of a physician's work, what I think of as my ministry. Seventy-five percent of patients coming to my practice have a psycho-social component to their problems and need empathy and understanding in the form of a good relationship with their doctor. Advanced technology and pharmacology alone will not be enough.

For me, it is this relationship to patients that makes it a privilege to be a member of the medical profession. But although medicine, as a responsible, serving profession, remains unchanged, the climate will continue to change. The difficulties of the current climate should not dissuade you from choosing a career that will be pursued for a lifetime: entering medicine requires a lifelong commitment and demands generous time and effort. As a physician, you will be entrusted with the duties and responsibilities described by Osler and Bartlett so many years ago, to "become a true and constant friend of the sick, to minister to their care and cheer the desponding and rekindle their lamp of hope," to be willing to lose sleep when duty calls at night.

Your prime concern will be the welfare of your patients, but you must become involved in the politics of medicine and be proactive in developing rules and regulations that create the climate of medicine for the good of your patients. In other words, rather than adapt to change, I have found it better to try to create change. The hassles of today are due in part to the failure of physicians to take responsibility for the culture of medicine and the provisions and effects of medicine on all in the broader culture. Keep in mind that physicians can no longer live in isolation as they once did. Nor should they, I have found. Today's physician responsibly preserves the dignity and true purpose of medicine.

It is up to us physicians to keep our profession from being lessened by forces that consider medicine just another business and that regard a physician as simply another health care provider. Regulators need to understand that medicine is a very different profession and is distinguished by its primary purpose of caring for sick human beings. You will find that caring to be a challenging, complex, and serious responsibility. The road to joy in medicine is long and difficult, but I hope you will find your duties most rewarding.

HOWARD M. SPIRO

Growing Old in Medicine

H ow long can one last in medicine? I doubt that anyone reading this book, high school and college students most assuredly, ever broods about that question and growing old. That is just as well: to face old age in your youth might be paralyzing and would be certainly depressing. Presumably readers of these pages, in your second or third decade, are civic-minded enough to consider entering a profession whose income must seem paltry in what has been a culture of under-thirty multimillionaires. Nevertheless, for those of you contemplating a career in medicine, it is worthwhile to think about how long a medical career can last in a world in which ever-changing technology and new discoveries send waves crashing down on what has gone before. Yet there is nothing new under the sun: while I may treat an ulcer patient in the twenty-first century with antibiotics rather than with milk and mush, that patient and I can talk with each other in the same way as we might have done a hundred years ago. Diseases may evolve, mechanisms may unfold, but "a man's a man for all that," and that is why Shakespeare and Plato can still speak to us so readily after so many centuries.

Doctors are human, however, and we must admit our weaknesses. I remember the unhappiness of a Yale pre-med student with Crohn's disease when I advised him to choose a field of medicine that would not be overly taxing and particularly one that would not make him get up at night. As a sophomore he was ambitious and his exuberance had no bounds until, some years later, a residency in internal medicine gave him a realistic view of what he could or should not do. Yet even as I write this, I am amazed at the advances in technology that seem to make it probable that even a physical handicap will one day not prevent a would-be surgeon from performing operations. So do not despair. Medical practice has many rooms, and there is a place for almost everyone.

"No living man has heirs," my father used to warn, mirroring Jonathan Edwards, who seemed delighted that any one of us sinners might fall into the fiery pit at any moment. No one can predict how things will turn out, but here I will tell you about some of the challenges that aging doctors face, at least at present. My friend, whom I will call Dr. Paul, nicely exemplifies how age limits what physicians can do. Trained as a general surgeon at Yale, he was at the top of his form for the first twenty years of private practice. He could carry out two or three operations every day and yet be delighted to come back to the hospital at night to cut out a stomach that was bleeding or to patch up a colon that had "blown out." Such nocturnal escapades gave him a sense of accomplishment and excitement that made his six years of residency worthwhile. Indeed, he used to boast that he liked working at night even more than during the day because then he felt like a general commanding all that he surveyed. In his fifties, however, he began to lose his enthusiasm, especially for the emergencies that had once so fulfilled him. The operating lists showed that he was doing routine hernias and gallbladders in the place of more taxing procedures. That is how it goes for many surgeons who can face up to the challenges of life-and-death emergencies for only so long; at sixty, most are ready to settle for a less frenetic way to be a doctor, although you may know an exception or two.

The story of another colleague, Dr. Fred we can call him, was quite different. A chess player, he wrote poetry for his college magazine, and he read voraciously. I was not surprised that by the third year in medical school, he chose to become a psychiatrist. After five years of residency training, and in those days psychiatrists often took psychoanalytic training as well, he too went into private practice. Fifty years later, he boasts that he still works four days a week, and he claims that he is better than ever, by which I think he means, wiser. But many of us are envious of him, for my generation defines itself by its work, while yours, wiser I hope, may not need the reassurance of duties and the identity of a career.

Such extremes emphasize how disparate are the choices of life-style. Of course, a lot depends on luck and on what kind of person you are; some surgeons, like Dr. Michael DeBakey, keep operating into their nineties surrounded, one hopes, by their residents. In the 1950s, women medical students, first braving the restrictions of a nigh all-male profession, often chose pediatrics or psychiatry or radiology as fields with free time enough to raise a family, but that is changing as women are often now as likely to become brain surgeons as gastro-enterologists. And, nowadays, some pediatric clinics are open long into the night.

If you choose to become a practicing physician, you may have to decide between private practice (now usually with a group of like-minded colleagues), a salaried practice working for an institution, or academic life. You might think academic life would be a cushy way to go, with no nights on call, free weekends, and luxuriously long sum-mer vacations. Think again. Even in the best of times during the 1960s and 1970s, to be a good academic clinician you had to enjoy doing clinical research. Moreover, it was prudent to get a research grant or two to advance medical practice by new observations. Happily, in those days research was not so rigidly defined as laboratory work, so that it was possible for an academic full-time professor to study patients rather than their tissues or, later, their cells.

Most of us were delighted to work part-time in the laboratory because it gave us the chance to bring clinical problems and questions to be solved, or at least explained, by measurement or experiment. In the twenty-first century, however, combining clinical care with clinical research has become less comfortable because of the financial pressures on medical schools and teaching hospitals. It is very hard for me to find any difference between what modern clinicians do in private prac-tice and what they do in academic clinical practice. There are theoreti-cal distinctions, but the financial pressures on clinicians in academic life are enormous. I hope that things will change and that by the time you become a doctor, there will be a place for clinician-teachers once again. Right now, the main difference between a clinician in private practice and one in academic medicine seems to be that the first is somewhat more independent while the second is more willing to live in a hierarchical society. Some of you may be dismayed at the attitude of older doctors, who now urge their children into other fields and who loudly complain that "clinical freedom" has been destroyed. Be kind and listen to them, but remember that fashions come and go, and that while medicine right now seems to be in a crisis, things change and develop, and there will be return to a stable, albeit different, state.

Academic medicine, however, has been one of the fields of human endeavor where the young rejoice to teach the old. That has come about because clinical and laboratory advances over the past few decades have meant that teaching clinicians have had to run fast to keep up with all the advances. Still, for people who like to keep learning and teaching it has been a lot of fun. But there comes even in academic life a time, with salaries slowly rising and young folks clamoring to take over positions, that the chair of the academic department in which you work may well suggest, delicately if illegally, that you move on. And there is no easy egress for old clinicians in academic life unless they have worked on the basis of their clinical prowess.

That may even be true of private practice in the twenty-first century. Dissatisfaction at the profession's change into a business has forced many clinicians into retirement. In the 1900s, private doctors usually worked until they dropped, as the phrase goes. They had built their own careers, gradually enlarging their practice by taking on associates, and after thirty years or so, they began to take more time off. In those days, when hospitals were places to study the sick and not the intensive care units they have become, it was easy for such physicians to stop admitting patients to the hospital. Instead they were content to give advice from behind a desk to increasingly older patients, and kept that up into their seventies or more. That always made sense, for I do not understand why the most recently trained physicians are now urged to go into primary care, taking care of relatively healthy ambulatory patients, when they have learned the latest technology, which is far more needed in the hospital. Older doctors, I am convinced, should turn to primary care because they have learned patience with time and wisdom from living and practicing. As they have found how many problems get better with time, they are better able to advise patients who are walking around, whereas hospital patients, nowadays much sicker, can benefit from what the young have learned and can do. That isn't the way it goes, however. Whenever an older doctor decides to cut back, his or her associates rise up in anger mixed with derision to demand that he or she leave the practice, or at least take a salary cut. There's no getting around the conflict between the young and the old.

What the future will bring I do not know. For myself, I still would choose to become a physician in the twenty-first century, though I might not get into medical school given the rigorous requirements and the MCAT scores required nowadays. I probably would not become a gastroenterologist but would choose neurobiology for the excitement that I believe the future will bring, and for the chance to muse about body, mind, and spirit.

I hope that I have not discouraged any of you, for as I emphasized earlier, technological advances are vastly expanding what doctors can do—and even who can become a doctor. Medicine is still a wonderful career: physicians have the chance to help people, to feel needed, and to enjoy the spiritual arrogance that comes from "doing well by doing good." That is a great feeling at the end of the day, and at the end of a life.

Practicing Medicine

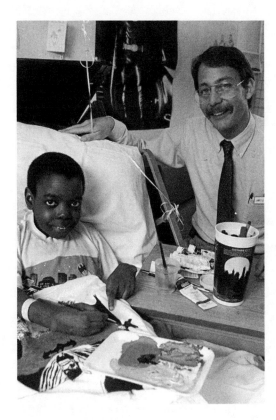

ifty years ago, a medical school class in America typically would have been composed of mostly white Protestant men, leavened by a few Catholic and Jewish men, one or two Asian or Hispanic men, and perhaps a few women. The Yale University Medical School of today has equal numbers of men and women from all over the world. They bring with them varied beliefs, habits, and cultural practices. But while those who practice medicine have become more varied, the practice of medicine itself has become more specialized.

David B. Melchinger makes vivid the almost frantic pace that the practice of internal medicine requires. In his downtown New Haven office he must deal with everything from ailing patients to faulty toilets. Yet he is content enough to predict that the future will continue to be fulfilling—and exciting—for those who care for patients. Cynthia A. Gingalewski and Dana K. Andersen describe with straightforward practicality the connections they see between everyday skills, well-rounded interests, and surgery. Charles McKhann describes what it was like to train in surgery at "the Hopkins" long ago, and he comments on what it is like to train in surgery now. The personal qualities which he suggests are necessary in the practice of surgery are, however, timeless. Morris Wessel praises mentors as he lovingly relates what made him the caring pediatrician he was for more than forty years. Ann Skopek, mother as well as family physician, relates the joys and difficulties women face in combining two careers. You will wonder how she gets everything done, but you will also learn why "motherly instincts" are crucial to patient care. Mary Jane Minkin, also a mother, describes her life in obstetrics and gynecology and has comforting words for men who still dare enter the profession. Malcolm B. Bowers, Jr., offers vignettes that gracefully illustrate what it is that psychiatrists do in an era of psychotropic pills. He and the writers preceding him share the joys and the problems of caring for patients.

In the last part of this section you will read how physicians must increasingly rely on other experts in their diagnostic endeavors. Bruce McClennan tells of the grand future for radiology, now frequently described as diagnostic imaging, and Brian West details the equally important role for pathology. They convey the extraordinary relevance of both specialties to twenty-first century medicine. Maurice J. Mahoney will rivet your attention with the intricacies—and even majesty—of genetics and the hope it presents to modern medicine.

DAVID B. MELCHINGER

The Future of Internal Medicine

This is a good time to think about becoming a doctor. The world seems to be changing daily, and medicine is no exception. Internal medicine in particular is in need of new understanding and new purpose from new minds.

A new vision of this purpose will depend on your vantage point. Your graduation date might be 2006. The year 1966 was mine, so my vision for the coming century grows out of a checkered, or widely experienced, four decades as internist, epidemiologist, "wet" bench clinical researcher, philosopher, and clinical teacher. This is perhaps a strange professional background, but I will lay out my biases by reciting my history in internal medicine from 1962 to 2000.

I started by watching Oscar Deutel, the eccentric and dedicated family doctor who ministered to my birth family. I remember calling Dr. Deutel when I was left alone at age twelve to take care of my seven-year-old sister when she was attacked by a dog. He seemed to arrive as I was hanging up the phone. For fifteen years, I watched how he enjoyed his work and the autonomy, skill, intellectual challenge, and interaction with children and adults that accompanied it. He told me stories that I now recognize were increasingly intellectual clinical and psychological exercises for him and for me. He was a traditionalist from Jefferson Medical School and wanted me to become a "Jeff boy." I suppose it was the same in his mind as my becoming a doctor. In college, while waiting for an angel with a flaming sword to appear at the foot of my bed to point the way for me in philosophy, I found I had only applications for medical schools on my desk. My interviews were unexciting until a canny Yale professor asked me to explain certain points about Wittgenstein that he did not understand. After the third question, I realized my answers were less adroit than his Socratic questions. I was accepted to Yale University School of Medicine, and as I entered the main building I read over the entryway large blue Greek letters suggestively recalling *The Republic* with "They shall pass their torches from one to another." The original is actually a question by a bored Socrates about night horseback relay races to friends trying to lure him back to Athenian Olympics, but I was happy to think I had been selected as a symbolic torchbearer.

Anatomy was cadaver-based, and information was in books. In an elective course in the history of medicine from Hippocrates to the 1960s, I learned that medicine was always changing despite my own attempt to hold it still for analysis. My philosophical romance with the mind and body was rapidly seduced to the investigative side. The academics who were my teachers in medical school were keen investigators and often "triple threats" in research, teaching, and doing clinical medicine. I was eager to find out what they were doing. On the wards in my third year, my new heroes were surgeons. A forceful senior resident's style impressed me most. He diagnosed appendicitis in silent four-year-olds with his "bed shake test" and used stairs rather than elevators on rounds to save time. He once diagnosed typhoid fever in a child who was thought by the pediatric staff to have osteomyelitis; he waved off their offended amazement by saying he had spent two years on a reservation and knew what children with typhoid looked like. His unassuming confidence and backhanded panache seemed worthy of emulation. Then fate changed my heroes and my timing.

In my junior year a medical intern died in a freak accident and a second intern developed severe ulcer bleeding and had to leave his post, so I was called back from Christmas vacation to take his place. For the next two weeks I was cosseted every afternoon by top professors who "just dropped by to help." I was a sponge for learning. Patients and their problems from that period are still heavily imprinted on my personal and clinical memory. Internal medicine was clearly the route for a philosopher. They wanted me, and I never thought of applying in another field or anywhere else. Professionally, I was home.

In the meantime, I worked at the blood bank to help defray my tuition costs and to support my student research in hematology. I was attacking the magic of coagulation with modern protein chemistry and I saw a life of wet bench, ward, and lecture hall. That life paled somewhat as I began to see the difficulties of academic infighting. My wife and I agreed that we wanted to get out of the country to reset our political and emotional bearings during that strange late-1960s period of turmoil and race riots, and we spent 1967–69 in West Africa with the U.S. Public Health Service, working toward the eradication of smallpox. In 1967 we felt right as a nurse-doctor team in Ghana with a Kennedyesque fervor of taking technology to the Third World. The ironies of such programs came to me later. Eradication was achieved more effectively with simple, individual vaccination needles than with our high-tech jet vaccination guns. Worse, we well-meaning techies may have been duped to make the world safer for biochemical warfare because the United States and Russia kept the variola virus alive "for research." In Ghana we saw the United States through foreign eyes. Children sick and dying in their mothers' arms waited in line at the Korle Bu Hospital Pediatric Clinic. Onchocerciasis turned from a poetic parasite disease studied in my second-year pathology class into "river blindness." Children not yet blind led blind thirty- and forty-year-olds through the villages to the banks of the expanding Volta Dam Lake.

I came back to Western internal medicine with a sense of the immense numbers of untreated tropical misery—even before AIDS—and I was aged before my time about life and death in my old professional world. Here in the temperate United States we were trying to save all lives in the context of the technological imperative. I had become chief resident and saw more of the good and the bad of academic medicine. I soon returned to my love of hematology in a research fellowship, but personal and professional incompatibilities eroded the love very quickly and I returned to clinical medicine, with heavy periods of clinical teaching at Yale.

Eleven years at Yale University Health Services taught me that physicians who do not administrate are doomed to be administrated by others—and the others will not be physicians! Doctors who say, "Don't they understand, I just want to practice medicine?" do not understand that they let others narrow that practice. Eventually, I tried for more freedom in private practice while remaining in the shadow of Yale. At this very point, Medicare and the rise of HMOs restricted physician autonomy with harsh rules and nasty language. The successes of medicine in the 1970s and '80s led everyone to expect medicine to solve everything. An arm cut off, polio, heart attacks, kidney failure, pneumonia—we could be expected to fix it all. The ancient awe for doctors was developing into an impatience with delayed delivery. And "delivery of health care" was the new catchword.

Where does this odyssey take me, and where might it lead you? All my experiences are facets of internal medicine. Internal medicine now is more a generalist part of medicine at large than the specialty it was in the 1960s. As "primary care" physicians, we are often the first physician a patient sees for an illness before referring the patient to the "specialist" who focuses on a particular, serious disease. I often refer to myself as a dinosaur. I have acquired hypersubspecialty skills in tropical medicine and eating disorders, but most of my daily work is "primary care." I do not bristle any more when my patients call me a general practitioner, but I confess I try to correct them. They don't really care much—they sometimes have an understandable confusion between "intern" and "internist." (In my more ironic moods I remark on the stunning similarity in paper work.)

The better part of my day is spent with patients I like, taking histories, listening to accounts of human problems, doing physical examinations, and trying to decide how far to carry diagnosis with potentially dangerous procedures and treatments. The intrusions from administrative requirements by the various regulatory agencies, recertification tomes from HMOs, precertification for hospital admissions and referrals, and the simple business of making sure the office has staff, working toilets, phones, and other wherewithals erodes my time with patients. Such problems may push many young internists into salaried jobs in managed care HMOs so that others can take care of the "nonmedical problems." Such physician/employee status can cost a lot in salary, job uncertainty, and autonomy, but it allows you to leave the building when your employer says your work is done. In a world ready to have doctors work forever, this may provide protection for yourself and your family.

Spend a day with me to see the flow in a general internal medicine office. The Tuesday schedule is long. I start at home at 4 A.M. and do notes, consult letters, and forms (two pages for Medicare's certification for a "quad-point" cane) until OJ and coffee at 7:00 before running to see two early patients for lower bowel checks with fiber-optic endoscopy. One is clear. The other has a large polyp likely to be cancer and will need further evaluation and possibly surgery. We go over this. By 8:00 I am doing ECGs and urines myself since the first of our staff doesn't come in until 8:30. I act as office manager, and everyone has my unlisted home number should they need to call in sick. I haven't heard from anyone, so I expect a full team today. By 10–11 A.M. I have seen six to ten patients, answered half a dozen phone calls, triaged someone with chest pain to the emergency room, and filled cancellations with patients who have acute problems ranging from colds and sinusitis to pneumonia. One of my colleagues asks my opinion about a woman whose mastectomy has left her with swelling that serves bacteria as a launchpad for invading her bloodstream. I respond that she needs inpatient IV treatment. Another in-office consult for my special interest in inflammation leaves another colleague and me wondering how the fourth finger of her right hand developed middle and then distal bands of redness. She is seventy years old and somewhat coyly admits to gardening without gloves and rowing daily on the Connecticut River. I surmise that she is doing something strange to her hands so I search for questions to bring some repressed habit to her mind. More of such intrigue until I force myself to go and check my hospital patients. I prefer to wait until evening to make rounds—all the lab work will be in—but the early afternoon hospital trip lets me see the interns and residents working on my three current inpatients. None of this has the exhilarating intensity, however, of my four weeks in July–August when I spend most of my time on the acute wards working with and teaching these sharp young doctors. They also teach me. Two afternoons a week, I try to leave time for patients with eating disorders or complex internal medicine consultations. This special scheduling lets me avoid the usual three to five interruptions per patient visit from phone calls and other troubles. It allows me the time, say, to sit on the floor of Exam Room 2 holding three-year-old Isabella's hand after her mother, who is here to check her Crohn's disease, tells me Isabella was bitten in school by a classmate and feels too traumatized to talk with me as she usually does. Many of my colleagues would regard this as beyond internal medicine, but my interpretation of internal medicine includes an element of family practice. I like to talk with children, and I have not infrequently held babies in one arm while examining parents with the other.

During the day I fit in office management problems: stuck windows, invading bees, running toilets, and sick staff. The intensity still can be wearing. Thursdays and Fridays I treat myself to Medical Grand Rounds and Cardiology Rounds. Fridays lately I spend time with students on Ethics and Critical Incidents Rounds. The talk is often very personal and very passionate. By 7–8 P.M. I go home, and my wife Chris and I review our day. I am on call nights and weekends in rotation with my three colleagues. Time off is important but hard to arrange. The paperwork is endless. I hit parity years ago when time with patients equaled time with paper. This burden would be very heavy for me without the joy of teaching.

Some of my most enjoyable experiences teaching medical students and house officers have been at Yale. Enthusiastic and dedicated students and doctors in training are always the best reward for the sacrifices modern teaching demands. In earlier times, patients stayed for one or two weeks and so much of the teaching was contemplative and unhurried. There were far fewer tests and procedures to consider. Modern teaching is more complex. Patients need to be moved in and out of the hospital very quickly for financial reasons. They may arrive with a vast array of data to be sorted, reviewed, and assessed. Or they may arrive with none. Time is always a pressure, and there is a sense of great urgency. Patients do not get into hospitals now unless they are very ill or about to have critical procedures. Patients in a teaching hospital such as Yale have multiple evaluations, and competition surfaces among students, house officers, and teachers to discover historical or physical exam information that others have missed. Yet, the cooperation within this competition among dedicated clinicians is sometimes strange and wonderful. At Yale the tradition in internal medicine is that students who find things their seniors have not yet seen gain approval and respect for their thoroughness.

Teaching may be the best experience an internist can have. It is the test of the *techne* of the profession. The Greek sense of *techne* translates as "art." *Techne* is also the root of our modern sense of "technical." The apparent dichotomy between technical skill and art is as artificial as the apparent division between *psyche* and *soma*. Yet many internists no longer go to hospitals because the time spent there is long and generally poorly compensated. Some specialists now even express surprise at finding general internists in hospitals. Hospital boards often have more specialist than generalist representation because only specialists have the income to support such time out of their offices. All these factors allow and even encourage a lessening of the traditional leadership role of internal medicine in the life of medicine and society.

Internal medicine for the next thirty to forty years probably will present basic training for evolving subspecialization in areas such as cardiology, infectious disease, transplantation, cancer, and the like. There should continue to be options for focusing on basic biochemistry and pharmacology in labs, primary teaching, or taking care of patients in hospital or office/clinic settings. Specific careers are hard to predict. One good vaccine against coronary artery disease would make major changes in cardiology. The developments in the last ten to twenty years almost make me dizzy imagining what can come next.

These times are exciting and run at a faster pace than *The Republic*'s night torch relay races invoked in those blue Greek letters over the Yale School of Medicine Cedar Street entry. Rene Dubos in *Mirage of Health* pointed out that wherever humans meet the changing niches of their environment they will find new diseases. The front line of diagnosis and treatment for these new diseases in 2030 probably still will be internists.

CYNTHIAA.**GINGALEWSKI**
and **DANA**K.**ANDERSEN**

Coming to Surgery from Many Directions

I t is hard, if not impossible, for a pre-medical student to know what surgery is like as a specialty, unless one of your parents is a surgeon. Some interests that you have discovered, or skills that you already have, may forecast a satisfying career choice in surgery. But the first challenge, of course, is gaining admission to a school of medicine, and you may have a better chance of being accepted if you have done well in an area you are interested in, outside of science, rather than feeling compelled to concentrate on science courses as a prerequisite for gaining admission. Although academic achievement is required, a well-rounded set of interests and a knowledge of different cultures are probably more important as predictors of success in medicine, and surgery in particular, rather than high grades per se. So our advice is to excel in the things in which you are interested.

There are some common regrets that are felt by many in medicine, and one of the most common is not having taken courses in college that were outside the "required" fields of study. More than just pleasant pastimes, music, art history, painting, photography, marine studies, geography, and history are all important aspects in the development of someone who will interact with patients from diverse backgrounds for the rest of his or her life.

Read lots of good books, and participate—perhaps even achieve a high skill level—in the arts, music, or sports. Learn about people

and civilizations and the artistry of cultures, in addition to the fundamentals of chemistry or biology. If you love biology and enjoy learning
of the relationship of molecules, structures, and organ function, take
the time to experience different people by traveling, joining clubs with
diverse membership, and taking courses that enhance your sophistica-
tion. In surgery, technical dexterity is a necessity, and advanced biology laboratories or summers spent in a scientific environment may
confirm your enjoyment of precise technical tasks. But so might video
games, fly-fishing, or archery! So do not be afraid to spend time on
hobbies, not just to pass the time, but to learn another area of endeavor in depth.

A lack of comfort in talking to others is shared by many students
despite high scholastic competence. Although all of the hands-on specialties require an ability to relate to people, the surgeon has to achieve
a bond of trust with his or her patient. This is possible only if you feel
comfortable talking with people. It is a good idea to volunteer at a
shelter or a children's care center, or to give music, sports, or math
lessons. You have to feel comfortable talking to people, and to learn
how to ask questions about others. If you are not sure whether your
people skills are as developed as you would like them to be, consider
taking a year off to work with people, to travel, or to spend time with
patients to learn what this is all about.

Are there technical skills or interests that predict satisfaction in
surgery? Certainly, the ability to handle surgical instruments is required, but for the undergraduate student this may mean playing the
cello, painting landscapes, or working as a laboratory assistant. Having
the hand-eye coordination to toss a basketball into a fifteen-inch hoop
twenty feet away, or to putt a golf ball well, might be equally relevant.
Understanding spatial relationships is probably the most important
underlying skill, and a student who enjoys activities that include an
awareness of spatial factors is already well along the way to discovering
surgery as a gratifying career.

Surgery is practiced in a windowless, high-tech environment, in
which a team of people has to function successfully. This collaborative
environment is as important as the surgeon's technical dexterity but
is an often overlooked aspect of the field. Skillful teamwork is the second most essential predictor of success in surgery, and the ability to

relate to, and manage, a team (which is perhaps more innate to women than to men) may be the next most important prerequisite after the enjoyment of handling delicate tissues precisely. So participate on a team, and take the responsibility for leading the team if the chance comes your way. The team may be academic, athletic, or social, but the focus of endeavor is less important than the experience of learning how to herd a group of enthusiastic people toward a common goal.

What experiences prepare the student for success as a surgeon? One of our favorite examples is the surgeon who, as a student, worked each summer as a bartender on a railroad bar car. There he successfully learned to be precise, efficient, punctual, aware of the principles of cleanliness, and able to relate to people (and listen empathically to their stories). Another predictive quality is stubbornness, at least in terms of devotion to a goal. Surgery is hard work and selects people who are willing to subjugate their own personal enjoyments for the privilege of operating on people. Whether you will love it enough to pursue it will depend on your experiences in medical school. The most important predictor is whether you want to help sick people get well, one on one.

Finally, an important quality is the pursuit of excellence. Not a presumption of excellence, but a lifelong willingness to try to do things better. In surgery, we meet weekly to discuss our mistakes and disappointing outcomes in something called a "mortality and morbidity conference." We may be the last clinical specialty to do so, but it underscores our awareness of the fact that a small error, or a seemingly trivial oversight, can have a devastating result. So we perpetually ask ourselves, how can we do things better? Or, put another way, surgery is the lifelong pursuit of outstanding clinical skills. If this does not interest you, you should not apply. It is very helpful if you realize this aspect of surgical culture early on.

Good advice is important, but not just from your pre-medical advisor. Talk to people who are in medical school, people who are in their training, and people who have practiced medicine for years. During vacation, visit with your family physician and ask about his or her interests and experiences in medicine. Find out what knowledge or skills that this individual wishes he or she had acquired, and spend time in the hospital with a physician to understand the environment.

Many, if not most, who eventually select surgery as a career, are uncertain of their career choice upon entry to medical school. They discover that the team environment, the emphasis on efficiency and technique, the thrill of participating in the surgical event, and the satisfaction of seeing people get well after their direct intervention describe the setting in which they see themselves functioning happily for decades. Some books that may help acquaint you with a career in surgery include *Century of the Surgeon* (Jurgen Thorwald), *Intern* (Dr. X), *The Making of a Surgeon* (William Nolen), *Mortal Lessons* (Richard Selzer), and *Human Hands* (Hardy Hendren). If one or more of these captivates you, chances are you already have the spirit and the devotion to the task, and that predicts success in a surgical career. We wish you good luck.

Surgery: High Stakes, High Rewards

The lobby of the hospital where I trained and worked as a surgeon for several years was the gateway to a different and wonderful world. Walking through it late at night reminded me of why I went into medicine, and surgery, in the first place. It was a large, impressive hall with a very high ceiling. In the wee hours of the morning I usually had it completely to myself, the only sound being the echo of my own footsteps. Like my other surgical colleagues under similar circumstances, I was there because someone was very sick or badly injured and I had every reason to believe that we could help him or her. The twenty-minute drive from home to the hospital gave me a chance to review what I had been told on the telephone, including the diagnostic possibilities and the various steps that would be required to deal with each one. After examining the patient, reviewing the laboratory studies and X rays to confirm the diagnosis, and explaining to the patient and family what needed to be done, I was ready to say, "I think we'd better take him to the O.R."

The operating room is the surgeon's workshop. It is the inner sanctum of the hospital, air-conditioned but windowless, where access is limited to keep outside traffic to a minimum and reduce the risk of infection in surgical patients. The drama popularized on television is in reality a quiet, understated drama. Its main participants are the patient, who has the problem, and the surgeon, who must solve it. The surgeon must provide leadership throughout the course of the patient's care, particularly so in the operating room, where he or she has responsibility for a large and complex team. Skilled people from a variety of medical and technical specialties, including assistant surgeons, anesthesiologists, nurses, and technicians, pool their efforts to provide maximum benefit for a patient in a very short period of time, usually just a few hours. Large operations, such as open-heart surgery or organ transplantation, may require as many as ten or more people working as a team toward a single goal, so it is understandable that a bond of camaraderie exists in the operating room between the surgeons, resident surgeons, and nurses. Medical students are often incorporated into this association very quickly; some who eventually go into surgery even date their attraction to the time they first experienced the sounds, emotion, and energy of the operating room.

Preparation for a career in surgery is a long process of graded responsibility. Four years of medical school are followed by five years of clinical training, or "residency," in surgery. This residency is a hospital-based experience; most teaching hospitals are associated with medical schools. The relatively easy operations that residents learn to do in their first year, such as biopsies and hernia repairs, are followed by increasingly complex procedures and much greater responsibility for decision making. By the end of the final year a surgical resident should have done all of the procedures that would be encountered in the practice of surgery. Moreover, surgical training is where it all begins, rather than where it ends. The life of a practicing surgeon continues to be stressful. The hours are long, irregular, and unpredictable.

Surgery is a manual activity in which you deal with things that you can see, feel, touch, and actually change. It is tangible, tactile, and technical, a direct, hands-on approach to the treatment of disease. As such, it appeals to people who like to use their hands, people who may have made things as children and enjoy repairing things as adults, and who see the technical aspects of surgery as a craft. Many who go into surgery are intrigued by the beauty of human anatomy, realizing that they will explore and treat areas of the body that few people ever see. Surgeons enjoy seeing the pathology with their own eyes, not just through an abnormal laboratory value or even on X ray. More important, they enjoy the practical solving of problems with a very direct connection between their medical knowledge and its help for the patient. In emergency settings this may require making important decisions with far less than complete information. Surgery is a dynamic and aggressive approach to disease that provides a nice balance between intellectual and technical skills. It allows one to think and then to act.

Although it is the product of a rich tradition and a colorful history, modern surgery is one of the most rapidly evolving disciplines in all of medicine, constantly being fed by new technology and techniques. Heart-lung machines that make open-heart surgery possible, artificial joints as large as hips and as small as those in fingers, and prosthetic grafts to replace obstructed blood vessels are a few of these. General surgery has been "made over" by the advent of laparoscopic surgery, in which major intra-abdominal operations are carried out through tiny incisions, using tubular ports into the abdomen and long-handled instruments, many smaller in diameter than a pencil. This is all made possible by having a tiny light source and a miniature video camera that can be moved around inside the abdominal cavity and provide surgeons with a greatly enlarged picture of what they are doing. The procedure is followed completely on a television screen. The advent of laparoscopic surgery required older surgeons to learn an entirely new set of manual skills and requires surgeons in training to learn these new skills at the same time they are learning traditional "open" surgery carried out under direct vision.

Not all medical problems lend themselves to surgical correction, but those that do provide a rich experience. Surgery usually deals with well-defined issues, most of which can be solved in a few hours in the operating room with immediately gratifying results. The impact of surgery on the life of the patient is prompt and dramatic. As a surgeon, you find out right away if you have helped the patient—or not. The very high yield of good results in modern surgery and the gratitude of the patients are certainly among the rewards most appreciated by practicing surgeons.

The responsibilities of a surgeon extend far beyond the operating room, before and after the operation. Preoperative evaluation of the patient is essential. A variety of studies may be needed to pinpoint the diagnosis, to be sure that the patient can tolerate the operation and that it will achieve the desired results. This may also require the humility to refuse to intervene surgically when such an approach seems inappropriate or too risky. Postoperative management can be even more complicated. One must treat not only the patient's underlying illness but also the frequently very serious physiological disturbances caused by the surgery itself. The patient who has just had open-heart surgery or been the recipient of a kidney, liver, or heart-lung transplant is a very sick person. While the minute details of the hour-to-hour management of such a patient are carried out by a team of physicians and nurses, usually in an intensive care unit setting, the ultimate responsibility rests with the surgeon who did the operation. This requires having a wide range of medical knowledge that can be applied to critically ill patients. It also requires knowledge of other medical disciplines, such as radiology, pathology, and cardiology, and the ability to interact with their respective specialists.

The surgeon has more independence, and with it more direct responsibility, than almost anyone else in the practice of medicine. The stakes are made higher by the fact that serious trauma is inflicted on a patient by the operation itself, trauma for which the surgeon must take complete responsibility. While they can usually expect to experience the joy of success, surgeons must also occasionally taste the bitterness of failure. One of my teachers had a disturbing way of putting this: "If you do it right, it works. If it doesn't work, ——." In this sense, surgery is also a self-criticizing and self-correcting specialty. Departments of surgery in teaching hospitals have weekly "morbidity and mortality" conferences, where all deaths and surgical complications are discussed, to determine if anything could have been done differently. Good conferences are critical of any error that may have been made in diagnosis, judgment, operative technique, or general management. Only when no such error can be found is the complication or death attributed to "patient's disease," implying that it could not have been avoided.

Coupled with compassion and empathy for patients, surgical skills open the door to a unique doctor-patient relationship. People place complete trust in their surgeons. When they are asleep under anesthesia they are helpless, and the surgeon's responsibility is absolute and extraordinary. At a time when they are most ill and vulnerable, patients literally put their lives and well-being into the hands of a surgeon who will invade the body to do whatever is necessary. The result of all of this is that surgeons enjoy very special interactions with their patients, for which both are grateful.

I took care of an elderly dentist a few years ago who came into the hospital because of bowel obstruction. At the time of surgery to relieve his obstruction he was found to have a cancer of the lower portion of his colon. When I explained to him the next day that he needed to have a much bigger operation to remove the cancer, he asked if he could survive it. His fiftieth wedding anniversary was coming up in a few months, and he and his wife were planning to have a big party and he wanted to be there. I told him that I would make a deal with him: he would be at his party if he would invite me. Everything went well and I forgot all about it until six months later when I received an invitation that actually took me a few minutes to understand. I was embarrassed because I had not been serious, but now he was. Under the circumstances I felt that I had to go. On a Saturday afternoon my wife and I walked into the ballroom of a hotel in downtown Minneapolis to see 200 strange faces and my patient. In the next few minutes, one by one, he introduced us to every single person in the room: "This is my surgeon. He saved my life."

MORRIS**WESSEL**

Practicing Pediatrics

I grew up in New London, Connecticut, and was acquainted with disease and medicine from an early age: my father died of influenza when I was eleven months old, and I was a sickly child—I had been diagnosed with leukemia, celiac disease, and several other rare conditions before I was eighteen months old. Only recently have I realized that my father's death and my early illnesses probably motivated my decision to become a pediatrician.

As a child with recurring health problems, I was fortunate to come under the care of Joseph Grover, a young pediatrician in Boston. He assumed responsibility for my care, believing I did have celiac disease, and supervised my care throughout my childhood. And he was the first in a series of caring and wise doctors who helped guide me throughout my training and career. In some ways, my experience with medicine is equally my experience with talented and kind mentors and colleagues.

Fifty years later, I sought my medical record at Children's Hospital in Boston, where I had been hospitalized in 1919. After a long search, the director of the record room returned with my chart. She appeared pale and ill at ease. I asked her if she was all right; as she pointed to the final note on my chart from 1919 she said, "Yes . . . are you?" The final note read: "Discharged against advice! Prognosis poor."

I did recover from my illnesses of childhood, and in 1935 I entered the College of Arts and Sciences at Johns Hopkins University. I majored in biology and anticipated a teaching career at a liberal arts college. But in my junior year I sought the advice of Dr. Tracey Sonneborn, a zoologist, about graduate training in biology. He was both a remarkable teacher and an extraordinarily perceptive individual. I recall his long silence following my question regarding further training. He responded, finally, "Morris, you don't like laboratory work. You like people who work in the laboratories. You should become a physician, where your talents will be appreciated." I wondered how he arrived at his conclusion!

But he was indeed quite correct. I applied to medical school and was fortunate enough to be accepted at Johns Hopkins and Yale. I chose to attend Yale, in part because I had heard of Dean Milton Winternitz's foresightful plans to broaden the Yale medical curriculum by adding courses in the social sciences and psychology. I was disappointed when I arrived in 1939 to discover that Winternitz had resigned the deanship. Many of his plans for expanding the curriculum were never implemented, though his conceptualization of what medical education should include was implicit in the curriculum. Despite my brief exposure to him, his ideas continued to influence me throughout my professional life as I thought about the social and emotional factors that affected my patients.

Nevertheless, my years at Yale University School of Medicine were relaxed and stimulating, despite the first moments of my first day. Those remain etched in my memory: my eyes burned and my stomach churned as I entered the anatomy laboratory and viewed twenty-five cadavers, each bathed in formaldehyde and awaiting the arrival of the first-year medical students. A gentleman in a tan lab coat, observing my discomfort, approached me. "Hey Doc," he said, "you look terrible! Take the weekend off—here are two tickets for the Yale-Brown football game."

This greeting impressed me—this man had called me "Doc," he recognized how I felt, and he gave me a gift. What a wonderful introduction to medical school. Only later did I learn that he was the Anatomy Department embalmer! But his kindness and advice was typical of encounters with other medical professionals throughout my training and career.

My first day in the pediatric ward rotation in 1942 I remember vividly. I reported at nine in the morning to the conference room, and Dr. Grover Powers, chairman of pediatrics, appeared promptly. He was a rotund individual with a shining, bald head. He wore a loose-fitting tan laboratory coat—he believed that starched white coats frightened children. A man of few words, Dr. Powers tersely instructed, "Come along with me." Four classmates and I followed along briskly to the room of a six-year-old boy, who was busily devouring his breakfast. Dr. Powers looked at the child for a brief moment. Suddenly, he turned and walked out of the room. Surprised, I remarked that I thought we were all there to examine the boy. Dr. Powers looked at me disapprovingly and said, "That child is eating breakfast! You wouldn't expect me to interrupt his breakfast, would you? We will return later." Indeed, I began to learn there is more to a person than merely the disease.

Dr. Powers always included discussion of the ways in which child and parent experienced the illness. He expected students to be acquainted not only with the course of a child's disease but also with the meaning of the symptoms and treatment. I recall how he would frequently say, "Tell me about how the child and parents are feeling."

Dr. Edith Jackson, a psychiatrist whose office was adjacent to the pediatric ward, was of immense value to me. I knew that after her graduation from Johns Hopkins Medical School in 1921 and a pediatric internship she had joined the staff of the New Haven Rickets Project. This group demonstrated that oral administration of Vitamin D in infancy would eliminate rickets, widespread among children in New Haven at that time. While working in this project, Dr. Jackson wondered whether there were measures that, if applied early in childhood, might prevent children from experiencing behavioral difficulties in later years. So in 1930, she traveled to Vienna to undergo psychoanalysis with Sigmund Freud and to participate in studies of young children. While there, she founded the Jackson Day Nursery in Vienna, the forerunner of the Hampstead Nursery in London. These day care centers provided the opportunity for children to have a place to attend amid the ongoing trauma of war. The observations of these children by pediatricians, psychoanalysts, and social workers led to classic understanding of how young children dealt with the horrendous wartime destruction of their communities. In 1936, Dr. Jackson returned to Yale, where she began providing psychiatric consultation for children in the pediatric clinic and in pediatric wards. She was the first psychoanalyst in the United States to have an office in an academic pediatric department.

It was in this office I found myself sitting one day and describing to Dr. Jackson my frustration in dealing with a seven-year-old child with a fractured femur and in a body cast. This little boy cried incessantly: he missed his parents, his siblings, and his home. He refused to eat hospital food. Nothing I could say or do consoled him, I complained. Suddenly I began to share with Dr. Jackson memories of my own hospitalization for a tonsillectomy at the age of seven, the same age as my patient! I left her office feeling much relieved and freer to care for this young patient. I realized that my intense frustration at my inability to comfort this child awakened memories of how I felt at his age when I experienced hospitalization and surgery. Recalling these memories increased considerably my desire to comfort this child. I hoped to provide for him what I had not experienced.

I met frequently with Dr. Jackson until I graduated. We discussed normal growth and development of children, as well as their reactions to illness, injuries, and hospitalization. Through these meetings, I learned that hospitalized children, in addition to suffering the effects of illness, injury, or surgery, also suffered from the very experience itself. The unfamiliar surroundings, including the food and bed, the care given by complete strangers, and the limited visitation by their parents all contributed to their distress. I would keep these important lessons for a lifetime.

I graduated from Yale School of Medicine in 1943, and after a nine-month internship in New York, I was drafted into the army. I spent three years in military service in Europe. Upon return to civilian life, I served an eighteen-month fellowship at the Mayo Clinic in Rochester, Minnesota, where I was fortunate to work under the guidance of C. Andrew Aldrich and Benjamin Spock, both outstanding pediatricians who were deeply concerned with the psychological well-being of children. I returned to Yale in 1948 as a Fellow in the Rooming-In Project, which was directed by Edith Jackson, now also at Yale.

Dr. Jackson had been increasingly drawn over the years to the "lying-in," or maternity, and newborn service. She concluded that rigid rules and the separation of babies and mothers interfered unnecessarily with the individual needs of infants. And so, in 1946, Dr. Jackson created a "rooming-in" unit on the maternity ward, where mothers and babies could remain together after the birth, and fathers would be encouraged to help care for the baby. Pediatric house officers in training were offered the opportunity to serve with this project. The "Rooming In Fellows," as we were called, interviewed expectant couples during pregnancy, provided pediatric care for the babies, visited the homes shortly after discharge, and followed the infants in a well-baby clinic. Although I signed on for one year as Fellow, I stayed for three!

During this time, I gained familiarity with the patterns of development in infancy and toddler years. I learned that growth is uneven and that some babies react more intensely than others to various life experiences. I discovered that parents were often unaware of the developmental changes that occur in the toddler years and that sometimes resulted in difficult behavior. A common experience is when an infant between six months and a year begins to demonstrate firm preference for care by the mother. This behavior is often misunderstood by parents. A mother often asks, "What did I do wrong? How did I spoil him?" My response would be to ask, "What did you do right? Your baby appreciates your care and wants you more than anyone else to take care of him." Indeed, many parents wondered at times what they had done wrong to produce this behavior.

In 1951 I began my career in my primary pediatric practice in New Haven, and continued in that practice for forty-two years. I discovered early that the many discussions with Edith Jackson and colleagues in the Rooming-In Project offered excellent preparation for my role as a primary pediatrician. I encouraged expectant couples to schedule a prenatal pediatric conference shortly before the anticipated date of delivery, a practice that was uncommon at the time. I also realized that the first weeks at home were often difficult for all members of the family. Mothers were likely to be preoccupied with caring for their infants and children, and husbands often felt neglected. More often than not, fathers were relieved to hear at the six-week visit that this was a normal phase.

I soon learned that when a child's sickness necessitated referral to a specialist, it was important for me as the primary pediatrician to maintain an ongoing and supportive relationship with the child, parents, and siblings. And through this relationship I could provide support to families during developmental challenges, sicknesses, injuries, family tensions, school experiences, or the losses of important individuals in their lives.

In 1969, Florence Wald, dean of the Yale School of Nursing, invited me to join an interdisciplinary group of colleagues to study terminally ill patients and their families. This group later initiated a home care program for terminally ill patients, and in 1980 we founded the Connecticut Hospice in Branford, Connecticut—the first hospice care program in the United States.

Participation in this study group stimulated as well my awareness of the needs in my own practice of families experiencing the loss of loved ones. I realized that I had given little attention to serving families at these tragic moments. As I thought about this, it became clear to me that these sad moments evoked memories of losses in my own life. Drawing on my early conversations with Edith Jackson, I realized that I could use those experiences and provide support to my patients and their families—and that providing support was an immensely important and ultimately rewarding duty.

As many of the children I had followed since birth entered adolescence, I found it was important to discuss plans for continuing care into the next decade of their lives. So I suggested to the parents that we arrange a conference to discuss details of the best ways for them to care for their growing children. I began by introducing them to the Academy of Pediatrics definition of the pediatric age group: children aged birth to twenty-one! I explained to parents and young patients that all patients have the privilege of a confidential relationship with the physician, and that as the children grow into adolescence, they mature into that confidential relationship with their pediatrician. I also explained to the parents and children, however, that if I felt it was important for parents to be involved in an issue, the young patient and I would discuss how to arrange this. Of course, this was not always easy. But when I retired from practice in 1993, I was pleased to receive many letters from adults who expressed gratitude for my having "been there" during their adolescent years. One woman wrote to me, "I liked to come to see you when I was a teenager—you always made my mother feel better about me!"

Now that I have retired from active practice, I serve as a developmental pediatrician at a local child guidance clinic. And, although I no longer see adolescent patients in a practice, I like to share with young adults who are entering medicine some of the history of the practice of pediatrics, some of the wisdom I've gained and the experiences I've had—and one way to do that is by writing articles like this one!

ANN**SKOPEK**

A Day in the Life of a Woman in Medicine

(The "XX Files")

4:00 A.M. The alarm goes off. If I can just push the right button I can lie here for another ten minutes.

4:10 A.M. The second alarm sounds and I know that if I don't move now, my day will already be thrown off schedule.

5:05 A.M. Dressed; lunch ready to go; school snacks packed for my daughter; oven timer set to warm the supper that was prepared two days ago—along with a few other meals so I don't have to cook each night. The ride to the hospital is ever so dark. I pass the ladies of the evening who are ending their shifts. Some have small children in tow and my stomach sinks. I think of my own two children at home, safe and warm in their beds. I remind myself how lucky I am and that I have nothing about which to complain.

6:30 A.M. Rounds at both downtown hospitals are completed. I'm now at the office for a solid two hours of paperwork—forms for various insurance companies, pre-operative clearance letters, correspondence from specialists to review, various lab data to check, patient letters, and phone calls. This is also the only time to discuss business matters with my practice manager, who helps hold this whole thing together.

8:30 A.M. Patient visits start, plus the seemingly endless stream of phone messages. Both are variable, ranging from simple mundane maladies that a little common sense addresses, to more serious problems that people have let slide for days and now require urgent attention, and to the acute and unpredictable symptoms and illnesses that surprise us all. And, of course, there are no more appointment slots to deal with this range of problems in a controlled manner.

Also through the day, there are times of frustration, and I dare say rage, trying to deal with a health system that often argues the necessity of tests with decisions being made over the phone by a nonmedical insurance person who has no idea what I'm talking about and can't possibly understand the agony of the patient sitting before me, or the seriousness of his or her problem.

12:30 P.M. Time for lunch, but there isn't any way that will happen. I still have two patients to see, and my afternoon schedule starts again at 1:00.

5:17 P.M. I've done all I can do for today and it's time to go home. At least supper will be cooked. Then it may be laundry or grocery shopping, not to mention making sure that homework is done and musical instruments are practiced. Bedtime will be by 9:00 P.M.—both my daughters' and mine!—so that I can start all over again tomorrow.

As I look at this schedule, it's hard to believe that I have wanted to do nothing other than practice medicine since seventh grade. My college years were spent during the height of the women's movement of the 1970s, and, although I was never a card-carrying member, I stayed on track toward my original goal in part bolstered by the fact that women everywhere were striving for a better station in life. The problem is that no one ever had the guts to say exactly how hard that was going to be. Everyone preached, "You can do it!" and "You can have it all." We didn't realize then the implicit question: "But at what cost?"

I recently hosted a small gathering of female physicians to welcome my new associate. This group represented multiple specialty areas and ages, but the main topic of conversation came down to one concern: how difficult it is to practice medicine, keep up with the business aspects of the practice, and also worry about all the other "stuff"—laundry, groceries, child care, school pickup, covering children's sick days, and how to attend various school musical productions that are invariably held in the middle of the workday! There was, in our conversations, a tremendous level of concern over these issues, but in the end, an unusual sense of relief in the realization that all of us are in the same boat. No one had a magic answer—we just shared the ways that each of us has found to cope and get everything done (or so we think!).

We did generally agree that as the days get more complicated and busy, we have to try to figure out how to remain sane—for ourselves, our staff, our colleagues, our patients, and (last, but certainly not least) our families. This has perhaps been the hardest thing for me to figure out. They don't teach you this in medical school; there are no guidelines anywhere. No one else can give you the answer. After more than twenty years of practicing, I am still in the process of working out this balance.

Over the past few years I have discovered that I have a real interest in (and maybe a knack for) gardening. With the usual intensity with which an internist tackles a problem, I have learned about perennials and have found that working with them gives me no end of pleasure and satisfaction. The dirtier I get and the more sore my muscles, the greater my sense of accomplishment. After a weekend with my family and doing my gardening, I come back to work refreshed and ready for another week of practicing medicine. The thought of how well a transplanted bush (a gift from the garden of a patient) has done truly reminds me of all the miracles that are around us but overlooked everyday. We must be better at recognizing these things and, in so doing, bringing ourselves back to this even keel, this balance.

The accomplishment of the daily work of a female physician draws not only on the years of schooling and the time spent in training. As a female internist, I find that I use my maternal instincts any number of times during the day. I believe that this softer, more motherly approach to patient care may be why not just my female patients confide in me, but some male patients do as well. I believe that patients many times wouldn't entrust a male physician with certain problems, but that the comfort level with a female physician is great enough even to let tears be shed while confiding these darkest secrets. I see this difference also in the hospital setting when I find myself doing the "little" things—searching out that extra blanket because someone is cold, or filling the water pitcher because someone's lips are parched—and I wonder if my male colleagues see themselves doing the same. I would like to think, though, that maternal instincts aren't the only driving force and that we would all help—and there simply isn't enough staff on the floors anymore to take care of these creature comforts.

I have also found that simply using good old-fashioned common sense sometimes makes you look like a genius. (Though I sometimes can't help myself and wonder why people don't think of these things themselves!) And, it never ceases to amaze me that if I say something as a DOCTOR, it is taken as gospel. My staff may tell a patient the exact same thing that I do, but the patient often doesn't believe it until he or she hears it from me. Even after twenty-two years, I find this hard to believe and have to keep reminding myself of the power we physicians have. We must be careful—this cannot be abused.

Even after many years of practice, it's vitally important to remember to listen to people—both their spoken words and their unspoken signals—and to be honest with them as you give them care. With our current state of medical advances, when we can do almost anything in the way of more testing or in thinking of "one more thing to try," there are times when the endless testing and experimenting will not change the outcome. Each of us really knows when that point is reached. The nurses, especially, often do—they have "been there, done that, and seen it all" and are great allies as we make very difficult decisions. If only we have the openness and courage to share this with the patient (who probably figured it out long before you and is just waiting for you to have a heart-to-heart talk). At this point, all they may need is our time—our very precious time. I believe this helps more than we can imagine. And, remember, sometimes it's the family who needs you even more at this point—the patient may no longer be aware and is at least comfortable. And while we're at it, we must also be honest with *ourselves* so that we can do what's right for the patient, not just go through the motions of a few extra tests or one last change in medication that will make *us* feel better. These are the things that really define dignity at the end of life, and I can tell you that they are truly appreciated.

At the same time, there will be times of great despair and guilt, usually at two or three o'clock in the morning when a sudden thought wakens you. You play the whole case over in your head to be sure you've done all you can do and have not overlooked something crucial or made any wrong decisions along the way. And I'm not talking about the worry of being sued—that can happen at any time and you learn not to dwell on it. What drives you is the closeness you develop with your patients after years of seeing them. Many will become like family to you. You will know who has a grandchild getting married; whose child is having trouble in school or going through a divorce; who is a proud new grandparent because you've taken a few minutes to look at the photos carried in their wallet. And, remarkably, during this whole process, the patient is actually interested in you as a person. Many will learn, as you converse, that you have a daughter with a chronic medical problem and will never fail to ask at each visit how she's doing, or that you have a son who is preparing for college. It allows a patient to see that you, too, are human and lends a certain comfort to your relationship. Many people are amazing and thoughtful—from the batch of homemade cookies that they bring to you during the holidays to the handmade crafts that are so proudly presented to you for your children. We must take time to appreciate these things. And at the same time, recognize that this is what gives substance to relationships that matter, and that it is, in part, what drives that 2 A.M. angst. It's not just the correct practice of medicine that becomes important. It is also that sense of responsibility toward human beings for whom you care.

For those of us who have chosen to have children in the midst of the fray and who have been fortunate enough to be granted that privilege, the practice of medicine can lend a positive parenting aspect despite the fact that it can rob you of time and energy to be a good parent. I hope that my kids see more than just the grumbling about the innumerable phone calls during my weekend on-call. Hopefully, they also see that I do have a deep and true interest in doing this, and that I really have a desire to help others and give back to those who have looked to me for help. And I think they do see that.

Recently, during a visit from my mother and father-in-law, who live in the Midwest, a story came on the news about the mosquito control efforts being implemented in Connecticut in an effort to control the West Nile Virus. My mother-in-law quizzed my twelve-year-old daughter about it and asked how much of a danger it really was for us. My daughter accurately recounted all that she'd read in the newspapers. Her summary of the situation was that it was certainly very dangerous . . . and that "not even my mom can fix it!"

I guess the moral to this story is that all women who dare to pursue this path need to be prepared for what lies ahead. You will be pulled in many directions, especially if you have or want to have a family. You will feel endless guilt if your child is sick and you cannot be the one to stay home with her or him, even though that's what any child would want. You will have feelings of guilt and sadness when one of your patients is facing a horrible illness—or loses that battle. You may even get choked up from time to time because patients and their families will become like your extended family and it's hard to see them go through pain and suffering, whether physical or emotional. But you will learn to do reality checks, remember the good things, and be thankful for all that you have, both professionally and personally, and you will return day after day to do the thing you are most and best qualified to do. You will strive to restore the art to, and preserve the humanity in, the practice of medicine. And yes, in spite of all the difficulties and challenges, if you had it to do all over again, you would choose the same course.

4:00 A.M. The alarm goes off. If I can just push the right button, I can lie here for another ten minutes . . .

MARYJANEMINKIN

The World of Obstetrics and Gynecology

One of my duties and privileges as a clinical professor of obstetrics and gynecology at Yale has been lecturing medical students every Wednesday morning for the last twenty-one years. As medicine has evolved over the last ten years, I regularly ask myself, "Am I being ethical in encouraging these talented young men and women to enter this profession? Would I enter this business now? Or would I have chosen a different profession that would have paid better and left me with less debt from schooling, and would not expose me to the risk of being sued despite practicing the best care I possibly could?" But the answer keeps coming up "yes," so I keep on teaching.

Despite these issues, the quality of students I teach has not fluctuated over the years. There is still a large cadre of bright and energetic people who really do want to help improve the public health. They may not all become wealthy, but a physician is unlikely to starve, either. They believe that the current crisis in HMO medicine must be resolved (no, I do not like having to waste fifteen minutes persuading an insurer that my patient with a precancerous condition of the uterus needs a hysterectomy—as I had to last year—but I think that this level of restriction may be passing). And tort reform on litigation against physicians is also in the works—my malpractice insurance premiums have leveled off from the constant escalations of the 1980s.

I had always wanted to be a doctor. Upon entering first grade,

I responded to the inquiry of "What do you want to be when you grow up?" with the question, "How do you spell pediatrician?" But by the time I entered medical school, I realized that dealing with sick kids would depress me too much, and besides, I wondered, who wants to deal with obnoxious parents and their questions?

What attracted me to medicine—not perhaps at the first-grade level, but certainly by my college years—remains my attraction even twenty-five years after my medical school graduation. I was always interested in science, the why of everything working, especially in the body. I took the basic high school "Blue Version" biology the year that Crick and Watson were awarded the Nobel Prize, and I really do believe that the first edition of *The Molecular Biology of the Gene* reads almost as beautifully as *The Great Gatsby*.

In addition to my attraction to the basic sciences, I really like to talk with people. Although LaRochefoucauld said that bright folks talk about ideas, not people, I think he got it wrong. To me, people are a lot more interesting. And in what other profession would I get to talk to thirty or forty people about their problems, or how to prevent them, every working day? In every interaction, I hope to have a positive impact on that person's life.

In obstetrics and gynecology I found the perfect niche. Gynecologists are among the few practitioners who not only can diagnose their patients' problems, but also then get to fix them. Internists can diagnose gallstones as the cause of their patients' abdominal pain, but they then have to refer these patients to the surgeon for therapy. When gynecologists see a patient who cannot conceive, we can prescribe medication to help her ovulate, and if her Fallopian tubes are blocked, we can operate and clear them. If you choose to go into gynecological oncology, you not only can operate to remove ovarian cancer, but you then can manage the patient's chemotherapy. Few other specialties allow for both medical and surgical skills.

In obstetrics, I found the opportunity, in caring for a pregnant patient, to care for two patients at once. Sure, you can help a pregnant woman in congestive heart failure by delivering her child, but what if that baby is still too immature to live outside of the uterus? The challenge is to save the mom and also deliver a healthy baby. Most of the time, we do end up with two healthy patients (and at least one of whom is usually quite happy). If I do my job well, that baby I deliver will probably live for eighty-plus years. I often felt that, sadly, no matter how good a job I did practicing my skills in internal medicine, many patients were gravely ill and could not live much longer.

I started doing obstetrics and gynecology at the time that the profession was becoming respectable. Until the 1970s, OB-GYN was considered the lowest of the low—that specialty for the "dummies" of the medical school class. Huge technological breakthroughs, such as fetal monitoring (invented at Yale, by the way), morning-after contraception (the same), radio immunoassays to measure hormones, and ultrasound (not invented, but obstetrical use in the United States pioneered at Yale) came into use at that time, and we could offer our patients increasingly innovative care. Also, the status of women in our society improved so that it was no longer acceptable for the less-intelligent doctors to care for women. And fortunately, it has become politically correct in the last few years to talk about women's health.

My profession has also changed dramatically in another way. The year before I started medical school, approximately 7 percent of the medical students in this country were women. The year I began medical school, 1971, that number jumped to 20 percent. The numbers have since climbed to parity. I was the second female resident in the gynecology department at Yale. As of two years ago, over half of the gynecology residents in the United States were women. When I started practice, many people asked my male partner (whom they thought was crazy for hiring me), "Do you really think women will want to go to a female gynecologist?" My practice now has two male physicians and five female physicians.

But many men believe that OB-GYN has gone too far for them to consider it as a profession; they are concerned that there is no longer a niche for a male obstetrician. To me, and, I think, to any rational female, the quality and humanity of the caregiver should matter, not the gender. My OB-GYN is a man, and not only I, but also my kids whom he delivered think he's terrific.

Residency directors strive to be gender-blind in accepting applicants. And fellowship programs are the same: among specialty areas, such as oncology, perinatology, and endocrinology, there is parity among the genders. It is true that in certain private practice situations employers do prefer to hire female applicants—but most groups, like my practice, which just hired a superb male chief resident, will go after the best-qualified person for the job, the one who will work the hardest and take the best care of patients regardless of gender. I no longer see new patients. But when my patients, acting on behalf of friends seeking a recommendation for an OB-GYN, ask which of my partners has the personality most similar to mine, I easily reply, "Steve, my new junior partner."

So what do I do on a daily basis? I spend most of my time in the office, seeing patients for routine checkups and problems. I see both gynecological patients and pregnant women. One day a week, on the average, I go to the operating room to perform laparoscopies or hysterectomies. As my group now has seven doctors, I am on call every seventh night and weekend, and, as is routine in a large practice, I spend much of my on-call time in the hospital. But one of the best parts of being an OB-GYN is that the labor floor is always the liveliest part of the hospital. So at 4 A.M. I am likely to be up with several friends, catching up on gossip and medical updates—OB-GYNs really like to do this. When I started in practice twenty-one years ago, my group had only two practitioners, so being on-call wasn't quite as much fun. But don't worry, most groups these days are fairly large, so the time required for on-call isn't as onerous as it once was.

Many students consider rejecting OB-GYN because of the fact that babies do like to be born at night, and they are concerned about taking care of their own children with those kinds of schedule interruptions. As long as you have a significant other who wants to be an active participant in child rearing, you can combine the two. My husband, a mathematician, devotes a considerable amount of time to our children, now ages ten and twelve. And my children are used to asking me how many centimeters my current laboring patient's cervix is dilated so that they can figure out if mom is coming home before they get to bed!

The advantage of a Yale education is that it encourages and allows you to remain flexible. Although I am primarily in private practice, seeing patients in the office, I will often have with me a medical student to whom I can introduce the fun of doing obstetrics and gynecology. Over the last twenty-one years I have become a "menopause doctor," and I spend a considerable amount of time lecturing both patient groups and physicians about new information on menopausal health. I enjoy attending medical meetings with my colleagues from other specialties, such as medicine and psychiatry, and learning about their perspectives. Because I didn't like any of the available books on menopause for lay people, I wrote my own based on what patients had taught me in my first twenty years as a physician. From that book grew an association with the health magazine *Prevention*. So when I write my "Talk to the Doctor" column every month, eleven million readers are hearing what I have to say—and I marvel at the opportunity to have an impact on the health of eleven million people! Hey, if I have stopped one more person from smoking, I have done some good. As I encourage all of my medical students, no matter what path of medicine you choose, do talk with people from the media, because for many patients that is the way they learn. I also have a weekly column on the Internet—I want to talk with as many people as I can!

My other avocation has grown out of a disturbing change in the practice of medicine, reflecting the litigious nature of our society. Many people seem to believe that no one in this country is responsible for his or her problems, so if a patient has an unfortunate outcome it obviously must be the doing of a bad physician or a bad product. Because of the growing numbers of malpractice suits (which were basically unheard of when I graduated from medical school) numerous physicians have left medicine or changed their practices.

So my avocation is that of reviewing and explaining medical details and events of medical malpractice cases. For example, I will try to convince a plaintiff's lawyer not to bring suit when a poor outcome resulted despite good medical care. And when an unjust suit is brought against a physician, I assist the defense attorney. Unfortunately, at times bad medicine is practiced, and in those cases I help the plaintiff/ patient attempt to gain some redress for injuries. I find those cases most useful as examples to the residents and medical students I teach how *not* to practice medicine. This review of various malpractice cases keeps me current on the practice of obstetrics and gynecology throughout the country.

My ultimate goal is to acquire as much experience in medical malpractice litigation as I can in order to help our legislators reform the system. It is possible, I think, to make these kinds of changes—

you just have to know your medicine well, and care about patients. I do believe that we are on the verge of tort reform, so I would advise you not to avoid medicine as a career because you might be sued. Besides, attorneys and accountants are sued, too.

With all of this entertainment and all of these rewards, how could I not have chosen wisely? For those of you who were avid chemistry clubbers in high school and who, like me, recited the chemist's creed at least once a week for years, I paraphrase: "Physicians are a strange class of mortals . . . that may I die if I were to trade places with a Persian king."

MALCOLM B. BOWERS, JR.

Practicing Psychiatry

I f you are giving thought to becoming a psychiatrist, let me offer some observations as a result of more than thirty-five years of experience in a unique and challenging field. I have, as you will see, taken seriously the editors' suggestions to be informal, personal, even idiosyncratic—and to give advice!

I think of psychiatry as a daring profession for two reasons. First of all, people understandably regard their personal, subjective life experience in a very special way. Whereas they may acknowledge ownership of, say, their liver or kidneys, their *mind* exists in a unique and private space. It has a special status. And anyone who would undertake to help someone *change* his or her mind is entering a very sacred realm. This is the work of a daring profession indeed.

Second, some individuals trust their lives to God or to fate or to some similar process. In other words, they believe that whatever happens, however the chapters of their lives appear to unfold, all things happen for a purpose, events are preordained and predetermined. Therefore, it may follow, one should not attempt to alter circumstances but rather accept the workings of fate. For such individuals, psychiatry or psychotherapeutic work represents going against nature and is therefore a challenge to their values. How dare you, they might inquire, criticize life as it unfolds?

How Dare We?

How dare we set about to ease the pain of lives, shoulder our own, yet take another burden on? How dare we hear the untold story, judge a passion or a joy that is not ours, or conjure up a vision that may be ours alone? I think we must dare, that the world as it is should have its critics, that we, like Job, should be fair.

Job suggests a basic value in our field: that one should take responsibility for one's life to the greatest extent possible, come to learn to trust and assert oneself, but maintain an open-minded humility in the process.

In considering psychiatry, you should know something about its history. Until recently, mental aberration was thought to be associated with external, supernatural forces or an undesirable mix of internal bodily humors. When it was not possible to rid a person of the controlling demons or to restore the proper internal vital balance, that individual was ostracized and frequently ridiculed. Slowly, elementary principles of psychology developed out of Greek and Roman philosophy, and mental life was generally characterized as a domain of the passions (desire, fear, joy, sorrow) that required control through the use of reason. During the Middle Ages, religion brought something of a humanizing influence into psychiatry, but many pagan and magical practices continued to survive. In many traditions the insane person and the religious prophet were often thought to possess a special knowledge and experience of the divine.

The arc of ideas began to bend slowly toward rationalism with the Renaissance. Institutions for the care of the insane began to appear, and attention turned increasingly to clinical description and to humane treatment. By the seventeenth century the origins of modern science and medicine can be more clearly discerned with Copernicus's challenge of the preeminence of earth as the center of the universe and Descartes's immortal aphorism, *cogito ergo sum*, declaring the primacy of reason and mental life. In the late eighteenth century, institutional approaches to the treatment of the mentally ill in Europe underwent a dramatic change. Under the leadership of Pinel, the concept of moral treatment began to emerge whereby physical restraints were minimized and a more enlightened approach to patient care was gradually adopted both in Europe and the United States, which established its first asylum in Williamsburg, Virginia, in 1773. The American Psychiatric Association was formed initially as a collection of asylum superintendents in the early nineteenth century. These pioneers of American psychiatry founded and attended hospitals that were first established with pride and optimism despite the overwhelming numbers of severely ill citizens suffering from a vast spectrum of illnesses including all the psychoses, general paresis (identified as syphilis), epilepsy, and the dementias of late life. There were no specific treatments, and etiological explanations were rudimentary. Concepts of stress and "nervous exhaustion" were proposed and were thought to be the result of maladaptive elimination of waste products by nerve cells.

There was also little consideration of the possibility that psychological *conflict* could lead to severe mental distress. It is interesting to speculate why, by the late nineteenth century, there was still so little place for the role of subjective mental life in the field of psychiatry. People were clearly aware of subjective experience and articulated their awareness in descriptions of the private life of thought and feeling. They may have regarded this realm of human experience as sacred, related to their religious life and their relationship to God—sinful, perhaps, but not sick in the sense that the body could be ill. But psychological conflict, as we think about it today, would have been considered a kind of blasphemy and almost unknown to most American psychiatrists at the turn of the twentieth century.

Gradually, through the contributions of such giants as Kraepelin, Freud, and Bleuler, modern psychiatry began to take shape. Over the past one hundred years a very rich and multifaceted scientific discipline has formed and includes major contributions from sociology, psychodynamic theory, learning theory, and neurobiology. There are many rooms in this mansion, many opportunities for those who are attracted to the subject matter and to its challenges.

My Own Story

During my college years, a wise English professor gave me Benjamin Rush as the topic for a term paper. Up until that time, I had little awareness of psychiatry and no idea at all how it had developed. Rush is generally considered the father of American psychiatry, and my professor characterized him as a "meliorist," that is, one who tried to "make things better." I was an English and philosophy major, but I also took pre-medical courses. Such a combination often leads to a kind of restless dialectic out of which an interest in psychiatry can grow. I have reviewed hundreds of applications for training in psychiatry and have been struck by the frequency of a dual interest in science and the humanities. In my case, I came into the field in the mid-sixties, just as the era of biological psychiatry was beginning. This new section in the symphony of the profession has sometimes led to dissonance but has also broadened the therapeutic reach of its practitioners in the most creative and exciting generation in the history of our field.

Most young medical students, however, do not go to medical school aiming to be psychiatrists. The field tends to grow on you as you find yourself mildly dissatisfied with the emphasis on biological mechanism rather than on the breadth of human complexity. Indeed, a psychiatrist's training is somewhat unique in that you must consider yourself both the subject and the object of your learning. You will find yourself to be your most important professional instrument. Becoming an informed and informing listener is one vital task. Learning self-examination and self-control is another. Additionally, for a psychiatrist, living and learning are intertwined; personal growth and development as a human being cannot be separated from professional maturation. The outcome of one's own struggles with intimacy, disillusionment, separation, and loss directly affect one's credibility and competence. Usually, however, as a young psychiatrist who has just begun to face the challenges of adult life, you may be asked to help people who are struggling with problems that you have yet to encounter firsthand. Humility and a commitment to lifelong learning and growth are essential to both your patients and yourself.

I am a general adult psychiatrist, and I am regularly surprised and excited by the clinical variety I encounter each day. To illustrate, let me give you an idea of a typical week in my professional life.

On the first day, I supervised electroconvulsive treatment in the hospital recovery room. The patient, a moderately depressed middle-aged woman who had been resistant to a host of antidepressant medications, had a satisfactory treatment that morning and ultimately was discharged after receiving six treatments over a fourteen-day period. Later that day, I consulted with the family of a twenty-year-old man who had been hospitalized more than twenty times within a five-year period for a schizo-affective disorder triggered by marijuana use. The young man was quite bothered by an uncomfortable restlessness, present for months as a result of his medication. I recommended a newer medication that does not produce these side effects, and I learned several months later that he was greatly improved.

The next day I received a call from a woman in her early sixties with manic-depressive illness. She had been my patient for over twenty-five years, and I had followed her through four hospitalizations as well as through numerous episodes of mania in her sister and an initial episode of this illness in her daughter. She informed me that her husband had been diagnosed with prostate cancer. We spoke over the phone several times that week, and she came to see me once as she tried to cope with this new stress in her life. I usually see her in my office every four to six months to discuss her life, her medication levels, and her general medical condition as monitored by an internist.

The following day I saw a young graduate student in continuing treatment. He had been hampered by obsessive symptoms and anxiety related to the completion of his thesis. We had been reviewing his somewhat overly disciplined lifestyle and searching for early developmental factors that could have contributed to this behavior. He had been short in stature as a child, and he recalled experiencing a great deal of teasing in school as a result; he may have learned to try to be "perfect" in his studies in order to gain respect from his peers. We explored this possibility and others at weekly meetings, and his symptoms slowly improved over a six-month period.

Later that week I saw a young faculty member whose fiancée of two years had decided just days before their wedding that she did not want to be married, and he had become suicidally depressed. I needed to be emphatic that he take antidepressant medication and see me twice a week for a period of time. After several months of therapy he thanked me for insisting that he get treatment. For about a year, we examined several relationships in his life that had turned out similarly and discussed ways he might guard against such choices in the future.

These vignettes, I hope, convey something of the range of problems we psychiatrists are called upon to treat. I hope they also illustrate how psychological treatments can work hand in hand with medication. Some observers, largely outside the field, conclude that psychiatry is hopelessly divided between those practitioners who favor psychotherapy and those who favor medication. This view, as my college philoso-phy professor might have said, is a "false dichotomy." Anyone working actively with psychiatric patients these days must conclude that both psychological and medical therapies are frequently required and that knowledge and skill in both areas are always necessary. I am talking about the demands of clinical problems, not about what insurance companies willingly cover. We must not allow reimbursement schemes to distort and disfigure our profession. Our task must be to clarify what patients need. How our work will be compensated is another and occasionally daunting problem, and we must not confuse the two. If you choose psychiatry as a field of study and practice, you will need to remember this admonition.

What We Value

I like to think about the fundamental values of our profession to help set my priorities. They may serve as one approach to letting you know what psychiatry is all about.

First of all, for me it is a privilege to be a psychiatrist. There can be nothing inherently more humane and sacred than living life as well as one can, and no profession is more privileged than one that aspires to assisting this goal.

Second, our knowledge base is evolving. Therefore, we psychia-trists must stay informed by reading and continuing our education throughout our professional lives. Because of our incomplete knowl-edge we will often need to push ahead with treatment while tolerating some ambiguity and uncertainty. And we must keep an open mind. If our knowledge base is always in progress, there are going to be repeated surprises, and we must be open to them. If we do not now have all the answers, we can always hold out the possibility of a better future.

Third, the patient's story is fundamental. Prior to all theory and all therapeutic action, there is the story that we must hear and we must understand. Learning how to hear these stories in full and to respond appropriately is the essence of psychiatry. For the work we do can easily lead to pessimism and demoralization for ourselves and our patients, and the ability to step back and see the human spirit at work in a life can, like a restorative ritual, reconnect us to our professional center.

Finally, a career in psychiatry requires a certain passion for the field. Perhaps the same can be said for any branch of medicine, but it is certainly true for psychiatry. You will need a compelling interest in human lives, a fundamental optimism and gratitude for the miracle of human existence, and a fierce determination to "make things better."

BRUCE**MCCLENNAN**

The Future of Diagnostic Imaging

Much of medicine today turns on what a diagnostic radiologist says and does. Preparing for this field, and understanding the importance that the modern radiologist plays in the detection and management of disease, requires a microglimpse at the end of the nineteenth century. Diagnostic radiologists took little more than one hundred years to become the purveyors of imaging and the practitioners of minimally invasive image-guided interventions designed to provide the highest-quality patient care.

Wilhelm Conrad Roentgen had an unconventional beginning to his Nobel prize–winning career in physics (not recommended for Yale students!). He never received a diploma from a *gymnasium* (high school), yet his perseverance and talent eventually won him the academic rank of instructor at the University of Strasburg, and three years later a professorship at the University of Giessen, both in his native Germany. His background in mechanical engineering and mathematics, as well as his aptitude for numbers, allowed him to create a variety of instruments to detect and measure physical phenomena much as researchers in biomedical engineering now use radiological tools for cellular and molecular imaging, tissue engineering, and developing biosensors. Roentgen abandoned mechanical engineering for theoretical physics, and after his discovery of the X ray on November 8, 1895, others brought his technology to the forefront of medicine. And there it will remain, though X rays are used in increasingly smaller and more focused and refined ways in the twenty-first century. Perseverance is still required for modern-day diagnostic radiology, but the skills are readily learned in the five- to six-year training period, which includes time in a fellowship. Graduates of radiology training programs today bring a broad background and perspective to this discipline—grounded in liberal arts and business as well as in chemistry, physics, and computer science.

Conventional X rays, or radiography, still make up the bulk of the imaging studies carried out by a modern diagnostic radiologist. However, direct digital capture devices and "dry" laser printers will soon send film and "wet" chemical processing to the History of Medicine Library archives. Cross-sectional imaging and three-dimensional (3D) display of complex data sets, viewed on high-resolution monitors at workstations, are replacing the classic film and view-box method for interpretation and diagnosis.

Another Nobel laureate, mathematician, and computer scientist, Sir Godfrey Hounsfield, viewed the human brain in 1972 with X rays that were directed from multiple angles and converted into digital data sets or "slices." These slices were then made available for viewing on Polaroid film. This process, called *computerized transverse axial tomography*—CAT or CT scanning—has revolutionized medicine as much as penicillin and other antibiotics have done. CT scanning, along with magnetic resonance imaging (MRI), account for another significant part of the modern radiologist's daily workload. The CT scanner, which is now able to image the entire body in a single breath-hold and generate one to three thousand (in the not too distant future) images, is used twenty-four hours a day. It has all but replaced the exploratory surgical operations of the past century.

What radiologists do today in hospitals, clinics, and outpatient centers as problem-solving imaging consultants and minimally invasive image-guided therapists has as profound an impact on patient care as that of almost any medical, surgical, or pediatric specialist. One of my professors once said that the radiology department is the "marketplace of the hospital where everything is bought and sold." This statement is more true today than when first uttered many decades ago. In the high-tech environment of multidetector helical CT, high field strength magnetic resonance (MR), color Doppler ultrasound, and biplane digital fluoroscopy, radiologists now harness the Internet to store and distribute massive amounts of imaging data that can be made readily available to referring physicians, nurses, physician assistants, and patients—simultaneously!

But thanks to the development of "interventional" techniques, radiologists are more than simply observers. In fact, sometimes it's difficult to tell a radiologist from a surgeon or a cardiologist or other specialist. Armed with myriad needles, wires, catheters, stents, coils, glues, and thrombolytic drugs, the interventional radiologist of today is in many ways the general practitioner or the general surgeon of the past century. A variety of technologies—computers, fiber or wireless communication networks including the next generation internet (NGI), and computer-aided diagnosis (CAD)—allow us to study, describe, screen for, predict, follow up, and report—and offer treatments for—the findings that represent real or potential disease. The same armamentarium will soon be used to detect vulnerability to disease that depends on one's genetic makeup.

Research directions are being forged using imaging for understanding of the normal or near-normal, including how the mind actually works. Techniques such as functional MRI (fMRI) for studying learning disorders in children (dyslexia) and neurodegenerative conditions in the elderly (such as Alzheimer's or Parkinson's disease) will result in earlier and improved diagnosis and treatment. The process of imaging from input to display now includes linking images with patient information, lab tests, and reports. This is done through the use of PACS (picture archiving and communication systems), making all such information available in real time, on line at multiple sites for multiple users.

Despite the impact of managed care, utilization of many radiological services is increasing, particularly as the baby boomers age, for they are accustomed to modern technology. Technology to help improve productivity is important for continuing education and training, which, in turn, are so necessary for research in diagnostic radiology. The financing of health care, a continuing political and societal issue, will require the attention of all physicians, but those in the high-tech specialties such as diagnostic radiology will need to follow it most closely. Funding for research for diagnostic imaging from the National Institutes of Health and other sources has and will continue to increase, but at the same time the baby boomers will demand faster, more accurate, less-invasive imaging options. Virtual 3D imaging to look inside the body, such as virtual bronchography, virtual colonography, and virtual cystoscopy, will continue to help radiologists replace other, more invasive diagnostic methods with imaging. These 3D methods will improve conspicuity and will be available twenty-four hours a day over wide-area networks. Such image and information transfer will be encrypted to ensure patient confidentiality. The methods to do all this are in daily use today at Yale. The display of human anatomy and pathology will soon seem almost passé compared with the imaging of molecules and metabolic processes, and most importantly, the earlier detection of genetically predisposed illnesses. Radiological evaluations will be necessary as genes are replaced or altered to improve human health.

A cascade of opportunities faces the student of today who considers a career in the field of diagnostic radiology. For the foreseeable future, armed with a host of ever-changing imaging technologies, including those emerging soon such as infrared-ometry and optical coherent tomography, the radiologist will have the responsibility of making and transmitting the diagnosis to referring physicians. If you become a radiologist, you will find new and rewarding sources of personal and professional satisfaction. Even more, given the current shortage of specialists and subspecialists in diagnostic radiology, employment prospects are bright for those who choose to follow the "digital brick road" to a career in imaging and intervention.

BRIAN**WEST**

The Role of the Pathologist in Clinical Medicine

"I'm a pathologist" can be as good a social conversation stopper as any. To most nonmedical people it conjures an image of a forensic sleuth like television's Quincy or novel heroine Scarpetta, someone who does gory autopsies or tracks down murderers and deals only with the dead. For most pathologists, nothing could be further from the truth: they are intimately concerned with the care of living patients and play a critical, though often not apparent, role in diagnosis and in monitoring of patient progress.

Most pathologists run hospital or other medical laboratories and are responsible for ensuring that diagnostic tests performed on blood, body fluids, and tissues are reliable, and in many cases they are responsible also for interpreting those results. A pathologist usually has overall responsibility for running laboratory services in a health care facility. This sounds pretty dull; in reality it is far from that, because in practice the pathologist has a firsthand opportunity to observe, visualize, and understand mechanisms and processes of disease at the molecular level, and to play a critical role in patient management. To illustrate this, I will outline the many subdisciplines within pathology.

Traditionally, there are two major divisions within pathology, anatomic pathology and clinical pathology. In health care settings with academic departments there is usually an additional division comprised of pathologists, most of whom are devoted to research. The anatomic pathologists deal with tissues, which they examine by microscopy in order to render diagnoses. The clinical pathologists perform chemical, micobiological, immunological, and hematological tests on specimens from patients, again to render diagnoses or to monitor effects of therapy or the course of disease. A new discipline, molecular pathology, is still in infancy but is growing fast. It overlaps extensively with both anatomic and clinical pathology, and may in the future force us to abandon those divisions.

It is a rule in most hospitals that all tissues removed from patients, with a few specific exceptions, are sent to the pathology department for examination. It is the pathologist's responsibility to report on what the tissue is, whether it is normal or abnormal, and if abnormal, what the diagnosis is. This is the sphere of the anatomic pathologist. Typically he or she examines the tissue specimen and then carefully selects samples from it for microscopic examination. This may be done while the patient is still asleep, if the surgeon needs an immediate intraoperative diagnosis to decide how the surgery should be completed, but most samples are used to make paraffin sections, which take a day or so to prepare but which provide more information.

Making a diagnosis is the first objective of this process, but it is by no means the only one. Take, for example, a breast lump that is removed. It will be critical to know not only whether it is benign or malignant (cancerous), but, if it is malignant, what type of cancer it is. Then a series of characteristics that have important implications for prognosis and treatment must be evaluated, such as the tumor size and whether it has been completely removed or has spread to lymph nodes, and whether it expresses receptors for the growth-promoting hormones estrogen and progesterone. This part of the anatomic pathologist's work is rapidly expanding, as increasingly the results of cutting-edge research are being applied using current molecular technology. These new applications will have a major impact on the treatment of cancer in the next decade. Experts in tissue diagnosis are central to these developments.

While much of the anatomic pathologist's work is focused on the diagnosis and evaluation of tumors, almost as much of his or her efforts is concerned with infectious and inflammatory conditions now that physicians can take biopsies of tissues as diverse as stomach, colon, liver, kidney, bladder, lung, and brain, in addition to the easily accessible sites such as skin and mouth. Many biopsies are only two or three millimeters in size, and as biopsy specimens have become smaller over recent years, the challenge for the pathologist has been to get more information from them.

When it comes to making diagnoses on really small tissue samples—often just a few cells—the experts are the pathologists who specialize in cytopathology. This branch of anatomic pathology developed initially from Papanicolaou's innovative application of using cells scraped gently from the uterine cervix and smeared on glass microscope slides to diagnose cervical diseases, including cancer and its precursor lesions. The Pap smear has had an enormous impact on public health, enabling cervical cancer to be either detected in a curable stage or prevented. Cytopathologists, however, are by no means restricted to evaluation of Pap smears: cells obtained from any body fluid are routinely used to diagnose cancers and infections.

A major development in cytopathology has been the fine needle aspiration (FNA) biopsy. This procedure provides a virtually painless way to sample lumps or cysts that can be either felt by the physician or visualized by radiologic techniques. A very fine hypodermic needle, attached to a syringe, is introduced into the lesion, and suction is applied to remove a few cells out of a solid mass or some cells and fluid from a cyst. The cells are then smeared onto a microscope slide, stained, and examined at the patient's bedside. For the patient, the opportunity to have a diagnosis made on the basis of a needle stick rather than an incisional biopsy is a real advantage; for the pathologist, it opens up a new avenue of opportunity for physician-patient interaction. Many cytopathologists perform their own FNAs, which enables them to take a history from the patient, locate and examine the lesion, obtain an adequate specimen, and, in some cases, give an immediate diagnosis to the patient.

Anatomic pathology is a very broad discipline and there is a trend in larger institutions to subspecialize, for example into gynecologic pathology, gastrointestinal pathology, pulmonary pathology, or genitourinary pathology, in much the same way as the medical and surgical subspecialties have developed. Such subspecialization within pathology will become more widespread as increasingly detailed, sophisticated, and site-specific information is required from tissue specimens. An example of this is hematopathology, already a subspecialty in most health centers.

Hematopathology is concerned with disorders of the blood, the blood-forming tissue (the bone marrow), and the cells and organs of the immune system (spleen, lymph nodes, thymus gland, etc). It is the area of anatomic pathology that, at present, is most influenced by advances in molecular biology, directly translated into patient care. In some cancers, for example, genetic defects can be identified whose adverse effects can be reversed by the use of certain drugs, thus preventing further growth of the tumor. The role of the pathologist in this is pivotal. This may well be the prototype for other areas of pathology to follow. Molecular assays will enable us to make more precise diagnoses and to improve treatment and outcome in all areas of anatomic pathology. This will be an exciting challenge for pathologists over the next twenty years, and it is almost certain that the nascent discipline of molecular pathology will grow to gigantic proportions during this period.

Autopsy pathology constitutes a very small portion of the work of most pathologists. Those who specialize in forensic pathology, and make their livelihood from autopsy work, undertake specialty forensic training following completion of a pathology residency. Their work is meticulous, demanding, and fascinating, and of great public importance. Hospital autopsies, in contrast to their forensic counterparts, are usually performed to establish the cause of death and the nature of a disease when these are not known with certainty, or to confirm established diagnoses.

The autopsy itself is the most complete examination possible and is performed only with the consent of the next of kin. Pathologists view it as a privilege to be given permission to perform an autopsy. Usually every major organ system is examined, and the findings are interpreted in the light of the patient's history and clinical record. Autopsies play an important role in quality assurance in modern medicine, and with current concerns regarding deaths due to medical errors, this role is likely to increase in the next few years.

Clinical pathology, sometimes termed *laboratory medicine,* encompasses the non-tissue-based disciplines of clinical chemistry, microbiology, immunology, hematology, and blood banking, all of which differ from anatomic pathology in that they have a much higher ratio of technical staff to pathologists and a much greater volume of tests per year. These subspecialties are highly automated—some laboratories are largely robotic—and the pathologist's role is usually that of director, with managerial support to oversee routine operations. Clinical pathologists act as consultants with regard to the interpretation of laboratory test results for their clinical colleagues, and in some areas, notably hematology, they may play a significant role in test performance.

Pathologists are also communicators. In terminology borrowed from the manufacturing industry, "Information is the product of pathologists." This information, whether the result of a pregnancy test, a breast biopsy, a blood test for hepatitis, or an analysis of a colon tumor, is critical to patient management. It must be effectively communicated to the patient's physician, who will, in turn, explain it to the patient. Not surprisingly, therefore, information technology is of key importance to pathologists. Equally predictable, pathologists spend much time communicating with their clinical colleagues, and they play a major role in informing and educating clinicians, trainees, and medical students at the numerous clinical-pathologic conferences that are routine tools for patient management in most medical centers.

For those of you who enter training, pathology will be different from what I have described here, but it will be exciting nonetheless. The next generation of pathologists will apply new tests based on advances in molecular biology and will interpret the results for better management of patients. You will need a strong general training in clinical medicine to enable you to communicate effectively with clinical colleagues on matters of patient management, a sound knowledge of clinical and anatomic pathology, and an up-to-date understanding of molecular pathology. You will also have to be conversant with the information systems that are becoming indispensable for handling the enormous amounts of data in this discipline.

Training in pathology is demanding but very rewarding. In medical school, the pathology course has traditionally been considered very tough, largely because of the breadth of the subject and its huge (and at that stage unfamiliar) vocabulary. Residency training in pathology is demanding also, but it constantly provides unexpected insights into mechanisms and natural history of disease that energize and stimulate the inquiring physician. Current training requires four years for the combined anatomic and clinical pathology residency (three years for either anatomic or clinical pathology alone), and most trainees take a subspecialty fellowship of one year following residency. Career opportunities are good: there are plenty of open positions at present and a severe shortage of American physicians both entering and graduating from pathology residency programs.

Pathology is a discipline that encompasses an amazing diversity of career opportunities. For the would-be sleuth, there is forensic pathology; for patient contact, there is cytopathology; for the computer fanatic there is the burgeoning field of pathology informatics. Those who wish to be managers can run clinical laboratories, the clinically oriented can go into subspecialties of anatomic pathology (where they have frequent interaction with the clinical specialists), and those interested in basic or translational research can take advantage of the fact that, as trained pathologists, they are expert in tissue changes in disease and are privileged among physicians in having both direct access to such tissues and the ability to confirm the diagnoses of the diseases with which they are working.

For me, the fascination of pathology has been to visualize at both gross and microscopic level the remarkable experiments of nature that constitute disease, to witness the presently unfolding panorama of knowledge about mechanisms of disease, to make diagnoses that enable patients to receive optimal treatment, and to interact with my clinical colleagues (including medical students and residents) to educate, learn, and improve patient care. If "I'm a pathologist" stops the conversation, my enthusiastic fascination about what I do usually gets it going again!

MAURICE J. MAHONEY

Genetics and Medicine

G enetic science has flourished over the past hundred years. The concept of a gene as a concrete entity that transmits information from generation to generation crystallized from the appreciation of Gregor Mendel's seminal experiments. Thrilling scientific breakthroughs followed: the recognition of DNA as the chemical molecule that codified this information; deciphering the code itself; learning how the code was read and how its information was transposed to the functioning proteins of life; and now a first working draft of the sequence of the genetic material, complete for the human animal. The basic place of genetics in the world of biology is secure and biologists continue to explore the role that genetics plays in their discipline. Increasingly, physicians, and even social scientists and nonscientists, have come to recognize the importance of genetics to their fields. It seems inevitable that this recognition will escalate and that insights from genetic principles will be a major foundation for future medical progress. Today, when one describes what naturally occurs (the physiology) and what goes wrong (the pathology) in a body system, that description is incomplete if it doesn't include the genetic information and processes that define normalcy and the changes (the mutations) that contribute to abnormalcy. There are still many holes to be filled in for these descriptions, but that is happening, sometimes at a dizzying pace, sometimes disappointingly slowly. No matter the speed, the excitement of genetic thinking is palpable in the medicine of our era.

If genetic science has leaped ahead in its contribution to understanding our world, what about genetic medicine and its contribution? Medicine strives not only to understand but to move beyond that base so as to prevent, to palliate, and to cure. First steps have been taken but the horizon is broad and distant. The foundation of genetic science is solid and ideas abound of how to translate insights into improved medical care. Major advances are few thus far, however, but a general feeling exists that we stand at the threshold of an era of genetics-based medicine. I hope an attempt to glimpse beyond that threshold will not be misleading.

An important place to start is to acknowledge the temptation to give too much credit to genes in predicting or dictating a biologic outcome (like a disease or a superperforming athletic ability), and to debunk that concept. Genetic determinism, or the idea that one's genes, if fully understood, would give a rather complete description of one's behaviors, one's diseases, one's future, doesn't fit the facts of our world. The environment in which those genes exist and act is just as important. Certain environments will not permit a gene to be read (that is, it will be turned off); other environments will let that gene be read (turned on), perhaps fully but perhaps only a little. Choice points, depending on conditions in the environment, abound to allow or deny the expression of a gene. A gene may be capable of directing the synthesis of different gene products. Which one is made, or the proportions of two possible products, will depend on the environment at any given moment. Because some choices are permanent, one result might be a malformed structure while the other choice would lead to a normal outcome. The environment that exerts control may be the microenvironment within the nucleus of a cell or it may be an environment of a much larger scale. Great complexity is likely to exist in these multiple gene-environment interactions. Some aspects will have more importance in controlling outcomes, and these will be targets for interventions. Many of these interventions will continue to be manipulations of the environment as when, for example, a patient is given a drug.

Another insight of modern genetics is that more than one gene, often several, will play major roles in the appearance or progression of a disorder. It's not one gene for baldness and one for a full mane, or one gene for cystic fibrosis and one for normal lung function, or even one gene for blue eyes and another for brown eyes. Almost always, reality is much more complex. Factor in important environmental variables and one has quite a goulash. This enormous complexity is daunting and yet it simultaneously provides many places to intervene and thereby control a disease. If we change our focus from our own genes and think about the genes of microbes, like the tuberculosis, anthrax, or malaria organisms, we find hope that there will be multiple targets of intervention through an understanding of their genes. Currently there are intense efforts to sequence the genomes of many microorganisms to find new antibiotics or other ways to stop their ability to cause disease.

Cancer has turned out to be a disease characterized and driven by many different genetic changes. Perhaps more correct, cancer has turned out to be many diseases, each type of cancer having its own set of changes. There are major overlaps, but strategies that will work with one cancer may well fail with another. Heart failure and hypertension, arthritis and dementia have similar complexities at the genetic level and, most certainly, at the environmental level as well. Each will require a step-by-step understanding and each will offer multiple opportunities for intervention.

What will those interventions be? Undoubtedly many, perhaps most, will be attempts to manipulate the macro- or microenvironment by pharmaceuticals or other means. But on the genetic side there will be new approaches. The fascination of soon being able to control our genes directly, to add new genes, to remove or silence extant genes propels the concepts of gene transfer and gene therapy. If we were born with a "bad" gene, maybe we can turn it off or even destroy it. Perhaps an extra dose of "good" genes can reverse a disease. Because gene action is very tightly regulated both in time (when the gene is turned on and when it is turned off) and space (genes are inside cell nuclei and mitochondria), progress in gene therapy has been slow. Nonetheless, efforts continue to expand and along with them, new hopes and dreams. When we do succeed in putting genes into cells, and have them work properly, we will immediately have new challenges. What is a disease and how severe must it be to think about altering someone's genes? Would we want to put "better" genes in even though the current status is considered normal or average?

For many people, understanding the operation of our brain and nervous system and being able to intervene in disease processes are the most challenging tasks for biology and medicine today. The decade of the 1990s was dubbed by some as the "Decade of the Brain." There was certainly progress, but our understanding of genetic control of development, function, and disease of our brains is very much in its infancy. We face most of our major mental disorders (such as retardation, schizophrenia), degenerative and progressive disorders of the brain (such as multiple sclerosis, Alzheimer's disease), and the impediments of "normal" aging with either no therapies or therapies of limited effect. It is hoped that genetic understanding of the brain will bring major improvements. It may be that a hundred years from now, we will label the twenty-first century as the "Century of the Brain."

For many, one of the fascinations is the way genetic information identifies an individual from all others. The corollary is that you will have more genes in common with those most closely related to you than you will with other people. This individual nature of our genetic makeup has led to DNA fingerprinting for use in postmortem identification and criminology. It is likely to facilitate learning about ancestral roots, for example, by those displaced by wars or slavery. Shared genes among more closely related people help the understanding of ancient human migrations. They also help predict the likelihood of certain disease states for an individual. This use of genetics will surely increase. Already, a field called pharmacogenomics has been born and is off to a well-financed start. It intends to define a person's genetic status with regard to drug actions so there can be a better decision about what drug to use or how much to use. Perhaps some day we will have "designer drugs" in a thousand different colors and flavors, each for specific individuals with a certain set of genes.

The excitement about genetics in the halls of science and in the corridors of hospitals has spilled into many other areas of the public's interest. Extrapolations feed movie scripts and sci-fi novels. Concerns about misuse of genetic knowledge have also been frequently raised; I have alluded to some of these. Genetic issues are now common subject matter for debates in bioethics. Issues exist from the newly conceived embryo prior to implantation in a woman's uterus through the last stages of life and probably beyond. Of particular concern at this time in the United States have been the privacy of genetic information and the use of genetic information by various parties. Among these parties are the government, financial institutions like insurance companies and employers, members of one's family, and even oneself. Many legislatures have weighed in on these issues. Concerns arise because there is a degree of predictive information, sometimes high, in one's genes. This information has not been available to past generations. The hope is that it can greatly benefit future generations. Many opportunities, many challenges, and many dilemmas define the excitement of genetics in medicine today.

Practicing in the Health Professions

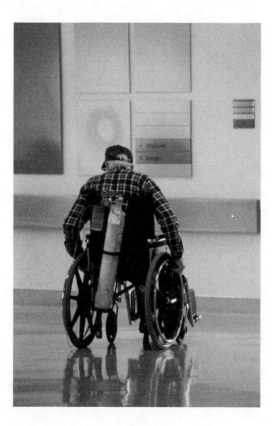

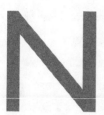ot so long ago, someone who wanted to be involved with medicine and patient care had little choice but to go to medical school and become a physician. Today, health care is no longer limited to the business of diagnosing and treating disease. Many aspects of society vitally affect health and disease. People with careers in such diverse fields as pharmacology, pollution control, epidemiology, ethics, and law are providing health benefits and services within our system of health care. Also connected to health care are careers related to occupational safety, consumer protection, injury prevention, food and drug safety, and environmental protection. Such diversity of effort translates into numerous careers in this broad field. Many college students reject a traditional career in medicine because of the years of costly training, the demanding work hours, the sometimes repugnant nature of the work, or the annoying regulations and paper work involved. If you believe that life as a physician is not for you but are still interested in entering the field of health care, you should find out more about the parallel careers. The careers described here certainly do not make up the full slate of possibilities.

The essays in this section provide a sampling of the career opportunities that lie beyond the realm of the traditional medical profession. Some of these involve providing care to individual patients. Others involve forming the strategies, policies, and programs designed to protect and promote health.

We begin with an essay written jointly by a former dean and the present dean of Yale's School of Nursing. Together, Florence Wald and Catherine Gilliss depict the nursing profession of a half-century ago and indicate how it has changed. Douglas P. Olsen addresses the special issues that confront a man who has chosen to become a nurse. Both essays view the complexities of the nurse-physician relationship in the care of patients and illustrate the variety of careers available in nursing. One such career is midwifery, and Deborah Cibelli, a certified nurse midwife, characterizes the modern version of this ancient profession. Angela Delisle, a physician assistant, enjoys taking care of patients but did not have to undertake the rigorous training of a physician. Sandra Alfano, whose life's work began with a job in a drug store, relates how she earned a doctoral degree in pharmacy and discusses the career opportunities available to pharmacists in clinical and academic settings. Angela R. Holder delineates her long career as a lawyer for an academic medical center and as a teacher of medical students. Kathleen S. Lundgren addresses the importance of the application of ethical and moral theory to medical practice, especially in her work in ethics of research involving humans, in particular with vulnerable populations. Michael Rowe describes the role he plays as a sociologist participating in an innovative program that makes mental health services available to the poor.

Evie Lindemann gives a vivid description of her professional development in international social work. The practical aspects of medical social work are found in Gail Korrick's essay. Those interested in a career in public health will find informative the portrayal by Susan S. Addiss, former commissioner of public health for the state of Connecticut. An essay by Nora Groce, an associate professor of public health and epidemiology, tells how she became a medical anthropologist. D. George Joseph points out the value of pursuing knowledge of the history of medicine and its application to issues of today. Peter Salovey and Kelly D. Brownell, professors of psychology at Yale, describe how they go about understanding and improving health behavior. Michael Cocco, a chiropractor, describes how an interest in holistic medicine led him to his career.

The section ends with Howard Spiro's examination of the burgeoning field of complementary and alternative medicine (CAM). Readers may be surprised that the editors have included an essay on CAM in this volume, but we are eager to introduce you to careers in all aspects of the health professions. CAM is contributing to the new shape of medical practice in the twenty-first century, but comments on its body of practice veer from the wholly adulatory to the sneeringly skeptical. We hope that this account, written from the standpoint of a mainstream physician who has great faith in the power of hope, intuition, and empathy will provide a balanced view of this approach.

FLORENCE**WALD** and CATHERINE**GILLISS**

Nursing
One Field, Many Arenas

The stories of a career are not always coherent. The careers of men are often said to be clear from the earliest days and characterized by specific goals and outcomes. But women more often respond to career opportunities that emerge along the way. In sharing our experiences, we will discuss what factors led us to our careers, how our career choices have been rewarded, and where our careers fit in our lives.

Our professional lives have spanned more than half a century. We've both served as dean of the Yale University School of Nursing, Wald from 1958 to 1968 and Gilliss since 1998. When Dean Wald left that post, Dean Gilliss was in the fourth grade. The nursing profession is vastly changed today from sixty years ago, and so is nursing education. But the core of nursing has been constant: helping individuals to recover from illness, to manage full lives despite illness, and to be well informed about sustaining health throughout life.

Florence Wald's Career in Nursing

I have been a nurse for sixty years. I graduated from Yale University, at that time the only university program that required a bachelor's degree on entrance and granted the master of nursing degree. The decision was made when I was nine years old; the inspiration came from a private-duty nurse who saw me through scarlet fever and the complications that followed. Because I became ill while on a family vacation in Washington, D.C., I was taken from the hotel to an isolation hospital. It was the first time I had been away from my family. My mother had nursed me through severe bouts of pneumonia. I knew she could help me get well. But the nurse, Eunice Biller, made me feel as safe as my mother had and comforted me through the long and painful complications when my mastoid bones became infected and had to be reamed out.

Quarantine in the aging Garfield Hospital meant I could only see my mother when Miss Biller carried me to the window to wave to her as she stood three stories down. Miss Biller and my mother were the role models in my favorite pastime—being mother and nurse for a large family of dolls.

My choice of vocation was reinforced by the values of my parents, who stood up for the rights of the disadvantaged. As the first generation born of German immigrants and New York City residents, they supported the work of Lillian Wald and the Henry Street Settlement at the turn of the century.

My father was reluctant to give me a college education, but my mother and brother insisted on it. So after graduating from Mount Holyoke College, I went to the Yale University School of Nursing in 1938.

For the most part, the three-year curriculum suited my expectations. It provided ample experience in hospital and home care. The focus was on the patient as a person. In the years 1938 to 1941 patients were bed-bound for weeks as they recovered from surgery, childbirth, heart attacks, and infectious diseases. This was a benefit to the student nurse: we had long-standing relationships with patients and a good opportunity to observe the course of each disease.

I was not prepared, however, for the hospital culture and the overprotective rules and regulations imposed on student nurses. Submitting to hierarchical domination and dormitory surveillance was chafing after life in a liberal arts college where I had learned to innovate and to think for myself. I didn't mind standing when a physician entered the room, but making way for him to enter the elevator first seemed a breach of common etiquette. This was just one illustration of the reality that the nurse was the physician's assistant. It was to be twenty-five years before that stance was challenged and changed.

Faculty included physicians as well as nurses, but student nurses were spectators, rarely expected to contribute. That circumstance enforced the reality that the nurse was the physician's assistant, a role I had not anticipated. Student nurses spent three of their thirty months in a visiting nurse agency, where I felt most comfortable. In a few instances a student could be part of a team—an obstetrician and nurse in a home care delivery of an infant, for example.

Six months after I graduated in 1941, the United States entered World War II. I was a pacifist. Several of my classmates joined the army, but this did not appeal to me. The effect of the war on civilian and military health care was profound. Both hospital nursing and home care nursing were constrained by the limited number of health professionals available to care for a growing population. The prevailing career path for nurses led to teaching or administration, but my expectation was to put my healing hands to use. The possibility of becoming an advanced nurse practitioner wouldn't come for another twenty-five years.

Rudderless, I found refuge for the next twelve years as a medical research technician. As technology developed during and immediately after the war, Columbia College of Physicians and Surgeons launched projects to expand diagnostic techniques and to transplant tissues from animals and humans in experiments leading to the development of cardiac surgery. I became knowledgeable about planning and carrying out clinical research with physicians. The physicians conducting the research treated me as a colleague: though I was not a principal investigator, I was a full-fledged team member.

In 1953 I was thirty-six. In the 1950s the research of social scientists in sociology, anthropology, and psychiatry had a major impact on the care of patients. Publications of Anna Freud, Erich Fromm, Abram Kardiner, Erich Lindemann, Robert Morton, David Riesman, and Leo Sroll were shedding new light on the relationships between caregivers and patients. Through my reading of the works of these thinkers, and my own psychoanalysis, I became aware of how human behavior can be changed—and of the potential of psychiatric nursing. So I reentered Yale, this time in the graduate study of psychiatric nursing, and received the master of science of nursing.

In the next ten years I met six mentors who were the greatest influences on my professional life. The most productive and satisfying years of my career began in 1956. My mentors and the tenor of the times combined to propel my professional growth. Now my skills and interests were compatible with the changes in the health care system, and in the culture. I began to learn how to assist patients who had inadequate ways of coping and how to teach students in clinical practice. After my graduation, as teaching assistant to Hilde Peplau at Rutgers University School of Nursing, my career finally took hold.

During the 1950s, Yale's School of Nursing became committed to revising its curriculum, and I returned to teach there. I lacked a traditional nursing career, but my recent experience at Rutgers gave me a vision of the future. And by this time I had enough confidence and courage to accept the challenge and to become the acting dean of the school at the request of Yale's president, A. W. Griswold.

The university asked its nursing faculty to redesign the curriculum for advanced nurse practitioners in order to study the impact of nursing care on patient welfare. Finally, the time was right for the vision that had inspired me to become a nurse—not only helping patients to cope with illness but aiding in their recovery of health and teaching them about how that process worked. Although the faculty and staff of the school was small in number, it was rich in the quality of its practitioners and social scientists: the midwife Ernestine Wiedenbach, the sociologist Robert Leonard, the public health nurse Elizabeth Tennant, the psychiatric nurse Ida Orlando. Physicians including Max Pepper, Morris Wessel, Edmund Pellegrino, and Ray Duff took interest in our studies. Virginia Henderson compiled an index of nursing literature published in English. As a research associate, she served all the faculty as a generous source of information, critique, and wisdom.

Next, a visitor from England, Cicely Saunders, came to Yale in 1963 to lecture. She had trained as a nurse, as a hospital social worker, and as a physician. She was creating a hospice called St. Christopher's in a London suburb where an interdisciplinary team was to care for cancer patients and their families through the patients' last phase of life. Her work struck a deep chord in me. At the School of Nursing, we had witnessed the plummeting quality of life among patients receiving intensive treatment for cancer, and her approach to caring for the suffering of the terminally ill patient and the patient's family responded to that need.

As my deanship entered its seventh year, the new curriculum was established and we were about to adopt a new curriculum for entering college graduates en route to advanced degrees. It was an appropriate time for new leadership. And so, after ten years as dean of the School of Nursing, I resigned the position and returned to the practice of nursing, with a focus of working with the terminally ill.

During my deanship I had married, and now my career shift drew my husband's heartfelt support. Henry had been a widower, and as his wife, I had become the mother of his two children, ages six and eight. Henry and I were partners in raising these children, and his pleasure in my career had made the dual role of mother and dean possible. He was right behind me again when, at age fifty, I took on the nursing practice of the terminally ill, determined to learn whether the model of St. Christopher's Hospice fit the health care environment and needs of the United States. Today we know that it does, and palliative care for the dying is widely available.

My uneven, disjointed progress can be an important example for those thinking of a career in nursing. As you test your talents and interests and think about your future, I offer you some advice, based on more than sixty years in nursing: know your dreams, know the society in which you live, know the characteristics of the school you choose, find mentors, expect dead ends, and be prepared to seize the moment. At the same time, always be open to new possibilities.

Catherine Gilliss's Career in Nursing

Having made a choice to study nursing at a university when I was in my first year there, I have often been grateful that I selected an option so well suited to my growth across a lifetime. In thirty-four years I have assumed many identities—from clinician to teacher, from researcher to speaker, from author to academic administrator. The flexibility within the field has kept my interest alive.

Like many adolescents, I wasn't really sure who I was in high school. Did I want a career? Did I have the intellectual power to drive me to the top of any field? One thing I was sure of, though: whatever career I might choose would reflect my strong interest in people and an early inclination to serve others. I remember my father's respect for the religious women who served as administrators in large Catholic hospitals. He described them as "smart businesswomen," though the world recognized them as nurses. I later found that nursing matched my personal and family values, and the intellectual match was clear to me before I earned my bachelor's degree.

But in high school, I knew only that I wanted to attend college, and I had a vague notion that I would be a social worker. Somehow—the details have grown a bit foggy over the years—I ended up at Duke University in a four-year nursing program. I still was unsure of my career path, or even whether I would have a career outside the home. With a relatively low grade-point average, I couldn't transfer easily to another major, so I remained in Duke's nursing program and began to look more carefully at what I was studying. And then I was twenty-one years old, and married to someone we thought was terminally ill. Circumstances had conspired, it seemed, to provide me with structure, a direction, and the promise of work for as long as I sought it: nursing.

By my senior year in college, I had studied in two areas of practice, psychiatric nursing and public health, in which I appeared to have aptitude and had begun to have some success. There is no incentive like success. Under the mentorship of several faculty members, I took on elective and supplemental work in these two areas. Professor Frances Smith Blackwell supervised an optional program at a state psychiatric hospital where several of us directed therapy groups. In my senior year, under Professor Smith Blackwell's supervision, I began to believe that I could help people change. This is a stage at which I have seen the careers of others "take hold," too. The generalization I offer you from the particulars of my life is more about age and the influence of mentors than about my choice of career. People learn about themselves through reflection, and twenty-one-year-olds are trying to see where they fit in. Mentors matter, and especially then. So be on the lookout for mentors who can help you answer your questions about yourself.

I became intellectually committed to psychiatric nursing early in my career, and I received a federal traineeship from the National Institute of Mental Health (NIMH) to support my undergraduate studies. In accepting this support, I agreed to continue my education in psychiatric nursing at the graduate level, which would also be supported by the NIMH. In fact, I might not have continued my studies without that support. I was still not fully committed to a career, and other opportunities in my life could easily have distracted me and lured me away. I was a college graduate in a field in which fewer than 1 percent hold an advanced degree. I was not particularly ambitious, though I was increasingly curious.

In the late 1960s advanced practice roles for nurses were just emerging. At Duke the nurse practitioner concept was proposed, professionally rejected, and subsequently replaced by the idea of a physician's assistant. The first nurse practitioner program was successfully launched in Colorado as part of a collaborative effort to improve the care of community-based children. The hospital-based clinical nurse specialist became the advanced practice nurse with specialty knowledge and clinical leadership. Models were emerging for the evolution of careers in nursing that did not require a lateral move to the positions of educator or administrator. I entered the Catholic University of America to study psychiatric–mental health nursing.

While studying for my master's degree, I was regularly supervised by a faculty member who was a Roman Catholic nun. The program content heavily emphasized one's perceptions and strengths, achieved through self-reflection and discussion. Sister Anna used those same ideas as she counseled me on my work with clients. It was clear then that I had to understand my own life experience in order for me to be successful working with others. Sister Anna was tolerant and accepting, and I, in turn, learned to know and accept myself better during our time together.

I entered nursing education immediately after I had earned my master's degree. For two years I taught registered nurses returning for an undergraduate degree at a large state school. I then returned to Catholic University and taught undergraduates for another two years. But in these four years I never had the opportunity to teach psychiatric nursing. Psychiatric concepts were now integrated into other clinical rotations, and my job was to teach principles of mental health within the practice of these settings.

I was soon ready for a change and applied to the Robert Wood Johnson Foundation to participate in its new Primary Care Faculty Fellows Program. The foundation accepted me and sent me to the University of Rochester, where, after a year, I earned a post-master's certificate as an adult nurse practitioner.

The year in Rochester exposed me to powerful people and to big ideas and whetted my appetite for more intellectual challenges. The mentorship provided during that program was unparalleled. I met regularly with Loretta Ford, then dean at the University of Rochester's School of Nursing, and Ingeborg Mauksch, director of the Robert Wood Johnson program in which I was a fellow. I was encouraged to pursue my dreams and assured that anything was possible. In particular, I was encouraged to begin doctoral study.

My personal life was also unfolding. Married, pregnant, and the mother of a two-year-old daughter, I was unsure how to pursue all my dreams. I was accepted for doctoral study at the University of California, San Francisco. Knowing that my husband was ready for a professional change, I told him that I intended to go to San Francisco in fall 1979, and that I hoped he would come, too. Fortunately, he did. We left the East, where we had always lived, and set out for the West Coast. To our surprise, we were to live in California for the next twenty years!

My doctoral study reinforced my enthusiasm for ideas and theoretical thinking. Dr. Susan Gortner had recently joined the faculty following a career with the Health Services Resources Administration's Division of Nursing, the precursor to the National Institute for Nursing Research at the National Institutes of Health (NIH). She advised me and mentored me in a beginning program of nursing research on families and chronic illness. In fact, she generously shared her own work to accomplish my launch. Her actions served as a powerful lesson about the role of mentors.

I completed doctoral and postdoctoral studies at UCSF and was ready for a faculty position to continue my research. Sadly, no positions were available in the San Francisco Bay area, and my transplanted husband, happily engaged in the practice of law, was not interested in another relocation. I found a faculty position preparing nurse practitioners and maintained my affiliation with UCSF for research activities. Eventually, I competed successfully for a spot on the UCSF faculty, where I remained for fifteen years, moving from assistant professor to professor and department chair.

My research by now was well established and I was chairing a study section at the NIH. The National Organization of Nurse Practitioner Faculties acknowledged my teaching contributions by awarding me the Educator of the Year Award. I was fully engaged as an educational administrator and sought opportunities to create an environment in which others could be supported to do their best work. One of my children was in college on the East Coast, and the other soon would be.

Yale University's School of Nursing was unknown to me. When I was invited to consult on the development of the school's new doctoral program in 1993, I agreed in hopes of spending more time with Dr. Margaret Grey, the doctoral program director. And this association offered the chance to return to my native Connecticut. My father and both my brothers were graduates of Yale College, and I admit that I was curious about the place where they had spent several years. I was pleased to experience a part of their lives at Yale, even if only as a visit, and I returned home to California with a warm familiarity with Yale.

After six years of chairing the Department of Family Health Care at UCSF, I was ready for a change, and Yale was looking for a new dean. Visits and discussions suggested that the fit was right, and I left California for Yale in the summer of 1998. I have been dean of nursing since then.

In looking back over these years, I see some patterns worth noting. First, I have never been ruled by the politics of the day. Rather, the contemporary culture and trends have influenced my thinking and my aspirations in a quiet fashion, under the surface. During the Vietnam War, for instance, I was not protesting with many of my student colleagues. I was studying and preparing to marry. I was concerned for the welfare of those around me, but rather than participate in the protests, I participated in student government. While at Duke, I served as class president and president of the nursing school. In issues of politics, I have generally been moderate and worked from the inside.

Given the positions I have held and the interests I have pursued, I am struck by the fact that many of these positions did not require preparation as a nurse. I have participated very little in clinical nursing practice. The substance of my teaching has been in theory building and social sciences; my research has addressed problems of families and chronic illness. Nonetheless, my nursing degrees have provided a nearly ideal preparation. The greatest barrier I now face is discrimination by those who do not understand the capacities or training of the contemporary nurse. The public assumes that a nurse has a limited intellectual capacity and educational background. Unfortunately, these assumptions contribute to the current difficulty in recruitment to the field of nursing, and they may limit the options available to those entering nursing.

Finally, I note the importance of my family across the course of my life's development. As I was growing up, my family instilled in me a commitment to service to others. They exposed me to business principles and the value of relationships; they taught me not to be afraid of conflict. As an adult, my family has anchored me in reality. Surely there were times when my commitment to them prevented me from fully participating in some professional activity. And there were times I felt crazed trying to meet the needs of my career and my family. But more often than not, they provided the stability and perspective needed to rebalance a life sometimes out of focus.

As we reflect on our careers, we observe several similarities. Our careers have developed over time and have been nurtured by others. We view our careers as significantly influenced by the social contexts in which they unfolded. Finally, despite the different time frames, we have each been able to undertake a variety of roles within our chosen career of nursing. We remain satisfied with our choice and encourage others to examine their options within nursing.

DOUGLAS P. OLSEN

A Man's Experience in Nursing

I suppose there are reasons why men who are nurses are singled out as "male" nurses. We are certainly in the minority. About 5 percent of nurses are male, and this figure has been remarkably stable since I entered nursing in 1979. But even beyond these demographics, the essential concept of nursing is inherently feminine. The words "nurse" and "nursing" themselves are associated with a uniquely female act. Members of the nursing profession derive our identity from the act of giving nurturing care to the suffering and sick. We make a point of distinguishing care from cure: nurses believe that the difference between our profession and medicine is that we focus on caring for patients while medicine focuses on cure. In our society, nurturing is closely identified with the female psyche, and nursing embraces this image. The experience of a man in the profession is inevitably colored by this philosophy.

In my experience, the feminine essence and feminist outlook of nursing have two facets: first, men are an awkward minority in nursing. Although we are a very small minority in this profession, men are generally held to be dominant, if not oppressive, in the society and the job market at large. And I find it a bit embarrassing that men are overrepresented in nursing's leadership positions as well. Yet I was pleased that the job ad I responded to at Yale said that men and other minorities were encouraged to apply. I know of no other nursing school that makes this modification to the standard formula. Ads for nurses that encourage women to apply have always seemed rather thoughtless to me. Still, it is disingenuous for a white man to make too much of his minority status in the nursing world.

Second, I sometimes feel awkward advocating essential feminist positions and ideals, yet my writing and research explicate caring, empathy, and relationships. No one has ever said I didn't belong or that I was misplaced as a man dealing with matters some think best left to women. But at times I have felt a vague sense of distance from my female colleagues and wondered whether others saw me as an intruder. Admittedly, this has been so subtle that the feeling may have been generated entirely by my own insecurities. Even if some of my colleagues do occasionally wonder what a man is doing advocating a version of bioethics generally seen to have arisen from a female or feminist perspective, such feelings have never influenced me in a material way, and certainly they have never discouraged me from continuing on my chosen path.

I have always tried to present myself clearly as a man, with a man's outlook, who is a nurse, rather than as a man who became a nurse because he has views like a woman. And so I have at various times in my career found myself as the representative and defender of the male sex. Sometimes this means acknowledging women's feelings about an issue and then reminding colleagues that men may feel differently. And sometimes this means acknowledging women's feelings and then reminding my female colleagues that many men have similar feelings.

One aspect of "doing something out of the ordinary," whether it's being a male nurse or a female firefighter, is responding to the reactions of others. While still in school, I learned to dislike hearing acquaintances and strangers say how marvelous it was that I was becoming a "male" nurse, how caring and brave I was, and so on. I often wanted to say that I went into nursing because I was "turned on by women in white," and then watch the reactions. But I didn't. On the positive side, I can report that I have rarely been subjected to what I feared to be the stereotypes of male nurses, that we were either sissies or gay. I can also say that in my experience, men in nursing aren't any more or any less masculine than men in any other walk of life.

I sometimes have heard my female nursing colleagues accuse certain male physicians of having "difficulty" with women, rather than simply saying these doctors were hard to get along with, as they might have said about a female physician or fellow nurse. Men so labeled often were patronizingly courteous, then turned irritable when deference wasn't shown them. Generally, I have found that I have an easier time dealing with these male physicians than do my female colleagues, and unfortunately, that serves to confirm their judgment. However, I feel a bit guilty having an easier time because of my sex.

As a man in a female-dominated profession, I have learned that women are more attuned to misogyny than most men believe. I have noticed that one sign of a staff in which members are comfortable and working well together is that people break up easily for conversation or social interaction along gender lines rather than along the traditional doctor-nurse division.

Nursing's identity crisis arises not only from its feminine nature but also from its historically subservient relationship to medicine. The perception of nurses as doctors' assistants really became clear to me when I planned to pursue my Ph.D. in nursing. A physician who was also a close friend once characterized the contrast of respect and subservience of the nursing doctorate with the joking title "Sir Boy." Another time I was interviewed by Tom Jerrel for the national network news magazine show *20/20* on a topic unrelated to my profession; following the interview he asked me how a nurse could be called "doctor." But I am certain that he would have no difficulty calling a person with a Ph.D. in history "doctor."

But negative stereotyping as a nurse or as a male nurse has been a rare experience for me. Overall, my sex has rarely been a factor in doing my job either with my patients, my colleagues, or my students. I can truly say that the decision to be a nurse is one that I have never regretted. Rather, hindsight has affirmed my decision again and again. Nursing provided me the ability to make a comfortable living while continually bettering my position through education and experience. I found further education very accessible as a nurse because of the flexibility in hours. In fact, my wife was also able to go back to school full-time after the birth of our son, and we never needed to pay for child care because I could easily tailor my schedule to meet our needs.

The real wisdom of my decision to pursue a career in nursing, though, beyond its many practical values, lay in the way it opened me to the rewards of being useful to others and of fulfilling my dreams.

I did not dream of being a nurse. As child I never told anyone that I wanted to be nurse, or a doctor, or any other health care professional. My career ambitions as a child ranged freely and changed often: astronaut, scientist, architect, lawyer. One theme that remained consistent in my aspirations was that I wanted to contend with ideas, and the bigger the better. A career in health was one of the few options I didn't consider. On entering college, at the last minute, I changed my major from physics to biology, and that change led to my career in nursing.

Rightly or wrongly, when asked about how I became a nurse, I am always sensitive that some people are really asking why I didn't become a doctor. I am especially sensitive when I tell people I was a biology major, for I fear that they might assume that I failed to get into medical school and opted for "second-best." But biology majors were very different folk from pre-med majors at Penn State, where I earned my first undergraduate degree. None of the biology majors I knew planned to go into health care. One friend dreamed of working with trout and another went to graduate school for entomology. My fantasy was that I would replace Marlin Perkins, the longtime host of *Wild Kingdom,* a popular nature show, before the days of cable TV and the Discovery Channel. My coursework emphasized evolution and population dynamics.

My third year in college I realized that I would be expected to turn my education into a career, and Mr. Perkins wasn't leaving his enviable job anytime soon. During that year, I became intrigued by my psychology electives, and at the same time, I was working nights as a nurse's aide at a nursing home. Although working nights while in school was difficult, I enjoyed interactions with the people in the nursing home and began to feel close to the nursing staff. I decided not to switch my major to psychology because I was gaining what I considered a more realistic view of human beings than the psych majors with whom I'd talked. I was beginning to think of human beings as full and rich organisms.

I decided to finish my degree in biology and then get a two-year associate degree in nursing. Even at this point I was not planning on making a career of nursing. With my nurse's license I intended to make a decent living with a flexible work schedule that would allow me to pursue a graduate education in psychology. And I would be gaining experience working in mental health.

Once I had my license and began working, I examined the roles of nurses, psychologists, and social workers. For me, the most interesting jobs with the broadest opportunities were all in nursing, so I stuck with it. Nursing has given me everything I wanted in a career, and it has taught me the value of what is really important in life and work.

I admit that I didn't become a nurse for altruistic reasons; that others might benefit from my actions was perceived as merely a nice side effect when I first contemplated nursing. It was in the practice of nursing, in the interaction with patients, and now students, that the touching of lives took on a primary position. Although I've largely devoted emphasis to the experience of being a man in a primarily female profession, make no mistake, nursing is the profession that affords one the greatest opportunity to touch, not merely influence, the lives of others. Of all the benefits a profession can offer, nothing provides a person with purpose and meaning like the sense that others gain from what you do.

DEBORAH**CIBELLI**

Modern Midwifery

Midwifery care is attractive to many women and families because of the personalized nature of the relationship and the philosophy that pregnancy, birth, and transition through life's stages are normal events. Certified nurse-midwives (CNMs) schedule ample time for each client visit and emphasize education and preventive care. As a midwife, you have more opportunity to get to know the woman, her family, and their plans for the birth. CNMs are often at the bedside with the family during labor and throughout the birthing process. You will have the privilege of ensuring that the woman's experience will be as safe and satisfying as it can be. For gynecological clients, midwives provide education about nutrition, exercise, and lifestyle, in addition to routine physical exams.

Recently, I attended a woman for the birth of her fourth child. Her first three had been born in a physician-only practice in another part of the state. She had been very satisfied with her care there and had given birth to healthy infants. When she moved to this area, she was uncertain about going to a practice with midwives. Why would she want a midwife to deliver her baby when she had insurance that would cover a physician's attendance? Her neighbor encouraged her to come to our practice and discover the difference. She was cautious at first. She asked a lot of questions about our training and experience. Then she started to appreciate the time we spent with her at her visits. She discovered there was a lot of information about nutrition and the emotional and physical changes of pregnancy that she didn't know, even though she had had three babies. When she came to the hospital in labor, she was relieved to see someone she knew well and trusted. She appreciated my presence and the fact that I never left her side as she labored and gave birth to her fourth child and first daughter.

I learned all of this only after attending her birth. Her husband told me that this was the first birth at which he didn't feel like "an intruder." He found it helpful when I guided him during her labor, instructing him to fan her, rub her back and support her head while she pushed. He told me how unsure they both were in the beginning about this "midwife thing," but that now he couldn't imagine why anyone would choose to have a baby without one. His wife smiled over her newborn daughter still lying on her abdomen and agreed.

During my junior and senior years in college, I volunteered at a community health center as a medical assistant, determining the reason for patients' visits, taking a brief history, checking vital signs, and performing simple laboratory tests. I was interested in a career in health care but unsure of which path to pursue. I enjoyed working with the children, but I found that talking to the women and teenagers who came seeking birth control or gynecological exams was definitely my strength. When a physician at the health center suggested that I become a midwife, I must admit I looked at her oddly. My image of that practice was of granny midwives attending births at home without any formal education or license. I had no idea that midwifery had become a recognized profession.

That was 1975. It wasn't surprising that I had never heard of certified nurse-midwives: there were only about seventeen hundred in practice in the United States. They attended fewer than twenty thousand births in 1975. There were very few midwifery educational programs—only one program in the country, in fact, that I could attend without being a registered nurse. Fortunately, I was accepted into the Yale University School of Nursing Midwifery Program, graduated three years later and have been a practicing CNM ever since.

Certified nurse-midwives are registered nurses (RNs) with graduate training in the care of essentially healthy women from menarche through menopause. Midwifery education emphasizes personalized, family-centered care. The focus is on patient education, wellness, and consumer choice. There are forty-three midwifery educational programs in the United States. Fifteen of them accept individuals who have bachelor's degrees in any field but are not registered nurses. Usually these programs are between one and one and a half years longer than for those individuals who enter as RNs. The student does basic nursing training, takes the RN boards, and proceeds directly into the midwifery aspect of the educational program. After graduation, one must sit for a national certification exam before practicing as a nurse-midwife anywhere in the United States.

All CNMs have a professional relationship with an obstetrician/gynecologist who provides consultation and collaborative care when indicated. As the health care system changes and physicians have less time to spend with their patients, many are incorporating CNMs into their practices. This ensures that the women receive the time that they deserve while freeing the physicians to care for the higher-risk patients. The American College of Obstetricians and Gynecologists reported in 1992 that 7.7 percent of obstetricians employed CNMs. By 1999 the figure was 17.7 percent. Health maintenance organizations (HMOs), family planning clinics, community health centers, and hospitals have had CNMs as part of their health care teams for a number of years. Birth centers are opening throughout the country. CNMs are opening their own practices. Employment opportunities for midwives continue to grow.

As a college graduate, you have a number of ways to pursue a career in midwifery. There are accelerated RN programs that provide a nursing degree in one to two years for those with a bachelor's degree. Registered nurses can apply to any of the midwifery programs in the United States. More than a third of the programs also accept applications from nonnurse college graduates. These programs incorporate the RN education into the CNM program. In 1994 the American College of Nurse-Midwives (ACNM) recognized the "direct entry" route into midwifery. There are now two educational programs in the United States—the State University of New York Downstate Medical Center in Brooklyn and Baystate Medical Center in Springfield, Mass.—that do not link a nursing degree to the midwifery degree. Graduates of these program take the same certification exam as CNMs and become certified midwives (CMs). Currently this certification is

accepted in only one state, but legislative efforts are underway to recognize CMs in several other states.

Midwives practice in a variety of settings. In 1998 there were
approximately 5,700 CNMs in clinical practice in the United States.
They attended nearly 280,000, or 9 percent, of the total births in the
country. The majority of CNM-attended births are in hospitals, with
fewer than 4 percent occurring in birth centers or at home. Most
CNMs practice in hospitals or clinics. Other sites include HMOs, private practices owned by physicians or CNMs, and birth centers. This
wide range of practice settings makes a career in midwifery very flexible. Some CNMs do only prenatal or gynecological care and work
regular hours without any time on-call. Some do clinic sessions as well
as births, but have regular hours as hospital or HMO employees.
CNMs working in private practices take call for their clients in addition
to their regularly scheduled office hours. Each work environment has
its strengths and drawbacks.

I have worked in the same private practice for twenty-one years
with one physician and one other CNM. Early in my career, I cared
primarily for women during their pregnancies and births. Slowly, as
those women gave birth and moved on to the next stage in their lives,
my days included more annual exams and pap smears, more birth control counseling and prescribing, and more treatment of minor infections. Nearly 40 percent of my office sessions now are occupied with
gynecology. Midwifery is a career that allows for this kind of expansion
of practice. Over the years, I have taken many continuing education
courses and expanded my practice to include more gynecology skills.
Working in a practice with a physician affords me this independence
because I have a collaborative relationship with a supportive physician
who is always readily available.

Small practices make sizable time demands because of the on-
call requirements. I have been on call for half of the past twenty-one
years. I have missed a number of family gatherings, movies, and holidays. In return, I have attended approximately two thousand births
and know the names of the majority of my clients, as well as the names
of their partners and children. I have cared for women from their first
gynecological exam through the birth of their children. Others I have
known from the birth of their children through menopause. Recently

there was a pregnant young woman in my practice whose own birth I had attended nineteen years ago. I cannot imagine a career more fulfilling.

Clearly, this type of time commitment is not for everyone. CNMs employed by hospitals or HMOs may not have the same personal relationships that I have had with clients, but they have more manageable schedules that provide them with more time for their families.

Midwives in midwife-owned practices or birth centers have more independence and are often providing care in a warmer and more homelike atmosphere but may be limited to caring for women who meet the strictest definition of "normal." Fortunately, there is a practice setting that can meet the needs of almost any midwife. Regardless of the employment setting, every midwife has the professional and personal satisfaction of having a positive impact on the lives of women.

ANGELA**DELISLE**

How I Became
a Physician Assistant

I
t was 1988, my junior year in high school. All my classmates seemed to know what they wanted to do with their lives, and a lot of them had already formalized their plans. Between cheerleading and studying advanced-placement biology, I hadn't given the rest of my life much thought. I was only sixteen—I could barely decide what to eat for breakfast!

Feeling pressured, I spoke with my guidance counselor ("There's a nice all-girls school in West Hartford you could go to"), to my parents ("We will support what you do as long as you are happy"), and to my friends ("Go to the best party school"). Ultimately, I combined the women's school with the support of my parents, in vague pursuit of some scientific endeavor.

Science interested me, but I wasn't sure just what venues were available. With the encouragement of my parents, I entered the traditional woman's route of nursing. The basic sciences kept my interest. I constantly wanted to learn the whys and hows of the human body. I was fascinated at how clever Mother Nature was at making things work.

Next came Nursing 101, 102, and so on, complete with accompanying clinical experiences. I got an A for effort, but I was constantly reminded by my superiors to look at things from a nursing perspective as opposed to a medical perspective. There is a distinct difference between the two approaches: those following the medical model diagnose and determine the treatment plan, while those who follow the nursing model understand and carry out that plan. As a nurse, I often inadvertently blurred the two models.

For the next two years, I grudgingly worked as a nurse, but I was hoping for professional satisfaction, and as a nurse I felt I wasn't playing the role that was meant for me. I valued the education that I received at that women's school, but I felt that I wasn't completely fulfilled in my profession. Looking back, I realize that I should not have been so quick to enter into the gender-accepted role and should have (despite my parents's advice) considered a direction in medicine. I soon became restless. I wanted to go back to school to advance my career, but I didn't know in what direction.

A logical choice would have been to become a nurse practitioner, but at that time I also learned about the possibility of becoming a physician assistant. And I was faced with a dilemma. I knew I wanted advancement, yet I was also in a relationship with someone, and marriage and children were not far down the road. I was still in a stereotypical mindset and felt that if I was accepted into medical school, what would follow would surely impinge on my being able to provide a good home for my then-nonexistent children and my still-not-yet-husband. I was tormented by my desire to go into medicine, but at the same time, I desperately wanted to be there for my family.

The program for becoming a nurse practitioner at the time was nonstructured and allowed for a highly individualized experience. It also permitted the student to focus on one area of interest and to develop highly specialized expertise in that one area. Good, I thought. But in the end I found that I would be doing my patients a disservice by being so highly specialized and not having a more rounded experience.

So I looked at the possibility of becoming a physician assistant (PA). There are many schools offering the program and most teach the basic curriculum taught in the medical model, diagnosis and treatment. Core requirements are universal: all programs include basic sciences and clinical rotations. The basic program lasts twenty-four to twenty-seven months, with degrees and certificates awarded upon completion (as opposed to four years of medical school, three to five years of residency, and three or more years of fellowship for physicians). In the PA program, I found something else important. There was an opportunity to train to assist in surgery. This opportunity is not generally available in nurse practitioner programs.

This was just what I was looking for, and I decided to practice medicine under the guidance of a physician; there would be no ambiguity about the level of my training, as most programs require core material. I could go into surgery or stay in medicine, and as a PA, I would be able to spend time with my anticipated family, because the position of a PA is generally more structured than that of a physician, allowing easier management of an "outside life."

I was accepted into the physician assistant program at Quinnipiac University the first year that I applied. I went through the rigors of classroom activities and clinical rotations, pouring myself into my studies and loving every challenging moment.

I was especially taken by the field of gastroenterology and sought a position in that area of medicine upon completion of my program. Unfortunately, though, there were no opportunities in that specialty. Undaunted, I considered the surgical side of gastroenterology: I would still have to understand the general disease processes and treatment, but the treatment would often involve a scalpel rather than a pill. To specialize in this area, I wanted additional training. I applied to a few postgraduate surgical residencies for physician assistants. I was accepted into the Yale University School of Medicine/Norwalk Hospital Postgraduate Surgical Residency for PAs. This was a one-year program, similar to that of a surgical intern. I would have monthlong rotations in various surgical subspecialties, learning to assist in surgery, take night call, respond to trauma call, and so on. It was a truly rewarding experience. It taught me how to prioritize, become confident in my knowledge, and sharpen my skills assisting in the OR.

Then came the real world. I had to find a job. While I was taking an elective rotation in cardiothoracic (CT) surgery and learning the basics of that specialty, a position became available. And so I progressed from being a student and became part of the team. The experience was memorable. I started my mornings by reviewing the cines— films of the cardiac catheterizations from the cardiologists—with the attending surgeon to get an idea of where the coronary lesions were. From that I would determine how much vein I anticipated needing for the revascularization procedure. During procedures, I would take the vein from the leg, prepare it by tying off its branches, and then close the leg before going "up top" to the chest to help with the grafts. Or I would assist in valve replacements, work in the step-down unit (where the patients go when they leave the intensive care unit), or work in the intensive care unit. I was trained to insert a chest tube, to insert a Swan-Ganz catheter and to interpret invasive heart monitoring, to insert an arterial line—in short, to do anything required.

After I had been in my CT position for about a year, one of the gastroenterologists in the area approached me with a job offer. Ultimately, my fondness for gastroenterology won out, and I was stolen away from the surgical arena. Since then I have completed a postgraduate fellowship in liver disease under the mentorship of one of the physicians in my practice. I have been here two years now, learning and practicing gastroenterology under the direction of some of the most accomplished physicians in the field.

It has been a long road, but I've loved every single step. I have benefited from every effort, including the initial steps in nursing, as all the steps helped me to my ultimate goal of practicing medicine in a capacity that allows for professional growth and family enjoyment. Oh, and remember that early relationship? We're married now. And the kids? Well, we still have time to think about that . . .

SANDRA**ALFANO**

The Art of the Apothecary

I can sum up in three words what has brought me to where I am today: introspection, opportunity, and knowledge. Alone, each offers some guidance to a productive life. Together, they point the way to a wonderful journey. Knowing oneself is an essential beginning, but mentors and leaders, as well as exposure to critical, creative thinking, also contribute to growth and development. So, the best advice? Get to know your strengths and weaknesses, your interest and talents, seek out leaders and even visionaries, surround yourself with the best, and you will learn from even the most difficult of situations.

My story in pharmacy begins at the age of sixteen, with my first job. Since then, I've come to believe that a first job can be a great molder of character, so I've always advised young people to choose a first job carefully. I was hired at the corner drugstore to sell cosmetics, cards, and candy. I wasn't much of a cosmetics and candy person, and people who know me will tell you that this still holds true today! Instead, I quickly became fascinated by the medicines in the back room. I was soon working side by side with the pharmacist-owner, Gus, who became my mentor and, later, close friend. He was highly respected in the community, and he instilled a sense of professionalism and integrity in his flock of students. I was one of a long line of high school students who worked there after school and on weekends and who later went on to become pharmacists. Gus would tell me that he kept up to date by spending time with students. Actually, he was quite knowledgeable, and always kept *us* on our toes. His methodology apparently worked—or maybe his steady involvement with professional associations, discussions with physician colleagues, and reading were the secret. But it was from his foundation that I observed firsthand the need for a commitment to lifelong learning in any health care profession.

Out of this experience, and motivated by my interest in the sciences, I chose to pursue a pharmacy degree. Finishing my bachelor of science degree in the late 1970s, I became intrigued by a movement called clinical pharmacy, designed to develop practitioners who are adept at functioning in a clinical environment and who provide pharmaceutical services that center on the patient. Heady stuff for a young, idealistic college graduate, and I charged ahead in pursuit of a graduate degree, the doctorate of pharmacy (Pharm.D.). That choice, at that time, brought me to work with the cream of the crop.

These pharmacists, leaders in this new specialty of clinical pharmacy, were striking off in new directions and developing novel practices that we still rely on. Examples of their ingenuity included developing formal drug information centers and serving as nutritional support consultants, pharmacokineticists, and ambulatory care providers. Following the shift to the consumer in the 1960s, pharmacy's focus also changed from product to patient. No longer was it enough to "count and pour, lick and stick." Now pharmacists were tailoring patient-specific doses based on kinetic values, counseling patients in proper use of their drugs, making rounds with medical teams, and contributing to positive therapeutic outcomes for these patients. This concept evolved during the 1990s into "pharmaceutical care," a movement that embodies a covenantal bond between the pharmacist and the patient, with the pharmacist committed to helping patients make the best use of their medications. Pharmacy was evolving, with a greater emphasis on care. The profession began to attract practitioners who were meticulous and detail oriented, critical thinkers who cared about patients, and who wanted to make a difference. This pharmacy model took the best from the medical and nursing models. The result was to focus the pharmacist on patient care and decrease the emphasis on the drug alone. Knowledge of ever-changing medical practice, good communication skills, and nurturing patient empathy became required skills.

My own training involved classroom instruction, clinical experience through a hospital residency, and completion of a research project and defense of a thesis. Yes, it's true when they say these are learning experiences—looking back, I can see just how valuable they were. I took call every fifth night and served as the main resource for a busy poison control center. I went on rounds with the medical residents and attending physicians. And I developed a research proposal in my area of interest, cardiology. I discussed the research with patients to get their consent, crunched the numbers, and defended my thesis, which examined the pharmacokinetics of a drug that regulated heartbeat and linked patients' blood levels to kidney function.

After graduate school I found that new positions in patient care were being developed at Yale–New Haven Hospital. These provided me a wonderful opportunity to develop as a practitioner in a challenging environment. I was originally assigned to practice in the cardiology units, the coronary care unit, and its step-down floor, where patients are treated after leaving the unit. Other pharmacists had similar roles in the medical and surgical intensive care units. Our mission was to promote rational drug therapy—selecting a drug on the bases of efficacy, safety, cost, and compliance. This became a recurring theme, and it captures the essence of what I've tried to accomplish in my various positions. I have especially espoused this theme in my long-standing dealings with medical, nursing, and pharmacy students.

In the past twenty years, I have had the pleasure of teaching in a number of settings, from formal classrooms where I taught pharmacology courses to undergraduate and graduate nursing students, to hospitals at which I counseled pharmacy residents and students on precepts of pharmaceutical care, to national professional meetings at which I made numerous presentations. I have endeavored to foster a rational approach to drug therapy in all of the health care professionals whom I've taught and mentored. It has been gratifying to run into practicing nurses and pharmacists who, years later, tell me that they learned critical thinking and problem-solving skills from my courses. Mentorship means a lot to me, and I value the opportunity to share my experience with new colleagues. Like my mentors, I have worked to foster critical thinking and intellectual curiosity in the students with whom I've spent time.

When choosing a career, you will often be encouraged to decide where you want to go and to understand how to get there. For a time, I was associate director of my department and spent a lot of time working on these planning skills as I counseled younger practitioners in their career development. I suggested that they develop a goal, then formulate a plan, and then achieve the desired results. As I've often told them, you will not achieve the results you intend unless you spend time thinking about your goals and your plans. This introspection should occur regularly and be an honest self-assessment of your strengths and weaknesses. Commitment to lifelong learning, including learning about oneself, has been an attribute that I have personally espoused over the past twenty years. I continue to work to foster this quality in all health care professionals I have the opportunity to influence.

I have also had roles as a wife and a mother, and I often juggle work, teaching responsibilities and child care. My husband has been a pillar of support, encouraging me to follow opportunities as they arose. This support was absolutely essential when I was pursuing positions with ever-increasing responsibilities. I grew up as a part of the generation that could "have it all": career, marriage, and family. But in all honesty, I don't think I ever quite figured it all out; I often felt like one or two of the three suffered.

My career took me into a midlevel management position when my children were still only eight and three years old. After several years of the stresses and rigors of this leadership position, an excerpt from Sylvia Ann Hewlett's *When the Bough Breaks* caught my eye. She writes that the qualities required for success in a career are long hours and one's best energy, mobility, a prime commitment to oneself, efficiency, a controlling attitude, a drive for high performance, orientation toward the future, and a goal-oriented, time-pressured approach to the task at hand. Yet she also writes that the qualities required to meet the needs of a child are time together as a family, energy for parenting, stability, selflessness and a commitment to others, a tolerance for chaos, an ability to let go, an acceptance of the moment, and an ability to tie the same pair of shoelaces twenty-nine times—with patience and humor!

For me, these lists are strikingly on target and reflect the sum of my experience. Anyone who hopes to combine a health care career with marriage and a family should reflect on these qualities—and on how often they are directly at odds! Balance is the key, and hard work trying to figure out that balance is necessary to do the best at all three priorities.

Currently, I am fortunate to be a member of the Institutional Review Board (IRB) at Yale, a committee charged with ensuring protections for human subjects of biomedical research. As the pharmacist member, I share with the committee my experiences with scientific design and investigational drugs. The committee is challenged to look at some of the science and all of the ethics involved with a wide array of research projects. We grapple with onerous government regulations and struggle with issues of risk, conflict, and consent. I always find the long discussions and struggles refreshing. The process of participating in these IRB discussions helps me clarify my own point of view. We have worked through many difficult issues, including research involving young children, research with individuals who are cognitively impaired, and even research intended to take place in other countries. Exposure to different viewpoints, and learning to understand this diversity, has helped me to articulate my own viewpoint and advocate the best interests of patients. This role once again flows from my experience in caring for patients and assisting with their medication needs.

I hope that my career reflects my personal motivation and burning passion for the profession of pharmacy in a collegial relationship with numerous other health care professionals. I encourage you to get to know yourself. And then seek out strong mentors with integrity, recognize and seize opportunities, and commit yourself to lifelong learning.

ANGELAR.HOLDER

A Lawyer in a Medical Environment

A lawyer who works within a hospital, medical school, or other medical environment has a bird's-eye view of the practice of medicine and a front-row seat at life's most important dramas. I wouldn't want to be anywhere else! After I had practiced law for fourteen years, primarily as a malpractice defense lawyer, I came to Yale Law School for an advanced degree in the Commonwealth Program in Law, Science and Medicine. This program helped midcareer practitioners of either law or medicine who wanted to teach in law schools or medical schools at a time when "the malpractice crisis" made many schools want to add faculty who knew something about the topic.

I went from there to open the in-house legal office at Yale–New Haven Hospital and Yale Medical School. That office (which now has three lawyers) deals with issues pertaining to the patient's relationships with health care professionals. The lawyers do everything from defending malpractice claims to helping draft living wills to getting court orders when parents refuse medical care for their sick children. It is the responsibility of in-house medical lawyers to know about the regulation of human subjects research, child abuse, access to medical records, informed consent, the right to refuse treatment—the whole range of legal issues in medicine. Each semester I also taught one course to law and medical students together, and I think Yale is the only school where this is done.

Since 1989 I have been a full-time member of the medical school faculty at Yale. I teach in and direct a required course for all first-year medical students on professional responsibility. In this course, we discuss legal, ethical, and economic issues affecting the physician-patient relationship. I continue to teach both law and medical students, and now I also teach a seminar in Yale College on bioethics and law.

In college, in law school and often in graduate school, one or two teachers teach an entire course. They make decisions about what the course will cover and what the reading will be; they also make up the exams and grade them. They are the people, if the class is small enough, who get to know you, the people you will most remember when you graduate from college. Medical school is quite different. Although an increasing number of courses are taught in small groups, with the same teacher or teachers every week, lecture courses during the first two years of medical school take a very different form. There is a course director, who may give one or two lectures and who organizes the course, but you may have a different lecturer each session. This means that there is less uniformity throughout the course than you may have had in college, but it also means that the person teaching you about the subject under discussion is an expert on it.

Lawyers who work for hospitals, other health care organizations, and physicians are involved in resolving claims that the care given by the doctor or at the hospital was so bad that it constitutes malpractice. To prove medical malpractice is not just to prove that somebody made a mistake. One must show that the person made a mistake because of insufficient knowledge, a lack of necessary manual dexterity or other physical skills, or (the usual claim) a lack of sufficient attention. The patient must prove to the jury that these failures would not have happened had the defendant doctor behaved as any appropriately qualified "reasonable physician" would have behaved under the same circumstances.

There are two reasons most people initiate malpractice claims, whether or not they are justified. The first is that the patient requires expensive care to recover from the accident (which may or may not have been somebody's "fault," but which unquestionably happened) and they have inadequate insurance or other resources to pay for it.

Thus they sue to force the physician or the hospital (and usually both) to pay for treatment of the injury. A young couple, for example, may sue if their newborn baby has such severe brain damage that they must pay an institution $100,000 a year to care for their child over a projected life expectancy of seventy-five years. The economic obligation exists regardless of whose fault the brain injury was, or whether it was nobody's fault. This explains the much lower incidence of malpractice suits in Great Britain and in Europe—where the national health insurance system pays for the rehabilitative care.

The second reason people sue for malpractice is that they are angry. They think that a mistake happened and that the physician and hospital personnel lied to them about it. None of the physicians and nurses seems to care about them and their extra stress and pain and worry. The role of the hospital lawyer is to try to eliminate the second problem as the cause of suits. When something goes wrong, the patient or the family is told the truth, immediate care for the problem is provided, and no bills are sent for the reparative therapy. Mistakes are inevitable, but a caring response can make a major difference in how the patient and the family perceive the situation. Aside from that, of course, there is the duty to be honest.

Hospital lawyers are also involved in such activities as teaching residents and attending physicians about patient's rights. Are there any limits to an adult patient's right to refuse treatment even if he or she will die without it? Do the parents of a horribly handicapped newborn have the right to let the baby die? Does a family have the right to insist that the pediatricians caring for their handicapped newborn provide treatment that the physicians believe to be futile and even harmful in causing pain to the baby? Does a family have the right to insist that a ninety-two-year-old woman with Alzheimer's disease have major surgery for cancer even though the anesthesiologist advises against operating on someone so frail? Hospital lawyers teach physicians and nurses about those issues and help in making those decisions, too.

Lawyers sit on institutional review boards (IRBs), the groups within research institutions that decide whether the rights and welfare of human subjects are adequately protected in research proposals. Should a new drug that will be prescribed for children be tested for safety on children, or is that using children as guinea pigs? Do parents have the right to consent to their child's being used as a research subject if the child will not receive any benefit from the research? Should a new drug thought to be of use in treating migraine headaches be tested against an inert substance called a placebo (since many people do respond favorably to placebos in tests of pain relievers), or should it be tested against the standard therapy available? Questions like these come up at each meeting of a busy IRB.

New technologies are first tried in research hospitals. When *in vitro* fertilization was first attempted, no one knew whether it would work—could an ovum and sperm meet in a petri dish, be implanted in a uterus and become a baby? If it could work, what was the risk that a child born after this procedure might have a major medical problem as the result of the way it was created? The only data available at first were from veterinary schools, which had been fertilizing prize cows *in vitro* with the sperm of prize bulls for years. None of the calves had problems related to the fertilization, but was that enough evidence to extend the same procedure to humans? Baby Louise Brown, now in her twenties, born in England, was the first "test tube baby." Fortunately the procedure was demonstrated to be safe, but how worrisome it was at first! How brave were the first human parents whose children were born after this procedure! All these scientific advances that so quickly become unremarkable also involve legal questions, and lawyers in the institutions where advances are first tried usually take part in their planning.

Not only are hospital lawyers interested in the theoretical issues of medicine, both in practice and in research, but they also enjoy being around physicians and nurses. The lawyers are there to help, whether there has been an accident to a patient or to explain the rules for research on human subjects to someone who may find a cure for a terrible disease. The work is immensely challenging because it requires not only knowing about law, but learning about science and medicine as well.

KATHLEENS.LUNDGREN

Applied Ethics in Medicine
Faith and Process

"**M**oral theories are useless unless they are developed in a way that eliminates and helps resolve real problems," says moral philosopher Baruch Brody. These words embody a principal tenet of my life as an ethicist—that is, moral and ethical theory must have practical application within real-life circumstances. So when the theory of ethics is applied to the situations and emerging issues in medicine—from caring for patients to cloning to end-of-life decisions—we are confronted with the increasingly relevant impact that the practice of ethics has on these most personal and crucial aspects of our lives.

We are increasingly interested in these ethical questions and their application to real life, both in the health professions and in the culture at large. In December 2001 I had an experience that suggested to me that you, the future generation of health professionals, are committed to expanding the application of ethics to the practice of medicine. At a master's tea at Yale's Berkeley College, several of us presented a panel entitled "Coming to Medicine?" We discussed the issues in this book and offered advice about the options and opportunities for students considering careers in medicine and the health professions. Eight or ten students approached me afterward to ask about topics I'd touched on—ethics, research, and education—and women asked about combining careers with family, still an important aspect of a professional life. If these young people are representative of their generation, clearly the issues in the twenty-first century will continue to center on ethics and its application to the medical dilemmas brought about by the increasingly more complex practice of health care.

My career development in bioethics has been, like me, a work in process, neither linear nor even obvious to me during the early years. In college, I majored in human development, with a minor in psychology. I did my field work in a program that paired college students with adolescents who had violated the law. I found myself giving girls in my care practical instruction in day-to-day living, time management, and goal setting, but not much of the counseling for which I'd begun training. There I first encountered the gap between theory and practice: the concrete problems of these girls' lives could not be addressed by the theory I had studied. So I began to think about the limits of theories. Something more was required—the circumstances of their lives had to be incorporated into my practice if I was to have any "just" understanding of their needs.

Shortly after college I married. As my husband and I started our careers and our family, each of my parents was diagnosed with cancer, and they began to need my help. With two young children and two very ill parents I ran headlong into the dilemmas of care and medical decision making. I thought a lot about the ways practical decisions are informed by values and principles, but at the time, I wasn't aware that a discipline existed for thinking about how practical end-of-life decisions can be informed by values and principles. Later, I would learn how to identify these questions and competing claims in terms of the balance of harms and benefits, autonomy, futility, and palliative care— and I would understand them as issues of bioethics.

The discipline of bioethics arose in response to shifts in medicine and in American culture during the 1960s and 1970s. The politics of those years, advances in medical technology and the diverse demand for its use, and the revelations and disclosures of research brought about a change in the physician-patient relationship. In response to these and other changes, medical ethics/bioethics was evolving theories drawn from philosophy, theology, and law that could be applied to the complex practical and moral decision making required in medicine.

Aware now of this shift, I wanted to translate my interests into this work and found bioethics (or, as it was called then, medical ethics) to be a natural fit for me. When my children were both in grammar school, I returned to school to begin work on a master of divinity degree at Yale. I was not interested in pursuing ordination, but I was drawn to the attention to spiritual aspects of life and to what I believe is our responsibility to join our Creator in trying to bring order out of chaos. Those influences, I knew, would contribute to the direction of my academic work.

I chose an interdisciplinary path and did coursework in philosophy, theology, social sciences, law, and medicine. I concentrated in ethics and history. That approach helped me to identify and evaluate tensions in medical decision making, and introduced me to a way of thinking about pain and suffering, including cultural and individual marginalization—the experience of living or, more often, merely existing at the edge of culture, whatever form that culture takes. Elaine Scarry's *The Body in Pain* and Dorothee Soelle's *Suffering* illuminated the important distinctions between pain and suffering. I became especially interested in Soelle's concept of "muteness": suffering so isolating, so extreme and so profound, as to render the sufferer incapable of speech. I thought about how to combine that concept with my work on identifying the emotional and social elements of life on the margin, in order to speak for those who could not. This study reconfirmed for me that understanding the concrete settings in which people live leads to understanding of the relevant issues in moral decision making.

With two professors who profoundly influenced me, I developed two reading courses. The first, "Institutionalization of Violence: Dehumanization in the Nazi Experiments" with Kathryn Tanner, focused on the history of research concerning human subjects; the second, with Margaret Farley, was on advanced medical ethics.

These courses, together with my previous work on understanding the social and historical experience of the marginalized, dovetailed with a clinical internship at the Connecticut Mental Health Center, where I worked on a research and treatment floor with patients who suffered from both substance abuse and psychiatric illness. My growing interest in the ethics of research crystallized in this setting. I became familiar with the ethical issues of research in psychiatry and with vulnerable people who have a diminished capacity to take "deliberate and free" action. In looking at how we recruit sick, substance-abusing, and other very vulnerable people into research studies, I began to think about the ethical concerns around the use of coercion, "pay," and continued drug use versus the subject's wish for abstinence: how much money should be offered for participation in research? Or, if a potential subject with a history of substance abuse wants enough money for a "fix," how much is too much "economic consideration" or "inducement" to offer for participation in research?

When the Special Olympics Games were held in New Haven in spring 1995, Margaret Farley and I formed a committee and arranged a symposium on ethical issues related to mental retardation, trauma, and (again) research with vulnerable populations. Through my coursework, my internship, and the symposium, I found that the work I was most interested in was the practical application of ethical and moral theory in research with human beings, especially in research with vulnerable populations.

As I graduated, my daughter was entering high school and my son was entering junior high. I focused again for a few years on my children. My husband is an attorney, and I was fortunate in a practical way that his support, both emotionally and financially, allowed me to have this flexibility and freedom, and later enabled me to do the work for the sake of the work. When I went back, I had a conversation with Merle Waxman, the ombudsperson at the Yale Medical School. She provided me with a great perspective on how I have chosen to live my life. Merle and I talked about the various paths of a professional life, and how there are periods when the professional and the personal do not fit in a life at the same time. Some people choose to interrupt their professional lives, as I did: children are born or their needs change, and parents (mostly mothers) choose to spend some period of time rearing and caring for their children. Some people interrupt their professional lives at major life events—for example, when an adult child must assist a parent in a "good death." And some people interrupt their professional lives simply because they want to or have to: Mount Everest beckons, and they must climb it while they are young enough.

Merle had a wonderful way of comparing these differing circumstances in the lives of developing professionals, and I pass it along to you. Many people, she says, climb ladders as they grow in their professional lives, others, like me, climb jungle gyms.

The goal is to make these circumstances work for you, and those around you, no matter what you climb. When I reentered professional life in graduate school, I found that the culture had changed since I had gone to college and the changes had given rise to a new profession for which I was ideally suited. I might have found my way to bioethics even if I had not interrupted my professional life, but I have been blessed by finding this work through those interruptions.

In climbing my jungle gym, I often find that I have to hold on to several different rungs at the same time—I write, edit, and serve on various committees. One of the most gratifying things I do is to serve as a member of the Human Investigation Committee (HIC), the institutional review board (IRB) at the Yale School of Medicine. The members of all IRBs are charged with evaluating the science, ethics, and federal regulatory compliance of research. Before any studies can begin, researchers must submit their protocols—that is, a description of their study—to the IRB. We discuss the protocol, and, using both ethical normative values (including religious, traditional, and cultural) and regulatory standards, we address issues within the research. Our approval requires evidence of sound science, compliance with government regulations, and adherence to the ethical principles of research—respect for persons, beneficence, and justice. To the extent that we, and other IRBs, are successful in careful evaluation of protocols, we achieve satisfaction of individual and societal needs by ensuring safe medical research.

Many other kinds of ethical analyses occur in medicine, and they are increasing in number and complexity. Education in ethics can enhance our ability to apply principles to real problems in addressing issues in medicine of social justice and amelioration—and prevention—of suffering.

When I began my education, the discipline of bioethics was in its formative years. By pursuing interests and values that were important to me, I grew with a discipline that will have increasing importance for years to come.

As you select courses and make career decisions, follow your interests, your intuitions, your inner direction. And be sure to take an ethics course or two. If you keep in mind the overarching themes in your life and make your decisions with those in mind, your choices will have cohesiveness. Whether you climb a ladder or climb a jungle gym, your professional and personal life will be solid and sound.

MICHAEL**ROWE**

Mental Health at the Margins of Society

I am a medical sociologist by training. This is not the same thing as being a medical social worker, who provides social services to patients and their family members in hospitals and other medical settings. Perhaps I can best explain what people like me do by telling you of my experience as the project director of a homeless outreach project for a public mental health center in New Haven, Connecticut, during the 1990s. The outreach project was one of eighteen in the country participating in research to test a relatively new approach called assertive mental health outreach. The approach is used with individuals who are homeless, have a mental illness, and are not receiving mental health care.

The difference between traditional, office-based mental health practice and assertive mental health outreach is dramatic. Assume that I am a homeless person with a mental illness. According to the traditional approach, I go to a public mental health clinic to seek help. After an interview with a psychiatrist, who determines that I am poor, have a severe mental illness, and thus belong to the clinic's target population, I meet with a clinician who talks with me about my problems and gives me a regular weekly appointment time. If I keep my appointments, the clinician treats my mental illness. Treatment may include my taking prescribed medications. The clinician is aware of my life circumstances and may make some efforts to help me with these, but my treatment focuses on decreasing the symptoms of my mental illness and keeping me stable while taking medications. If I start missing my appointments, the clinician calls me (if I have a phone) or writes to me (if I have an address) to remind me that I need to be in treatment. After a few futile attempts to reach me, the clinician discharges me as a "noncompliant patient."

Assertive mental health outreach to homeless persons turns traditional office-based practice on its head. It assumes that I will not come into the clinic, for any of several reasons. I may have had bad experiences with mental health treatment and treatment providers in the past. I may find the idea of going to the clinic and dealing with the building, the people, and the routines to be intimidating. I may not believe that I have a mental illness in the first place or may be opposed to giving out personal information to people I don't know. The exigencies of homeless life, such as getting to the soup kitchen at a certain time if I want to eat, or to the shelter at a certain time if I want to have a bed for the night, may not conform to the routines of mental health clinics. Outreach workers, knowing of my reluctance but convinced that I need help even if I refuse to ask for it, leave the office in teams and go out to look for people like me on the streets. They have a healthy respect for my strength as a survivor of homelessness. They accept the idea that I may not want the services they offer, at least not at first. They realize they must start small and with the basics, such as offering me a cup of coffee or a sandwich, buying me some warm clothing, or even helping me get into an emergency shelter, if I'm willing to trust them that far. They understand that they must take things slowly in order to build trust and must make a connection with me as a person, not a patient. They do not push mental health treatment on me at the outset, but they do hope eventually to persuade me to accept treatment. And finally, because it's likely that I need more than just mental health treatment, outreach workers offer me an array of additional services, including substance abuse treatment, medical care, access to housing and social support, and help in applying for a job or for disability income support.

In the 1990s there was an air of excitement among the staff of the emerging mental health outreach project in New Haven. As an administrator with experience running social service programs and as a sociologist experienced in studying them, I believed that the project's success would depend in part on its developing an organizational flu-idity and esprit de corps that are hard to achieve within large public bureaucracies. I was interested in how or whether innovative programs and approaches that draw a good deal of their identities from their newness can survive when they are located within traditional service organizations. I still think it was a good question, but I soon learned that the heart of the matter was the meetings that were beginning to take place on the streets between homeless persons and outreach workers. Over the next several years, I learned about homeless people and outreach workers by accompanying workers on their rounds, standing in soup kitchen lines, and visiting emergency shelters. I also interviewed homeless people and outreach workers and participated in the day-to-day work of running the project.

I was attracted to the potential of this work and the sense of moral urgency it carried. Outreach workers felt a special sense of per-sonal and collective mission about their work with those who were considered treatment failures. Moreover, the accompanying problems of these individuals—chronic homelessness, poverty, lack of social sup-port, and occasional serious physical health problems—made the res-cue and salvage operation of the outreach teams seem doubtful at best. The team was interdisciplinary and included an attending psychiatrist, social workers, case managers, public health nurses, and housing and vocational specialists. All staff members, even the psychiatrist, did some outreach work. They went out in teams of two or three and sought out people under highway bridges, in abandoned parking ga-rages, and on the New Haven Green, as well as in soup kitchens, drop-in centers, and emergency shelters. Key elements of success for workers were consistency, patience with repeated rejection, and the ability to develop a relationship with the core person, apart from his or her pa-thology, dirty clothes, or bad odor. Also essential was helping home-less persons tap available resources. In addition to assistance in ob-taining housing, those who were able to work got help with job placement, and those with disabilities were encouraged to apply for entitlements like Supplemental Security Income (SSI).

Work at the boundary calls for surrendering some of the institu-tional power that accompanies the traditional clinical encounter. In the early stages at least, workers must relinquish control over their potential clients' time and location, which they are accustomed and trained to control in office-based treatment settings. The ability to rethink and adapt one's own training applies to all disciplines, including the practice of medicine in the form of psychiatry. One psychiatrist who worked with the outreach project talked about his own learning process: "I look at homeless people with more respect now. Talking with and treating homeless people has reversed my understanding of psychiatric care. The usual approach is to medicate the person and then talk to him. In the work we are doing this has to be reversed. First talk to the patient. First try to engage the patient. First try to address his feelings and his personality, and after you do that, then you can possibly talk about medication."

Of course, sound professional judgment is at least as important to mental health practice at the margins of society as in a more traditional environment. Dori Laub, another psychiatrist with the New Haven project, has observed that unconditional patience with a reluctant client might make real contact impossible. He used the example of a meeting at an emergency shelter between a homeless woman named Andrea and an outreach worker named Jack. Andrea had rejected Jack's plea that she spend the night at the shelter rather than at an abandoned parking garage in the midst of winter temperatures that began to drop to zero. This was a life-threatening situation. After continued attempts to provide shelter, Jack simply but emphatically walked out. Andrea reconsidered the offer and changed her mind. Now she was ready to move into an apartment. Dr. Laub commented on the risk that Jack took by withdrawing his unconditional support for Andrea: "To say 'no,' to set limits, to refuse to participate in the ritual of offers that are perceived as rejections and repeated offers that improve the self-image of the generous giver may mean 'being real.' There is no engagement without risks."

The inherent tensions and contradictions of assertive mental health outreach represent part of its appeal for me. Homeless persons often weigh the outreach worker's offer of tangible services and help in finding their identity through housing against giving up the difficult but known life of homelessness. The prospect of crossing the border from homelessness into housing may arouse deep fears. For example, the social networks of homeless individuals may be thin by normal standards, but homeless persons do have contact with their peers. This may change dramatically when they move into their own apartments and experience a new form of social isolation, in which apartments and residential programs can be dead ends of routine and dependence.

Outreach workers are simultaneously client advocates and gate-keepers who operate under the aegis of institutional rules and pro-cesses. Street-level work forces outreach workers to look beyond cate-gorical or clinical perspectives to see the social environment in which people struggle. But bureaucratic demands, such as endless paperwork and categorical program criteria, assert themselves in outreach work as well. And outreach work has a contradiction at its core: while work-ers try to persuade individuals to accept their alternative form of help, they know that they must eventually get these individuals into more traditional office-based programs. Finally, although outreach workers hold up the ideal of a partnership with homeless persons, the two par-ties have unequal power. There are people who can dispense services and people who can accept them. Can the outreach worker make an offer that does not force the homeless person to accept the identity of a patient or client? Do outreach workers offer homeless people a ticket to the second-class citizenship of the barely housed in exchange for a loss of freedom?

As a medical sociologist, I have learned that essential questions underlie these encounters on the street and in emergency shelters: What efforts should we as a society make to help people at the margins? Where should the effort stop? What social obligation do we have to the disenfranchised to achieve what level of enfranchisement in ex-change for what mainstream responses of work, gratitude, and behav-ior? Beyond the interpersonal encounter and the individual outcome, these are questions that we ask when we send representatives to our social borders. The results of these encounters, on a large scale, are a measure of where we will set our social boundary and what standard of living we will accept for those who live at that boundary.

Despite its contradictions and dilemmas, assertive mental health outreach represents a hopeful new direction for mental health practice. While it is true that the idea of a partnership between worker and client belies differences in power, it still brings a shift from workers' orches-tration of services to clients' involvement in shaping their own destinies. And it's true that working with the whole person within his or her own environment may eventually hit a brick wall if the worker cannot deliver the resources of work or income or decent housing, as well as treatment, that are implied in this holistic ideal. Yet assertive mental health outreach can build a foundation for helping the individuals to make the best use of these resources when they are available. In a time when managed care and cost containment impinge on attempts to build new kinds of patient-provider relationships, assertive mental health outreach also harks back to an older form of medical practice in which doctors were able to see patients within their home environments. This new-old work may be critical for linking marginalized individuals to mainstream services and resources. For those who are disillusioned with the too-often impersonal practice of mental health and a reliance on medications as cures, this approach can be invigorating and enriching, allowing practitioners to exercise intellectual and empathic muscles they didn't know they had.

A final thought: In spite of what I've said about the contribution that mental health outreach can make, this work at the margins of society may seem too marginal within the practice of contemporary psychiatry to be of much interest to those who are contemplating a career in medicine. Yet marginal practices and practitioners can work their way, like the Trojan Horse, inside the fortress and become the new model for the next generation. Time will tell whether the kind of outreach I've described here will work its way back into the office-based clinics that workers had to leave to find those who weren't making their way through its doors.

EVIE**LINDEMANN**

Three Rules of the Road
A Social Worker's Lessons

P ersonal experiences and career choices are linked, normally by core values, life experiences, and education. I will tell you about the ones that shaped my decision to work in the health care field.

My personal philosophy evolved naturally. It was clear to me that if I trusted my basic instincts, the right decisions would follow. I decided, after graduation from college in California, to travel abroad. The image of a journey, both literal and figurative, best describes what influenced my career choice. My travel experiences allowed me to develop three "rules of the road" that have helped me to find balance, perspective, and inspiration.

Without a particular plan in mind, I began my journey in Europe. In Spain I met two Canadians who planned to work on a kibbutz in Israel. We had different itineraries, but we agreed to meet within two months at a kibbutz south of the Sea of Galilee, in the Jordan Valley. After my arrival there, I learned that my two friends, concerned by the proximity to the Jordanian border and the element of risk, had stayed only briefly at the kibbutz. Still, I decided to remain there. Bomb shelters were a regular part of life, and we routinely took refuge when the kibbutz was shelled from across the border. Being twenty-two, and still having some inflated sense of myself as being immortal, I did not feel frightened as much as curious: how did community members cope with living in a danger zone? Sometimes in the dining hall at breakfast, I would overhear someone telling about a kibbutznik who had gone out to tend the banana plants but died after stepping on a land mine. The kibbutz community described these incidents matter-of-factly, and took practical steps against such incidents; and they continued the daily tasks of growing eggplant, grapefruit, and bananas. They possessed an unusual combination of passion and detachment, which helped them to cohere as a community and to absorb the loss of a community member while still moving forward. The entire community supported the family that had experienced the loss, both emotionally and financially. This helped me to discover my first rule of the road: in the midst of seeming adversity, look for opportunities for growth. A solid sense of community can help with the healing of grief and loss. Seek community, rather than isolation, and learn to be a team player.

A few months later, I traveled overland by bus through Turkey and Iran and into Afghanistan. Because my travel companion became very ill, we were required to stay in the capital city of Kabul until he recovered some six months later. I was able to find a job as an artist and illustrator of children's stories with the Department of Education of Afghanistan. The government was attempting to develop new ways to teach children to read and hired me to travel with officials to various places in the region, drawing pictures of familiar sights and domestic scenes. The job allowed me to meet women who would otherwise be behind the veil, within the intimacy of their own homes. During these months, I also taught English at a private school, befriended by an Afghan family with boundless hospitality. This was how I learned my second rule of the road: no matter how different another person seems from you, be open and unjudgmental, and try to understand and share his or her worldview. Your life will be enriched by it. Allow others to give to you, and be willing to reciprocate.

Another lengthy bus ride along the perilous curves of the Khyber Pass took me through Pakistan and into India. I was exposed to Yoga, Indian music and dance, and the philosophies of Eastern mysticism. Through a series of contacts, I discovered the writings of an Indian mystic Meher Baba. He had written extensively while keeping silence for many years. He developed a community in the 1930s that was grounded in the spiritual principles of selfless service and compassion;

yet it also incorporated practical programs that improved education and agricultural management, as well as providing social work and health care to rural Indian villages. I vividly recall my first visit to the hub of this powerful philosophy in action. A bumpy red and beige state transport bus dropped me off at a dusty curve on a rural road. On one side was a reservoir; on the other side, I read a sign in Marathi: Meherazad Road. I later learned that this name signified "bountiful compassion." Both sides of the road were lined with well-developed shade trees, from which came the occasional sound of a birdsong. I followed the curves in the road for a while, until my footsteps led me to a simple compound, neatly maintained, with stucco buildings that included a meeting hall, a veranda for shelter from the brutal noonday sun, and a medical clinic. It was here that I met the people who inspired me, by their personal example, to return to the West to continue my education and find a career that would allow me to be not only skillful, but also heartful.

Later, when I returned to the United States, I went to graduate school and earned an advanced degree in psychology. I developed skills that permitted me to work with various populations that needed help. After six years of working as a psychotherapist with prison inmates, runaway teenagers, abused children, and families in crisis, I felt a need to return to India for additional learning.

Back in India, I interned in the medical clinic at Meherazad for six months. I studied enough of the local language to make myself understood some of the time. My mentor was a doctor whose gentle, supple hands were attached to one of the most compassionate human beings I had ever met. On one of my first days in the clinic, Dr. Goher warned me that I would be seeing medical conditions that might repulse me. The lack of access to health care, combined with poverty and inadequate education, made the people vulnerable to extreme physical pathologies. This internship confirmed my calling to be on the mental health side of health care, rather than in the physical treatment of disease. Although I could tolerate almost any kind of mental anguish expressed by a patient, I had more difficulty with the direct physical treatment, even though I had learned some basic skills for wound care and the giving of injections.

One day, Dr. Goher pointed out a woman in a pink sari who was in a long line of patients awaiting treatment. She outlined for me, in great detail, the context of this woman's illness: the death of her husband, cruel treatment by her in-laws, and extreme poverty. It struck me in that moment that I was witnessing a profound kind of medical treatment, one that attended not only to medical issues but also to the whole fabric of the patient's life. Dr. Goher described these conditions with a warmth, concern, and kindness that she later showed in treating the patient. The medical clinic also provided a uniquely integrative approach to patient care, offering Western medical practice as well as ayurvedic medicine, homeopathy, and acupuncture, all under one roof. No one seemed to be concerned about which approach was superior. The only concern was to find the best approach, or combination of approaches, for each patient. It was here that I learned my final rule of the road: Once you choose your path, follow it 100 percent. Be authentic, and find the part of you that wants to improve both the world and yourself.

After I returned to California, I accepted a hospital position that combined patient care ethics, social work, and human resources. I worked in the emergency room, dealing with traumatic incidents and sudden deaths, and helping families absorb the news that a beloved family member had died. I studied medical ethics and forged an effective alliance with physicians, nurses, administrators, and chaplains. I learned that advances in medical technology do not entitle health care professionals to treat patients without compassion. I found that an integrated team that uses the finest skills of each participant best addresses the most serious problems.

I moved to New Haven a few months ago, after my marriage to a faculty member at Yale. Although leaving my family, friends, and interesting work in California was personally challenging, I am continuing to master my three rules of the road. I currently work at the Yale School of Nursing with Margaret Grey, a diabetes researcher. Using my psychological skills, I help to organize groups for adolescents with diabetes and for parents of school-age children with diabetes. By learning coping skills, these teens and parents can more effectively communicate and solve problems. The beauty of this approach lies in offering learnable skills and emotional support, two of the cornerstones of self-empowerment in adapting to a serious medical condition. One of my finest moments this year came when a shy thirteen-year-old in my group announced at our final meeting that she has a summer job as a teacher's aide. She had pursued some leads at her inner-city school and followed up with the proper paperwork; now she has an opportunity to continue her own journey of learning and self-care.

If you feel drawn to medicine, there are many different ways to be involved. I wish you success in your career choice. Remember that life is a journey, and it is not always a direct path that takes you where you need to go. Develop your own rules of the road by searching for the core values that inspire you, and you will surely find your way.

GAIL**KORRICK**

My Life in Medical Social Work

When I was asked to write on the role of the clinical social worker and how it relates to the medical profession, I had to sit back and think about the past forty years.

I first thought of becoming a social worker when I was an adolescent living in Boston. During the 1950s the city funded facilities, called settlement houses, where neighborhood children would go to play, do activities, and socialize with other children. The settlement houses of those years are the community centers of today. At our settlement house, I came in contact with a social worker who gave me a wonderful feeling because she was very caring and tried to meet all the needs of the children, both emotionally and socially.

My desire to be a social worker grew all through high school and into college. In graduate school I was exposed to the different settings for social work, and I decided that I wanted to work in a hospital, where I would have contact with people who had many problems complicated by their illnesses. I thought I could be most helpful in those circumstances.

Then, as now, to be a social worker, one must receive a master's degree from an accredited program in social work. The training requires two years of study consisting of specialized courses in the fields of human behavior, psychology, and problem solving. During those two years of graduate study, one must also complete two years of supervised clinical internships.

And even after the coursework and the internship, the would-be social worker's "apprenticeship" continues. In most states, social workers must be certified or licensed to practice in their field. To accomplish this, they must serve under the supervision of a licensed social worker in a public or private agency, a hospital, a substance abuse center, or a school for another two years before being eligible to take the appropriate examination.

A clinical social worker often is asked to help solve a patient's emotional problems. When the emotional problems create or worsen medical conditions, the social worker can help the physician treat the patient. The clinical social worker becomes an integral part of the treatment experience, working with the physician in dealing with the medical problems and their emotional effects on the patient.

I have found through my many years of experience that no two persons will react emotionally the same way to a physical event, not even to the same illness. One must realize what a threat a physical illness can be to an individual, and the many ways in which it represents a loss of control. This perceived or actual loss of control may affect a patient's whole manner of living. One of the most important tasks that faces a social worker is to understand the patient and the disease—in particular, what the experience of illness means to that person and to his or her ability to cope. In our busy medical world, physicians, even if they recognize nonphysical problems, often feel helpless to do more than offer sympathy or advice. They just don't have the time. The clinical social worker can take the time and provide the expertise to help the patient deal with these problems without impinging on the patient-physician relationship.

When I came to Yale–New Haven Hospital in 1963, three years after earning my master's in social work, I wanted to do more than get patients placed in nursing homes or help them obtain financial aid. I felt that as a clinical social worker, I could assist a physician in the evaluation and treatment of the patient as well. I approached the chief of the gastroenterology department about the use of a clinical social worker in his treatment of patients with gastrointestinal diseases. I intended to convince him that the social worker could be valuable in treating these patients. The physician was somewhat skeptical, but I encouraged him to see how social and emotional factors could affect treatment. Soon I became an integral part of the medical team in gastroenterology.

My role as a social worker with the gastroenterology service evolved because I saw an opportunity to be an advocate for the patient to the physician. In this way, I helped the physician to better understand the patient. Patients often felt more comfortable talking to me because I wasn't threatening. They would tell me how they felt and whether they were adhering to the medical recommendations. Many times patients answered physicians' questions as they thought they were expected to answer, not necessarily the way they were really feeling. So I acted as the liaison between the patients and the physicians to convey patients' concerns and fears, and to express how they were dealing with their illnesses. I made it easier for the physician to care for the patient as a whole.

My work as a social worker helped the physician more clearly understand the "what and who" behind the complaints of the patient. I always paid close attention to such identifying information about the patient as age, marital status, educational background, and occupational level. This information might give clues to some factor that had triggered the symptoms. A good clinical social worker is interested in the patient as a person and willing to listen to the person's problems— sometimes that in itself is therapeutic. To achieve that kind of therapy, the clinical social worker tries to determine what precipitates stress in the patient's life. Because people usually cope with illness and disability in the same way they coped with earlier stressful situations, the social worker's interview often provides information for dealing with current illness. For many patients and families, it is a unique experience to talk to someone who listens with a nonjudgmental understanding. Many people readily respond once they are convinced of the social worker's sensitive understanding—once they know that the questions are designed to help the physician deal with their symptoms more appropriately and effectively. The confidential nature of the relationship is conducive to the patient's talking about problems related to his or her illness and concerns.

Since leaving Yale–New Haven Hospital, I continue to use these skills in my practice when I evaluate the precipitating factors that bring an individual in for counseling. In my office I see people who have been referred by physicians, school social workers, and employee assistance programs, as well as some who are self-referred. I listen to the issues and try to help the individual resolve the issues through problem-solving techniques and psychotherapy. Some of the treatments are geared to improving self-esteem. Improved self-esteem promotes changes in behavior, which can then further improve self-esteem. A clearer understanding of what's causing the conflicts and how to develop coping skills to deal with the issues can set this positive cycle in motion. I may see people with anxiety, depression, or problems related to various sources of stress, like family issues, divorce, aging parents, and work- and school-related struggles. In my work, I try to help people feel that they are not alone in resolving the issues that have interfered with their ability to function in their lives.

The role of the clinical social worker has changed markedly over the past forty years. Some of the changes have been positive, but some have driven the field backward, restricting the role of the social worker. With the advent of managed care, the fields of psychiatry, psychology, and social work have been restricted in deciding how many times someone should be seen for treatment. A team of psychiatric nurses, social workers, and marriage and family therapists are employed by the managed care company contracted by an insurance company to oversee the mental health treatment components of an insurance plan. These gatekeepers review the clinical information about a patient and inform the treating therapist whether an individual's problems warrant further treatment. If further treatment is indicated according to their standards, they also specify what the frequency and length of the treatment should be. Because of the restrictions imposed by the insurance companies—restrictions I feel are based on economic considerations, rather than medical or mental health considerations—the patients are being shortchanged in their mental health treatment.

Because of the economic crisis and the resultant change in delivery of mental health services, paraprofessionals have been employed to meet the patients' needs. Paraprofessionals play a vital role in helping a vast mental health population receive the services it needs In many pediatricians' offices today, for example, the clinical social worker participates in the daily care of the patient, provides valuable insight into the child's family life and factors that may be contributing to the child's problems, and then suggests ways to improve that life.

The clinical social worker can also help a school or day-care facility investigate a child's behavior for possible clinical problems. Social workers will always be an integral part of the child's care in these settings because the pediatrician must be involved with the whole family and not just with an illness.

Medicine cannot be practiced alone. All of the paraprofessionals play an integral and additional part in the delivery of good health care. I continue to look for ways to be an advocate, to be a liaison, to be a team member. As I care for individuals who are dealing with medical problems, I use my skills to reduce the impact of those problems on these individuals' ability to function socially and emotionally. And I look back and feel how much I was able to add to the treatment of patients with gastrointestinal disease because of the training and experience I had as a clinical social worker.

SUSANS.ADDISS

A Career in Public Health

Have you ever thought that you might like to work to promote the health of an entire community, rather than that of a series of individuals? Do you ever find yourself thinking about health problems that affect whole populations or particular neighborhoods? Are you more interested in the prevention of disease than in its treatment? Are you a team person, one who likes to collaborate with others? Do you consider yourself an educator? Do your values center on social justice and equity?

If so, then you might want to investigate a career in public health. It involves all the characteristics cited above, and many more. Back in the 1960s, I found myself thinking and talking about these issues. A friend and neighbor, Dr. Bill Kissick, suggested that I pursue a career in public health when I was ready. (I had two small children at the time.) Before too long, I was able to follow his suggestion, and he helped me get into the Yale School of Public Health in 1966. I needed all the help I could get, as I had majored in music as an undergraduate at Smith and had been out of college for fifteen years. I persuaded the school officials to let me take three years, instead of the usual two, to obtain a master's degree in public health. This permitted me to pursue a second master's degree in urban studies at the Yale School of Art and Architecture.

Three years later, with two master's degrees almost in hand, I began to look for my first job in public health. The director of health at the New Haven Health Department was looking for a health educator, the track I had chosen for my M.P.H. With a recommendation from my faculty advisor, I was hired. It was an ideal way to begin my career, because, as health educator, I also served as an informal deputy director and represented the department on some of the many committees and boards that the director was supposed to attend. I also had to deal with all the divisions of the department, so I learned quite quickly how a local health department was organized and how it functioned in the community.

My first assignment from the director was to apply to the city for a grant to screen children for lead poisoning. This turned out to be a wonderful introduction to public health work. In the process of applying for the grant, I learned about the problem of lead poisoning, developed a plan to address the problem, identified the people who would carry out that plan and the resources to implement it, and developed an evaluation process to tell us whether we had been successful. This was a process I was to repeat in many different ways for many different health problems over the next twenty-five years.

In 1972, with two children approaching their teen years, I began to feel constrained by one of the drawbacks of public sector service—a salary considerably lower than that for a comparable position in the private sector. At about this time, a professor from the School of Public Health, John Thompson, told me that a new position had just come open in the Lower Naugatuck Valley, where four towns had decided to form a public health district. They needed a full-time health director who would establish and manage a health department. This meant that I would recruit all the staff, set up inspection and permit programs, handle communicable disease reports, develop a community health education function, and, in general, conduct the public health affairs of the district's four towns. To encourage Connecticut communities to provide full-time public health services for their residents, the state legislature had established a subsidy of one dollar per capita to towns that earmarked at least that much for public health in their local budgets. There had not been many takers, in part because state statutes still required that local health directors be physicians, and most physicians considered the salaries that communities could pay from a budget of two dollars per capita to be inadequate. Acknowledging this, the legislature had removed the physician requirement and permitted people with public health degrees to be directors. One year later, the Lower Naugatuck Valley Health District was formed.

At that time, the Valley towns were blue-collar manufacturing communities with patriarchal cultures from Europe—not the sort of folks, I figured, who would choose a woman who was not even a physician to head their new health department. But I applied for the position, and, to my surprise, I was hired.

The next four years were challenging and rewarding. Building a health department from scratch is a rare opportunity, and I was aware of how lucky I was to be such a pioneer. I hired a secretary, enlisted the part-time sanitary inspectors who were already working in the four towns, recruited a director of environmental health from the state Department of Health, and together we made a health department.

The very first complaint we got on the first day was about a serious drainage problem in Ansonia. The affected homeowner had been calling City Hall about it for more than a year, with no effective response. We took on the problem. It took two years to resolve and involved two state agencies, the mayor's office, and two Ansonia agencies—immediate proof that these communities needed a full-time health department!

Four years later, in 1976, the department was running more or less smoothly, staffed as fully as our meager budget would allow; the four towns we served had become accustomed to us. Some of their citizens were even grateful that they now had a place to call when a public health problem arose. Some friends involved with the new nationwide health planning system approached me about seeking the position of director of health planning in Connecticut's Department of Health. At first I was reluctant, but my friends convinced me that this was a new challenge worthy of exploring, and I sent in an application. After several months, Governor Ella Grasso interviewed me, and I was appointed chief of the Bureau of Health Planning and Resource Allocation. For the second time in my career, I had the rare opportunity to create something that had not previously existed.

The bureau was structured to include the Division of Vital Statistics (births, marriages, deaths, and adoptions), the Tumor Registry (the oldest cancer registry in the world), and data processing. A Division of Health Planning was created, staffers were hired, and we set about developing a state health plan as required by the federal government, which funded health planning systems across the country. Connecticut was divided into five regions, each served by a health systems agency (HSA). Each HSA developed its own health systems plan, and the bureau then consolidated these plans into a single state health plan. The process required heavy collaboration among the agencies, mediation of disputes, and a steep learning curve, facilitated by federally sponsored regional workshops.

Unfortunately, our ascent of this learning curve was not deemed swift enough by Congress, which discontinued the entire program in the early 1980s on the grounds that it had not saved enough money for the health care system. Never mind that citizens had been educated about the ins and outs of health care and had been brought to the table where decisions were being made about the future directions of health care. The bottom line reigned, as it seems to now, and health planning virtually disappeared. There was a renaissance of sorts in the 1990s as communities became involved in assessing their health needs and charting directions for their futures.

In the midst of this slow demise of health planning, I served in 1984 as president of the American Public Health Association (APHA). In my news columns and presentations I focused on two issues: antitobacco efforts and the slow disappearance of federal data programs under the Reagan regime. Many of us thought that these programs were being abolished or attenuated so that the administration wouldn't have to "kill the messengers" who brought bad news about the effects of the cuts being made in health and social programs. No data, no bad news for the messengers to bear.

The APHA position involved quite a lot of out-of-state travel, so I wasn't really able to deal with the deteriorating health-planning situation again until 1985. Then I decided to accept an invitation to return to the local level as director of the Quinnipiack Valley Health District. I served for six years, presiding over programs like the ones in the district I had built in the Lower Naugatuck Valley and adding an AIDS curriculum guide for the schools, a cholesterol screening program, and an exercise program for the elderly. We were able to expand the staff because the state subsidy had increased. In a lucky coincidence, the director of environmental health I inherited was the same person I had hired for the Lower Naugatuck Valley Health District—a person with whom I worked well and whom I respected greatly.

In 1990 former Senator Lowell P. Weicker was elected governor of Connecticut. The statutes had been changed to allow a nonphysician with public health training to be commissioner, and I had for some time wanted to be the first woman state health commissioner, so, recognizing it as a very long shot, I went after the job. After months of interviews, letters, phone calls from supporters, and, finally, a big plug from my mentor Bill Kissick, I was offered the position, which I accepted with alacrity. This was the only position that I had ever actively and intensely campaigned for. In fact, when Governor Weicker was later asked how he had chosen his cabinet, he said of me that I had pestered him until he gave in.

During the next four years, the Department of Health met many challenges with varying degrees of success. Because the governor strongly supported both community health centers and school-based health centers (SBHCs), we received funds for dramatic expansion in both these areas. For example, the number of SBHCs increased from eight to forty-five in four years. For me, ten- to fourteen-hour days were the norm, political and media pressures were extreme, overall stress was always high, and dealing with the state bureaucracy was like slogging through a mud pit. Nevertheless, those four years were intensely rewarding, and it was a privilege to work for Governor Weicker, a man of complete integrity who seemed to believe that being governor really meant taking responsibility for running the state in the best possible manner.

When the governor decided not to run for a second term, all the commissioners knew that the future of their jobs was uncertain. For me, this wasn't much of a problem, for I had accumulated enough years in local and state pension plans to retire. The new governor, John Rowland, did indeed remove almost all of us within a few weeks after his inauguration. I retired from state service and became a public health consultant for a few years. Then I retired completely, and now serve as a volunteer for a number of health-related causes and organizations. How nice to be able to choose what you want to do, instead of having to confront whatever problems present themselves!

But I would maintain that I am really still practicing public health. Our mother science is epidemiology, our workforce is multidisciplinary, the problems we address are multifaceted, and we work for the good of the community. In 1988 the Institute of Medicine defined the functions of public health as "assessment, policy development, and assurance." This has been the framework for all my professional and volunteer activities. And within this framework, I have had a most challenging, rewarding, and productive career.

You might, too. Public health professionals practice in many and varied settings. Besides local, county, and state health departments, there are community health centers, school-based health centers, the federal Centers for Disease Control and Prevention (CDC) and other federal agencies, insurance companies, managed care plans, health policy think tanks, and academia, just for starters. For those with joint degrees in law, medicine, nursing, or social work the practice opportunities are even greater. The current public health work force in the United States is about 500,000, a number deemed insufficient by those who worry about the infrastructure of public health. So there's lots of room in the field, and a definite need.

NORA**GROCE**

Coming to Medicine
Through Anthropology

Wh"hen I was asked to write a brief account of how I found my way to a career in medicine, I realized that I could respond in two ways. I could describe in general terms how I now come to find myself doing work far different from my initial expectations. Or I could describe specifically how one starts off in anthropology and finds oneself involved at midcareer with health care practitioners and health policy makers.

What seems like a coherent career path is, in fact, the result of a series of choices, chance encounters, and unintended leads that seem only in retrospect to fall together. I will recount it here briefly, because I think it might be encouraging to others to know that one can sometimes benefit, even when plans go strangely awry. I suppose if there are lessons to share with younger professionals, they are these: first, while unanticipated opportunities may arise, having a solid foundation—being broadly educated and perhaps a bit curious—is a prerequisite for much that can follow; and second, look beyond your own discipline and ask the basic question, What contribution can this research make to broader questions and to the needs of a population?

I was always interested in anthropology, but it would be misleading to say that I always wanted to be an anthropologist. As a child, I read anything I could find on history, other cultures, evolution, and archaeology, and I thought wistfully about being an archaeologist in some distant land. I had no idea that one field of study could encompass all these stray interests, and anyway, by the time I was in my midteens I had long since given up my dreams of archaeology. I had plans, instead, for a career in classical music. I was a third-rate oboe player, but because oboe players are rare, I found myself in fairly august circles at an early age—I studied at Interlochen in Michigan and finished up high school dividing my time between my local school and the Juilliard School of Music in New York.

My parents encouraged my interest in classical music but worried about my ability to support myself as an adult with only a conservatory training and so I applied to college. (Cleverly, I ultimately earned a Ph.D. in one of the few fields that usually has less job security than classical music). I entered the University of Michigan in 1970 as a music major, but on the first day of that winter semester, my roommate walked into our room with a stack of books for her class, Introduction to Anthropology. I was amazed. Not only did these books cover everything I'd always found to be interesting, but it turned out there was a field that included all those childhood interests. One could actually do this for a living.

By the following semester, I had become an anthropology major, specializing in archaeology, still far from medicine. I worked at a number of archaeological sites during college and following graduation. I was, for a time, a "dig bum," going from site to site, eventually finding myself in the highlands of rural Oaxaca, Mexico, working on an archaeological site that overlooked a small Indian village. The village had only twenty or thirty houses, but it had a small church and graveyard. Frequently, from that hillside dig, I could see a small group walking slowly to the church, carrying a tiny coffin: the child morality rate in the region was high. While living in Oaxaca, I came to be more interested in talking to living villagers than in digging up the remains of their ancestors, and I wondered how I might best help the living with the knowledge and skills I had.

At the time, the field of anthropology was still largely academic and theoretical. What has come to be called applied anthropology—using information and insights gained by researchers in the field to effectively change policy for populations—was just emerging. The field of medical anthropology, in which both theoretical and applied aspects of health care and beliefs would be studied, was in its infancy, and I knew little about it. I was aware that anthropologists had begun to work in such fields as international development policy, but these experts were also still few and far between. Today, of course, many anthropologists work in all these subdisciplines.

Following my stint as a dig bum, I returned to the United States and began a doctoral program in anthropology at Brown. I still wanted to be an anthropologist, but I was also eager to make a difference with the knowledge I had. I concentrated in cultural anthropology, with a minor in folklore and oral history. This combination ultimately led me to medical anthropology. During my first year in graduate school, my new boyfriend, Larry Kaplan, invited me along on a day trip he was making to Martha's Vineyard, a small island off the coast of Massachusetts. He was going there to speak to an elderly islander, Gale Huntington. Larry thought I'd enjoy meeting Gale because of my interest in oral history and Gale's knowledge of the island's history. Gale turned out to be both island historian and island fiddle player. He and his wife, Mildred, took a liking to Larry and me, and we to them, and we returned to the island a number of times to visit. It was during the course of one of these visits that my dissertation topic appeared, quite by accident.

Gale's idea of a good time was to get his guests in a car and to travel around the island at speeds never exceeding twenty miles per hour, while pointing out spots of local interest. I loved it, and in the course of one of these jaunts "up-island" Gale mentioned that a number of deaf people used to live in this area. I knew nothing about deafness or about disability, but I vaguely remembered from an undergraduate course in evolution the idea of "founders effect," the increasing occurrence over several generations of a genetic anomaly in a small population with high rates of intermarriage. I recall thinking, "This might make a good five- or ten-page paper for a graduate class." Four years later, it had mushroomed into a doctoral dissertation. I had stumbled across a community which, for three hundred years, had had an unusually high rate of hereditary deafness. Hereditary deafness in small, inbred communities was not unusual even then—there were already almost one hundred such documented communities in the genetics literature. What was unusual was that I was an anthropologist, not a geneticist, so the questions I asked, over and above the obvious lines of descent, had not been widely asked before.

The questions were basic to anthropology, almost embarrassingly so: How did you communicate? What did people think about the deafness? How did those who were deaf fare in the wider community? The last deaf person had died in 1952, so I resorted to oral history to get the answers; over the course of about a year, I interviewed everyone I could find on the island who was more than seventy years old and who remembered the community's deaf citizens.

The answers I heard from these people were unanticipated. I was able to trace the deafness back to a small community in England and to a boatload of settlers in the 1640s. The islanders' adaptation to deafness was also unanticipated: many of the hearing people had adapted to the high incidence of deafness in the community by becoming bilingual in English and the local sign language. (This would be comparable to the benefit of speaking Spanish if one lived on the Mexican border today). Because of hearing islanders' ability to understand sign language, there were no barriers to those who were deaf, and they participated in all aspects of society. Using Vineyard Sign Language seemed like the only logical choice to the pragmatic old-time Yankees whom I interviewed, but it was a markedly different reaction to a disability than had been recorded in the literature up to that time. The research I was doing was not straight anthropology, nor even what was then found in medical anthropology. Nor was it straight genetics, history, or biology. The study I was doing could best be described as an oral history of a genetic disorder. Indeed, my professors at Brown did not really know what to make of my research; while encouraging me, they left me largely alone to sort it out for myself.

Like all graduate students, I hoped my research would have some significance to a body of scholars, but I feared that my work would make little real difference. Making that difference had been important to me as a scholar ever since my time in Mexico. I suppose that is why it came as such a shock when I published the first paper on my research, a short piece in *Natural History*. I got hundreds of letters and cards in response and even more responses to the book that I published with the full study. It seemed that while I was working away on the island, a new social movement, the disability rights movement, had gained momentum, and research such as mine, outside of formal clinical studies and structured settings like schools and medical institutions, was rare. I was pleased to find my research used by those who were trying to rethink and rewrite current national and international policy on disability from a human rights—not a medical—perspective, and I became involved with many of the people and groups who were part of this emerging movement and the accompanying new field of disability studies.

The rest of my history is fairly straightforward—on the basis of my work on disability, I was asked to do a postdoctoral fellowship at Harvard's Boston Children's Hospital. There I did research on domestic violence toward children and adults with disability, and I worked on issues of health care and delivery of services to ethnic and minority communities. I began working increasingly on disability issues and in international health development, consulting regularly with international agencies, groups within the United Nations system like UNICEF, the World Health Organization, and a number of organizations concerned with disability. This work helped bring me in 1993 to the Yale School of Public Health, where I continue my work on disability and have expanded my work with ethnic and minority health and with health in international development. Today I serve in a variety of roles: I teach students of public health and medicine about international health and development, cross-cultural aspects of health, and qualitative research; I consult on issues of international health; and I do a good deal of research related to international health issues.

In retrospect, my career path does seem to make some sense. Training as a social scientist allows one not only to ask specific questions about health beliefs and practices, but gives one—or should give one—the broader ability to look at issues of health beliefs, health practices, and health care systems in the context of family and community. Deep understanding of such systems goes further. Individual health and community health can themselves only be fully understood in the context of the social, political, and human rights frameworks within which they exist. If the leading cause today of global ill health is poverty and a lack of access to adequate care and to resources such as food and clean water, then approaching health issues from a social science perspective has validity.

There are numerous possibilities for doing significant work today as we learn to combine medicine and social science. This is so, in part, because fields like anthropology have come to accept applied knowledge and theory. Many in the clinical sciences also are more aware than ever that understanding sickness, health, and well-being has non-clinical components that must be understood and addressed. Combining questions from both disciplines often yields unanticipated but important results.

So in thinking about careers, I return to the advice I gave at the outset: be broadly educated, learn lots of things beyond the confines of your specific discipline, and always ask the very basic question: What difference does this research make and how does it contribute to our knowledge about the human condition? You may not always get the answers you seek, but the attempt is usually worth the effort.

D.GEORGE JOSEPH

Lessons from the History
of Medicine

P erhaps more than any other professionals, those in medicine care about its history. Ask an accountant or an engineer or a lawyer what they know about the history of their field, and you are unlikely to receive the kind of answer that you would from a physician. Medicine is a discipline immersed in its history. Most physicians have recited some variation of the Hippocratic Oath (originating in fifth-century BCE Greece), dissected a cadaver in anatomy class (a practice dating to Erasistratus in third-century BCE Alexandria), and donned the white doctor's coat (first worn by French surgeons in the late eighteenth century). Some of these physicians might be able to tell you that Hippocrates, a Greek healer, is considered the "Father of Medicine" or that the symbol of medicine—a staff entwined by a snake—originated with a school that followed the Greek healer-god Aesculapius. All physicians can tell you that the field of medicine includes thousands of diseases, anatomical structures, and conditions named for the physicians—Alzheimer, Graves, Pick, Wernicke, Parkinson, Hodgkin, Broca, and so on—who discovered or described them. A recently published dictionary of medical eponyms has nearly 15,000 entries. Others might know something about renowned physicians and surgeons such as Robert Koch, William Osler, or Harvey Cushing, even if they have encountered the names only by way of Koch's postulates, Osler-Weber-Rendu Disease, or Cushing's Syndrome. And in the form of oral history, most physicians have personal stories of influential teachers and mentors, illuminating patient encounters, perplexing diagnoses, or difficult surgeries.

But to suggest that the history of medicine and healing is merely a catalog of dates, names, and discoveries diminishes the important role that a basic knowledge of medical history can have for practicing physicians and for medical students. Physician and historian Owsei Temkin once wrote that "the history of medicine comprises all that is historical in medicine, as well as all that is medical in history" (from John Blake, *Education in the History of Medicine*, 1968, p. 55). As you begin your medical training, you should take advantage of the formal opportunities to explore the history of medicine that many of you will have. Some medical schools have required or elective courses in the history of medicine; other schools and hospitals have extracurricular societies or lecture series focusing on medical history. At some schools, the history of medicine will be bundled into a course on the medical humanities or social medicine, and will include explorations not only into medicine's history, but perhaps also into ethics, art, literature, sociology, economics, and public policy. One of the leading American departments of medical humanities described its curricular objectives this way: "To become sensitive to and to review some central moral, philosophical, and social issues in medicine and health policy; to reflect on physicians' traditions and responsibilities in developing and implementing health care delivery; to develop critical skills for evaluating the moral and philosophical claims, arguments, and goals frequently found in medicine; to formulate, present, and defend a particular position on a moral issue in health care; to reflect on the relationships between moral, professional, and legal obligations of physicians" (*www.ecu.edu/medhum/curriculum/Curriculum.htm*; Department of Medical Humanities, Brody School of Medicine, East Carolina University).

A life in medicine will not always leave much time and energy for nonmedical pursuits. Medical students are occupied with absorbing and mastering voluminous amounts of medical information and being introduced to patient care; interns and residents spend most of their time on hospital wards caring for patients; young physicians work to balance the demands of their patients, their career, and their family life. During all this, studying history or literature or art will not seem very practical to one's professional life, and will seem very far removed from one's immediate priorities. As students work to learn anatomy, pathology, physiology, microbiology, and the other basic medical sciences, the added task of attending lectures or reading in the medical humanities might seem irrelevant. After all, how will your knowledge of how healers a century earlier cared for their patients help your patients in the technology-intensive, fast-paced world of twenty-first-century medicine? The answer is that it will not help you directly. No one is suggesting a return to bloodletting and therapeutic purges, but there is value in understanding why healers at one time advocated such measures and what profound medical and social consequences those decisions could involve. In the end, an appreciation and an understanding of medicine's past and its humanistic dimensions will help you be a more thoughtful and more perceptive healer in any of the health professions.

Prior to the mid-1970s, medical history was a discipline dominated by physicians, typically retired physicians with avocational interests in the important events, figures, and discoveries of medicine. These physician-historians produced scholarship that emphasized the achievements of the "great doctors" and that did not consider the contributions or roles of patients, of women in general, of racial, ethnic, and economic groups, and of other minorities (as either patients or healers). Generally, these early medical historians were unconcerned about the social and cultural contexts in which medicine was practiced. Beginning in the early 1970s, this internalist approach to medical history began to be criticized by historians who were trained in history but who were not physicians. Such social and cultural historians of medicine argued that medical history is an important vehicle for interpreting broad social and cultural phenomena. They proposed that diseases and attitudes toward diseases and their sufferers are not value-free, but rather reflect their social, cultural, and historical contexts. A thorough study of medicine's history requires considering how medicine has been shaped by forces, institutions, and events outside itself. The vast majority of medical historians practicing today are not physician-historians but social and cultural historians of medicine who are broadly trained in the tools of social and cultural analysis. Scholarship in the history of medicine today is sophisticated, highly learned, and of immense potential to practicing physicians and other health care professionals as well.

My own decision to pursue graduate study in the history of medicine was one that I reached slowly while an undergraduate. Even before entering college, I had strong interests in literature and history, and, while in college, I worked to incorporate humanities courses into my largely premedical course of study in the sciences. During my first two years of college, I struggled to include history and literature courses into a schedule dominated by the science courses that were required. By the end of my second year of college, my passion for the humanities was being stifled by what seemed to be the dispassionate sciences. One professor at the university's medical school occasionally taught an advanced seminar in medical history. I approached him about the possibility of doing a tutorial of directed readings with him during the summer. Even now, I remember the first three books I read in medical history: Henry Sigerist's *The Great Doctors* (1933), Richard Shryock's *Medicine and Society in America* (1960), and Charles Rosenberg's *The Cholera Years* (1962). Reading and discussing these and other books that summer introduced me to a discipline where I could cultivate my disparate interests in the humanities and the sciences.

For many students, studying the history of medicine, or literature and medicine, or any of the other medical humanities, is one way to bridge seemingly different interests. But such a reason is rarely enough to motivate someone to pursue a career as a medical historian, either exclusively or as a practitioner-historian. My reasons for wanting to study medical history have changed many times since that summer when I was introduced to the field. I am now sure that the history of medicine is a powerful way to study the most basic and most universal of human conditions—sickness and death—and one of the most important of human interactions—caring for those who are sick. I have grown to learn that how we treat those who are sick reveals much about society because diseases and their sufferers are canvases onto which we project our deepest—often unexpressed—human emotions. Our attitudes toward the sick can be expressions of compassion, courage, hope, and understanding, and of fear, disgust, despair, and intolerance. This is why I believe the humanities matter in a medical education and in a medical career. Courses in the medical sciences prepare a student for the technical aspects of medical practice, but exposure to the medical humanities prepares a student for the equally important human interactions that are central to the work of healing. The death of a friend who was also a distinguished physician and medical historian reminded me that the virtue of physician–patient interactions has been diminished. When asked if he had any good doctors during his hospital care, he replied, "I have had many good technicians, but no doctors," a reminder that technically competent medical practice is a prerequisite to good patient care, but that technical competence alone should be never mistaken for caring medicine.

The value of medical history in particular, and the medical humanities in general, in day-to-day medical practice is intangible. The common response from students required to take a medical history course or encouraged to attend a lecture on medicine and poetry is "Why?" When one has to prepare for anatomy lab or complete a genetics problem set or simply catch up on sleep, it is difficult to take medical history seriously or to take the time to sit through a lecture that is not required. What could be "useful" about it, and what does one stand to gain?

Many people are quick to point out that history teaches lessons. For me, the history of medicine offers three unique lessons for medicine and the health professions. First, history connects these students to the rich legacy of healing that is being passed on to them. The decision to pursue such a career and the training and preparation required to realize that decision can be daunting. New choices, new experiences, and new ways of thinking will have to be confronted. Medical education, for example, is focused on training to become a physician, and it will not afford many opportunities to reflect and to think about the process one is going through or about one's place in the larger world of medicine. History gives one some sense of that larger world and allows one to gain some understanding about one's place in it by connecting personal experiences to the history of healing.

Second, history teaches humility. While the process of becoming a physician can be overwhelming, it can also be an empowering one that instills a sense of authority, privilege, and even superiority. History lends a sense of balance by offering perspectives not necessarily encountered in medical training. History, literature, ethics, and other medical humanities disciplines explore the complexity of medicine's culture, question medicine's objectivity and authority, probe the physician–patient relationship, and maintain the possibility that medicine is not an infallible institution. More important, these fields expose physicians to the perspectives of individuals who are not healers and who have experienced medicine as patients.

Knowledge of medical history instills humility and a sense of proportion in another way. Given the immense technological capabilities of medical science to prolong life, alleviate suffering, and identify and redress illnesses in ways that could have only been imagined decades earlier, it is natural for physicians in the twenty-first century to believe that their medical tools and capabilities are better and superior to those of the past. Many physicians who practiced in the mid-twentieth century, however, speak of that period as a "Golden Age" and believe the many advances that medicine now enjoys came at a profound cost to the physician–patient relationship and to the trust patients once vested in the health care system. In considering "The Usefulness of Medical History for Medicine," Owsei Temkin wrote of how history "helps us to see beyond the limits of prevailing theory and may even sometimes reward us with a new comprehension of an old truth" (*The Double Face of Janus and Other Essays in the History of Medicine*, 1977, p. 80). History reaffirms for physicians the many advances that medicine has undergone, but it also questions their sense of progress, by asking what of value has been lost or altered as the price of advancement and by what measure can one claim that the medicine of their time is superior to that of an earlier one.

Finally, a knowledge of the history of medicine can help physicians and medical students cope with medicine's ever-changing nature. At the start of the twentieth-first century, American medicine stands at a watershed moment: medical practice is highly sophisticated and technologically intensive, and, in turn, the American public regards physicians and medical care as impersonal and harried. Physician autonomy has eroded dramatically as health care financing by thirty-party health maintenance organizations and federal agencies impinges on physicians' abilities to provide and patients' abilities to receive necessary medical care. Nearly fifty million Americans have inadequate or no health insurance. Despite the fact that the United States spends more money on health care (in absolute and relative terms) than any other country in the world, thousands of Americans do not have access to quality health care. In the industrialized world, the United States ranks only eighteenth in overall infant mortality. The advent of newly emerging infectious diseases and the return of antibiotic-resistant strains of once widespread diseases pose new challenges for public health. As medical researchers utilize the knowledge obtained from the Human Genome Project, profound social, economic, and ethical implications will need to be addressed.

Medicine has confronted these issues before in other forms: before the mid-nineteenth century, the American medical profession was not held in very high regard, as medical therapy was largely ineffectual and as professional rivalries divided physicians. Similarly in the mid-nineteenth century, physicians and the public were critical of the increasing role of science in medical practice. The public felt that healing was becoming undemocratic, accessible only to a privileged few who had mastered the specialized knowledge of science. Epidemics of cholera, smallpox, and tuberculosis raised concerns about who should be responsible for protecting the public's health and how to balance preserving the rights of individual sufferers with protecting the larger public. During the twentieth century, the United States government repeatedly considered the issue of the national financing of health care. Issues such as how to contain the cost of medical care and how to provide care to all Americans are not unique to the present day. Rather, they are questions that have been considered and reflected on before.

Medicine in the twentieth-first century will be marked by a search for answers to urgent and complex questions. New scientific knowledge and medical technologies will pose perplexing ethical dilemmas. The inadequacies of the present American system of health care financing and delivery will require fundamental and genuine reform. Medicine's capability to sustain and to prolong life outstrips society's acceptance of the ethical, economic, and social consequences. The emergence of new infectious diseases and the resurgence of antibiotic-resistant strains of once controllable diseases will require physicians to have a broader understanding of, and engagement with, public health and social issues. And within the medical profession, the erosion of physician autonomy, the diminishment of the patient–doctor relationship, and the decline of physician job satisfaction will all need to be addressed. Medicine does not allow its practitioners sufficient opportunities to think about their profession and the issues it confronts.

As I write this, I am considering and reconsidering what my own role in the culture of twentieth-first-century medicine will be. Do I want to be solely a historian of medicine speaking largely to other historians or do I want to pursue a career in academic medicine as a physician and as a medical historian speaking particularly to medical students and colleagues? Is the quality of studying medicine as an outsider to its culture different from studying it from within? Will my perspectives about medicine be perceived and received differently? Those questions about whether I wanted to pursue a medical career or an academic career as a historian that filled my late college years with anxiety have never left me. What has changed is that I am not asking "What is it that I want to do with my life?" I long ago decided that I want to be a historian. What draws me to the possibility of a medical career is a belief that history can be more than a cognitive, "armchair" activity, one where I can use my training in history, ethics, and the social sciences—training that has equipped me with the analytical tools to explore the complexities of medical life and medical culture.

Adding to these questions is the knowledge that our world has changed in ways we might only begin to appreciate and to understand with the perspective of time. The terrorist attacks on the United States on September 11, 2001, the global military response against terrorism, and subsequent threats of biological, chemical, and nuclear terrorism have introduced uncertainty, anxiety, and insecurity into the lives of Americans, in turn placing new obligations on the medical profession. The confidence with which physicians entered the twentieth-first century—helped by an impressive array of drugs, machines, and techniques and assured in their abilities to help the most critically ill—has been tested, if not eroded. The specter of biological terrorism underscores the fragility of the American medical and public health systems to cope with new challenges posed by diseases relegated to history. The threats of anthrax and smallpox outbreaks were confronted with sophisticated new technologies, but the human and social responses to even the possibility of their outbreak—expressions of fear and panic—did not change appreciably from centuries earlier. A poignant image that remains with me after the terrorist attacks is that of physicians, nurses, and emergency medical personnel waiting at the New York City hospitals to treat the injured survivors. As the hours and days passed and they came to realize that far more people had died than survived, their skills and resources seemed powerless to help. In these circumstances, many turned to physicians with their concerns and fears, but these were experiences for which answers, comfort, and meaning had to be sought outside of medicine. No medical school lecture can teach a student empathy or caring. No medical textbook can prepare or instruct a physician how to respond to the human emotions that accompany this age of uncertainty. And that is part of my message: the daily experiences of healing, not only in times of crisis, are fraught with uncertainty, and physicians will not always be able to give meaning to their experiences without reaching outside themselves as physicians. Art, history, literature, and music are some of the many ways to mark one's experiences in medicine with meaning, to better understand those experiences, and to attempt to make sense of it all. The nature of medicine in the twentieth-first century is such that you must actively seek to infuse your experiences with meaning.

The attacks of September 11 reminded many Americans of the special duties and obligations the United States holds as an economic and military superpower and as American culture and mores pervade the globe. In the twentieth century, American medicine enjoyed remarkable advances while much of the Third World continued to lack the basic medical personnel, facilities, technologies, and other resources that Americans had grown to expect as ordinary. Today, when the United States and Western developed countries are the primary centers of biomedical research, patent owners and manufacturers of pharmaceuticals and medical technologies, and financiers of international health programs, what is American medicine's obligation to the world? This might seem a rhetorical question, but the events of September 11, after which the United States reiterated its global leadership, make the question's answers anything but academic. The question also might seem irrelevant and inappropriate in an essay on the medical humanities. But the answers will require the American health care system and medical profession to probe its humanistic mission, and a critical and workable answer will require physicians to have some understanding of the diverse perspectives of those who do not enjoy the sophisticated, high-quality basic care that Americans enjoy. Anthropology, economics, ethics, history, literature, sociology, and other humanities and social science disciplines will be all the more necessary to inform the direction and the role American medicine will play in an increasingly complex and divided world.

The humanities can serve you to negotiate the complexities of the medical world and the larger world of which it is a part. Interpretation and perspective are central to the task of the humanities, as they challenge you to see issues and situations through the eyes of another person and to refine your views. The time when medicine was essentially the highly personal relationship between a patient and his or her physician is over. In its place is left a medical system that is burdened with perplexing issues raised by the potential of new technologies, by questions of financing and equitable access to medical resources, by the international character of medicine, and by the changing role and authority of physicians in society. To evaluate such issues and to formulate an informed personal opinion without retreating to positions that are extreme, defensive, or unworkable, you will need critical and analytical skills that medicine alone cannot provide you.

The importance of cultivating the humanistic dimensions of healing and medical care has grown. Medical students and physicians in the twentieth-first century cannot practice medicine without facing the many crises and challenges confronting the American medical profession. If the past century is any indication of what can be expected, the medical profession you are now entering will be a very much different one when you retire. Perhaps as much as any time in the history of medicine, change will be the cardinal feature of medicine during your medical careers. Knowing something about medicine's past will inspire, challenge, and help you to adapt to the changes you will face.

PETER**SALOVEY** and
KELLYD.**BROWNELL**

Coming to Medicine Through Health Psychology

The field of health psychology is committed to identifying the links between the way people think, feel, and behave and their physical well-being. Health psychologists also attempt to improve health and ameliorate illness for individuals and for communities. Through their efforts to influence the behavior of individuals, health psychologists expect to address many of the major causes of premature mortality in our society.

Health psychologists hold the view that health or illness is the product of the interaction of biological factors (for example, genetics or pathogens), behavioral factors (lifestyle, stress, beliefs), and social conditions (family, social support, cultural practices). Many health psychologists came to work in this field because of their belief in the central importance to an individual's health of such behaviors as diet, exercise, smoking, alcohol consumption, and adherence to recommendations for disease screening.

Individual behavior plays a significant role in the top five causes of death in the United States—heart disease, cancer, stroke, chronic lung disease, and unintentional injuries. For instance, if every smoker in the United States quit tomorrow, there would be a 25 percent reduction in cancer deaths and 350,000 fewer fatal heart attacks each year. The HIV/AIDS epidemic provides another example. When vulnerable populations have been encouraged to change behaviors related to infection, such as reducing unprotected sexual intercourse or the sharing of syringes used to inject drugs intravenously, transmission of the virus from person to person has decreased dramatically.

If changing behaviors such as these and others relevant to health and illness were easy, health psychologists probably would not be necessary. But as our failed New Year's resolutions demonstrate every year, merely becoming informed about behaviors that affect health, or even promising to change them, carries no long-term guarantee. Consider the following:

- College students are well aware that by far the surest way for a sexually active person to prevent the spread of HIV is to use a condom. Yet less than 50 percent of sexually active college students report that they consistently use a condom during intercourse.

- Only about 55 percent of women over the age of fifty get screening mammograms regularly, even though it is the best way to detect breast cancer early, when it is more easily treated.

- The overwhelming majority of people who successfully complete weight-loss treatment programs are unable to maintain their change in weight over several years.

- Even when strongly motivated to prolong their lives, some people with HIV fail to take their protease inhibiting drugs as prescribed, which then increases their vulnerability to a drug-resistant strain of the virus.

- Even though people recognize that alcohol impairs their driving ability, many individuals maintain that they can drive safely after drinking.

- People purchase cellular car telephones in order to call for help in the unlikely event of an emergency; however, many use the phone while driving, which increases the risk of traffic accidents as much as driving while intoxicated.

- Regular physical activity is known to be one of the most effective means of reducing risk for the major chronic diseases, yet a majority of the population is inactive.

So why is behavior relevant to health and illness so difficult to change? Behavior related to health is not necessarily guided by the kind of rational analysis of costs and benefits that, according to conventional economic theories, underlies most decision making. Although people may often act based on a desire to maximize their "expected utility," there are times when they will act in the service of other psychological goals. Thus they will minimize effort, maximize immediate rather than long-term pleasure, or act to distinguish themselves from others, conform to others' expectations, or increase their acceptance by others.

These goals may change from moment to moment depending on the immediate social situation in which people find themselves. Although one individual may be willing to assume the personal risk of engaging in unhealthy practices, when hundreds of thousands in the population do the same, the burden to society can be unacceptable. Thus an analysis of these goals—both how they are represented mentally and how they are influenced by other people and social institutions—provides the grist for the health psychologist's mill.

Neither of us entered the field of health psychology as an alternative to a traditional medical education. We were interested primarily in research careers, and felt that Ph.D. programs within departments of psychology were the best way to acquire the background in theory and research methodology that would help us study psychological aspects of health and illness. However, our careers as health psychologists have included extensive collaborations with others in medicine, including clinicians, public health experts, epidemiologists, physiologists, exercise scientists, and other allied health professionals. For example, Brownell has extensively studied the interaction of biological, psychological, and social factors that contribute to people's inability to lose weight and keep it off. Salovey studies the role of emotions in health behavior and has used the principles of social psychology to maximize the impact of community-based interventions designed to encourage behaviors that reduce the risk of cancer and HIV/AIDS. In these activities, we have worked alongside other medical professionals, often bringing to the table a unique psychological perspective and particular expertise in experimental methods and the analysis of quantitative data.

If you are considering a career in health psychology, you should know that there are many different kinds of careers you can have in this field. In general, health psychologists may conduct research, provide assessment and treatment in clinical settings, or even help shape public policy relevant to entire communities. Some health psychologists engage in all three of these activities. The settings in which health psychologists work can also vary enormously. Most research is carried out in departments of psychology or epidemiology and public health, or in schools of medicine. Health psychologists also may engage in clinical work in primary care programs, general hospitals, or specialty programs concerned with pain management, cardiac rehabilitation, cancer prevention and treatment, smoking cessation, and the like. Health psychologists may work as part of a multidisciplinary team, provide a consultation liaison function, or act as sole providers.

Most individuals interested in the best training for a career in health psychology obtain a Ph.D. in clinical psychology from a university-based program accredited by the American Psychological Association. It is also possible to become a health psychologist with a Ph.D. in a different program of study, such as social or personality psychology. Some graduate programs provide explicit training in health psychology, either as an organized program or, as we do now at Yale, through work with individual faculty members who share this interest. Often specialized training in health psychology is acquired during the predoctoral internship for clinical psychology graduate students or in postdoctoral positions.

The present turmoil concerning the costs of medical care has given health psychologists—with their emphasis on prevention or lifestyle change—increasingly important roles in traditional medical settings. According to the American Psychological Association's Division of Health Psychology, medical centers have greatly expanded their employment of psychologists in recent years. In addition, colleges and universities, medical schools, health maintenance organizations, rehabilitation centers, and public health agencies also employ significant numbers of health psychologists. We believe that the most significant future role for health psychologists in medicine and health care will be as translational scientists. Translational research in health psychology addresses how information about basic biological, cognitive, emotional, social, and behavioral processes can be used in the prevention, diagnosis, treatment, and delivery of services for physical illness. As we write this, the director of the National Institute of Mental Health is calling for an increased focus on translational research with implications for improving the nation's public health. Health psychologists seem uniquely poised to deliver on this request.

Health psychologists will also play a major role in prevention of disease. Prevention may be the only hope for halting the spread of some infections (for example, HIV/AIDS), is logical to consider for diseases that are difficult to treat (like obesity), and is almost always more cost-effective than treatment. Because prevention relies largely on behavior change, the importance of knowledge from health psychology is obvious. Even when medications are developed to prevent disease, health psychologists can help to convince individuals that benefits outweigh side effects and costs, and persuade them to stick to their medication regimens over the long term.

The work of health psychologists is finding its way into medical school curricula, and increasing numbers of physicians are seeking training in health psychology. Our field is interdisciplinary both by necessity and in its conceptual foundations. As medicine, health-care, and psychology converge, rapid advances in the areas of disease prevention and health promotion are likely, and those advances will in turn assure that individuals and organizations with varying disciplinary backgrounds and perspectives will find themselves collaborating to address the health challenges that face our society.

Why I Chose Chiropractic

As I look back, many experiences in my life contributed to the development of my holistic attitude about health care. The most important experience occurred when I was seventeen years old. I lost my father to heart disease. He was only forty-seven. At that time, I believed that my father's lifestyle choices, as well as the medical establishment's lack of focus on such behavior, ultimately led to his disease and early death. Many years later, I still believe that to be true. My father's illness and my enduring concerns about the circumstances of his death still motivate me to try to influence my patients, family, and friends to choose a better lifestyle. By studying the holistic approach to health care, I have been able to encourage them to apply new and different ways of achieving and maintaining better health, and understanding what health is.

During my late adolescence I discovered nutrition. My oldest sister was determined to cure me of being a "junk food junkie." She referred me to a nutritionist, who diagnosed hypoglycemia—low blood sugar—resulting from poor diet and excessive exercise (I was a distance runner). After making dietary changes and taking supplements, I was amazed at how much my energy and overall health improved. And so I began to think seriously of becoming a nutritionist.

I began researching careers in nutrition, as well as medicine, naturopathy, and osteopathy. While home from college, I came upon a chiropractic brochure that my stepfather had brought home from a recent treatment. He shared his experience with me, and I was intrigued, yet skeptical. I had heard the stories about chiropractors. My impression of them at that time (the late 1970s) was that they were all "quacks." But the brochure outlined a holistic approach to health care that immediately impressed and interested me.

I started to obtain information on educational prerequisites, length of education, costs, location of schools, areas of specialization, and available student loans for chiropractic study. I discussed my interests with family, friends, and academic advisors. One of my professors, Dr. Gary Gesmonde of Southern Connecticut State University, had always recognized my interest in nutrition. He encouraged me to pursue a career in health care. I also met with three chiropractic physicians and became a patient of one. Now my interest expanded to include not just nutrition but all aspects of the chiropractic philosophy: structural, emotional, and nutritional. My decision to pursue a D.C. (doctor of chiropractice) degree was a practical one, based on the holistic scope of practice, popularity, and a general sense that most chiropractors were successful.

Throughout my chiropractic education, I took every opportunity to meet with practicing chiropractors. Doing this enabled me to gather ideas and open some doors to my future. After graduation, I briefly considered accepting an associate position, working as a salaried employee for another chiropractic physician. But ultimately I felt that starting my own private practice was the best choice for me. Still, as is true for many new chiropractic graduates, it was not financially feasible for me to open an office. So I decided to accept an offer to share office space with another D.C. Sharing space with an established practitioner for one year gave me the opportunity to develop a following as well as the confidence to open a private solo practice. While continuing to treat patients in my first office, I renovated the small practice space where I eventually worked and lived for about five years. This home/office provided me with a relatively low-overhead practice that allowed me time to create a professional reputation for quality service and results.

Over the next five years, my practice grew enough to move it to a larger space, where I've practiced for the past ten years. Five years ago, I was able to offer a space-sharing opportunity to a younger practitioner, and we've formed a partnership. This has allowed a sharing of clinical issues, growth of the practice and improved quality of service.

A typical day for me begins at 7:30 A.M. and ends between seven or eight at night. Most of this time is spent treating patients, with paperwork and staff meetings often consuming 25 to 50 percent of the work week. Additional time is spent outside the office at seminars and studying. The typical day is fast-paced and physically demanding. The treatment techniques that I use in my practice require a lot of deep pressure pushing and pulling on patients to help restore mobility to joints and muscle. The course of treatment for some patients is straightforward and routine, while for others it is complex and stressful. On a typical day, I treat thirty to forty patients and examine two to three new patients. A new patient history and exam usually requires sixty to ninety minutes. The actual treatment time varies from five to thirty minutes or more, depending on the type and severity of the condition. Some patient interactions are very friendly, even fun, while others can be emotionally draining. The most gratifying aspect of being a chiropractor is the thrill of helping patients to get well—especially when all else seems to have failed. (Chiropractic is often considered the last resort for many patients.)

Patient age varies from infants to the elderly, and every individual requires a specific approach to his or her condition. The typical patient is between twenty-five and fifty years old and requires some type of adjusting (joint manipulation). For some patients, such procedures as massage, acupuncture, heat, ice, ultrasound, and electrical stimulation are also considered, and attention may be given to nutrition as well. Some form of exercise is almost always recommended and instructed. In every visit, the patient is examined and symptoms are assessed. During the acute phase of care, it is not unusual to see a patient three to four times per week. Some patient conditions require only a few visits, while others may take weeks to respond to treatment.

Throughout the past sixteen years, the quality chiropractic care and service I have provided has helped my practice grow. The bottom line is to have the knowledge and skill to effectively treat a variety of patient conditions. Continuing education is a very important part of my career. I began taking additional seminars while still in chiropractic college. Over the past eighteen years I've taken multiple seminars.

Most of my postdoctoral training has been related to chiropractic neurology, in which I have earned a degree. In the past few years, I have received certification in acupuncture. I've also taken additional courses in exercise rehabilitation, nutrition, foot orthotics, various soft-tissue massage treatments, motivational, and business-related topics. For many years I participated in a monthly brainstorming group for chiropractors. Six to eight of us met monthly to share knowledge and discuss various professional issues.

Maturing in my career has been a slow, steady process, shaped by many experiences. Literally, every interaction with a patient, every journal I've read, and every seminar I've attended has contributed to my career development.

Probably one of the more difficult challenges has been to deal with prejudice toward chiropractic. Developing relationships within the medical, legal, business, and insurance communities is a slow, arduous process. Over the years I've had some success in being accepted by the community as a whole. But even now chiropractic is often misunderstood and unfairly discriminated against.

Being a chiropractor has its challenges. Besides the emotional stresses of operating a small business and being a practitioner, it is an extremely physically demanding job. But the enthusiasm within the chiropractic community is fueled by the joy and excitement of having helped many people, especially when no one else could.

I would advise anyone considering chiropractic as a career to meet with a few chiropractic physicians. Try to work or volunteer in a chiropractic office. Gather information from many sources, and discuss your goals with supportive family members, friends, and advisors. Attend state chiropractic conventions, visit chiropractic colleges, and meet with students while you are there. As with any career, you should spend some time with someone who is already doing it—learn firsthand what it will be like to be a chiropractor. Your commitment to your education and career will be greatly enhanced.

Once you've graduated, look at all the opportunities available to you. Consider some that are outside your comfort zone, such as positions overseas or out of state, associate positions, teaching, partnerships, buying an existing practice, sharing space with another chiropractor or a different professional, or starting a new practice. The better your research is, the more accurately you will make decisions that suit your personality and lifestyle. Your success depends on making good choices and being consistently motivated to pursue excellence. Continue your education forever, make a commitment to a subspecialty, and use various treatment approaches.

Now, after sixteen years in practice, I am in another stage of my career. Learning the newest in neurological applications and nutrition continues to be important. But it has become equally important that I apply to my life the same holistic philosophies that I recommend to my patients. I now have a family, and striking that balance between career, family, and play is a constant struggle. Maintaining my personal health and fitness is also a major focus. But for me, being a chiropractic physician is a way of life.

HOWARD M. SPIRO

Some Musings About Complementary and Alternative Medicine

As a college student thinking about a career in the health professions, you may already be aware of two main currents in medical practice. One accurately calls itself the mainstream, while the other is relegated to a "complementary" or "alternative" position, now often abbreviated CAM. These two streams, one depending on reason and science and the other on emotion and intuition, can be traced back loosely to Hippocrates and Aesculapius in ancient Greece. Hippocrates taught his acolytes that they were trained and rational practitioners who knew more than their patients knew. The priests of Aesculapius, in contrast, tried to help the sick by plying them with wine enough to make them sleep and then by whispering to them over and over again that they were better. The Enlightenment and the Counterenlightenment offer later examples pertinent today, when medical practice still veers between relying on science for the treatment of disease (what the physician sees or can measure) and art for soothing illness (what the patient feels or suffers).

Each way of practicing medicine has achieved considerable popularity at one time or another, although during the nineteenth and twentieth centuries, with the ascendancy of science in medicine, alternative therapies often had less appeal. However, the alternative methods during the past century and a half have not been completely dismissed. Medical students tend to think that neurobiology is new, and of course it is, but "mind-body medicine," popular one hundred years ago, traces its practices back to those priests of Aesculapius.

The dominance of mainstream medicine has come about over the past 150 years, thanks to the victories of science over so many diseases, particularly those of bacterial origin, and thanks also to the 1910 Flexner Report, which established the hegemony of scientific medicine. To some extent, throughout the twentieth century, what Isaiah Berlin called the scientific fallacy has spawned a growing belief that the tools of science can be used to explain everything, including morality, religion, and the very meaning of life.

In addition, during the past fifty years, technology has so amplified medical victories that doctors have begun to regard themselves as powerless without the aid of science and technology—that is to say, without their medications and instruments. In so doing, they have forgone the powers of persuasion, admonition, and helpful words, on which alternative practitioners rely. Modern doctors treat disease very well, but too often they ignore the patients who have the disease.

The pendulum always swings. Or, as a scientist might put it, there is always "regression to the mean." During the social upheaval of the 1960s, classes of previously marginalized, submerged, and powerless minorities began to claim their previously denied human and political rights. By the 1990s, these social revolutions brought a new diversity to our institutions, including the populations of medical students, physicians, and other health care professionals in the United States. In our "postmodern" era, the gradual realignment of the white Western male from his position of dominance and privilege to one of equality has been accompanied, paradoxically, by a growing interest and delight in the many notions that were disdained in the previous "modern" era of scientific medicine.

The growing rejection of white, male dominance has brought a new regard for CAM, especially in primary care, where physicians, nurses, and other health care professionals are inclined to think about patients as persons rather than as merely carriers of disease. CAM, or, as it was called for a while, holistic medicine, is usually defined as any therapy that focuses on mind-body relations and, more important, does not fit into current mainstream medical thinking. CAM does not include every therapeutic program that defines itself as outside the mainstream or is not taught in medical schools. (In fact, many medical schools are now teaching CAM.) "Unconventional" is only one of many labels applied to CAM by both supporters and detractors. Like the position CAM holds outside the mainstream postmodern medical practice, the very definition often seems porous enough to include everything but that core curriculum and practice of medical science.

Alternative practitioners are a very heterogeneous group: Westerners and non-Westerners, acupuncturists and iridologists and chiropractors, Christian Scientists and other faith healers, physicians and nonphysicians practicing homeopathy or aromatherapy, and various other practitioners. Commonly, and at their best, practitioners of CAM spend a lot of time talking with—and listening to—their patients. Much like placebos, most alternative methods seem to depend for their benefit on patients' expectations and belief—hope, some might say—that they will feel better, an approach praised by skeptics like Montaigne, who otherwise had little good to say about physicians.

Indeed, many mainstream medical physicians believe that placebos, with their very beneficial effects, may be taken as a substitute for CAM. A major problem in evaluating CAM is the faith that its practitioners have in the efficacy of their specific approaches, few of which have been rigorously and scientifically tested, and most of which seem to this cautiously dispassionate mainstream observer to benefit symptoms but not diseases. Unfortunately, practitioners of CAM have no tradition of clinical research and usually claim that, because they individualize therapy, clinical trials are rarely possible.

One kind of alternative practice, herbal medicine, really must be distinguished from the rest. Herbals or botanicals have been used and winnowed from the experience of thousands of years by all sorts of healers, from mainstream practitioners to shamans. Herbals and botanicals have become quite popular in the United States over the past two decades, but unfortunately an act of Congress classified them as nutritional supplements, and thereby removed them from the purview of the Food and Drug Administration (FDA). For that reason the FDA cannot require research on these supplements, and cannot determine through regulated research both their adverse effects and their efficacy.

Many of these compounds bring important, sometimes dangerous, side effects along with their undoubted therapeutic benefits, because they are pharmaceutical agents whose botanical origin alone, incongruously enough, classifies them as "alternative." They should be studied thoroughly, and the FDA should regulate them, at least for safety in human consumption.

An important distinction from the mainstream is that alternative medicine aims at "healing" by making patients feel better, whereas mainstream medicine aims at "cure," by eliminating a disease. Healing is often directed at mind and spirit, so that a patient may be healed and yet end up in the proverbial pine box. Healing often refers to a spiritual transformation which improves the quality of life and puts the patient at peace, even if the disease becomes worse. I often say that mainstream medicine relies on the eye, what the doctor can see with instruments and technology, whereas CAM relies on the ear, what the physician hears when the patient complains. Yet then I think of the aphorism "The eye is for accuracy, but the ear is for truth."

So what is conventional in one society and culture will be unconventional in another; remedies vary even from one European country to another. What passes for a "liver crisis" in France goes by the name of "cardiac insufficiency" in Germany. One has only to think of homeopathy or acupuncture, unconventional at one time, mainstream at another, and coming back in vogue at present.

The public spends billions of dollars on CAM, in part because physicians in the United States, and in much of the rest of the world, are trained as scientists—or at least are trained to think of themselves as scientists. They have been so seduced by science and technology that they have run the risk of ignoring patients. Modern doctors are very good at treating acute diseases, but they fare less well in relieving chronic complaints. Mainstream physicians are realists, however, so the very popularity of CAM has led to a melding of alternative and conventional practices. Still, none of us should forget that mainstream medicine, underpinned by science and technology, cures many diseases for which CAM can only relieve symptoms, what has been called the illness. Trials to evaluate the two have foundered on this distinction.

The popularity of CAM in large part depends on the time and

interest that such practitioners give their patients. Empathy is one of many lessons from CAM for mainstream doctors who stick so faithfully to their technology. If it is true, as so many studies have suggested, that 80 percent of complaints have psychic, social, or economic origins, we can understand why such healers are so effective. They teach self-help and personal responsibility, and they engender an optimistic attitude and a listening support that brings about "healing." As William James wrote one hundred years ago, "The world can be handled according to many systems of ideas. . . . Religion in the shape of mind-cure gives to some of us serenity, moral poise, and happiness, and prevents certain forms of disease as well as science does."

Science provides the basis for mainstream medical treatment, and the claims of CAM should not be taken as undermining mainstream medical practice. The mind may turn out to be a program of the brain, but it could be more like smoke from a burning log, wood in a different form obeying different laws. After all, chemicals can lull depression, but sorrow does not yield to antidepressants, nor love to antioxidants. CAM provides the piers for a bridge between the cultures of science and art that make up medical practice. CAM reminds us that suggestion, which plays such a big role in the benefit of placebos, comes out of the therapeutic alliance between patient and physician. I will believe the current claim that there are too many doctors when patients complain, "I just couldn't get out of the doctor's office, because the doctor wanted to spend so much time talking with me."

Words can be used to exhort the healthy and they may be equally helpful to the sick. As I have already suggested, modern science has made too many physicians fear that they are mere conduits of power, of pills and procedures, that they are helpless without technology. The managed care industry reinforces that notion by treating patients and physicians as standardized modules, and current "standards of practice" and "clinical pathways" do much the same. Still, if you choose medicine as a profession, as I hope you will, sooner or later you must remember that not all pains come from disease, that many result from sorrow and tribulation. CAM brings the focus back to the patient as it reminds doctors of the importance and power of healing words and empathic listening. CAM assures us that our patients are more than their diseases.

PART SEVEN

Conducting Biomedical Research

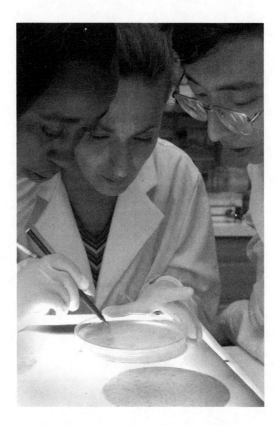

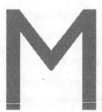Medicine depends on its academic enterprise to renew itself and to survive. Without research and development, the medical progress that fuels the practice of medicine would come to a halt. And without the education and training of physicians, no one would be available to carry on that practice. In the United States the academic medical enterprise resides largely in university-based academic health centers and in the federally funded National Institutes of Health. Important as academic medicine may be, one does not settle easily into a career as an academician; the path is long and rocky.

The essays collected in this section portray various careers in biomedical research and teaching. Leon Rosenberg, a distinguished investigator in human genetics and a former dean of Yale University Medical School, tells what it means to be a physician-scientist and how he came to be one. Physician-scientists bring to biomedical research a perspective that is directly relevant to human disease. Moreover, important discoveries about normal human biology often result only from an understanding of disease. To participate in this important work, a physician-scientist must possess an affinity for the scientific approach, a desire to solve problems, and—above all—persistence.

The oversight of research involving human subjects is a matter of increasing importance to biomedical research. Robert J. Levine pioneered our understanding of the ethical issues of research involving human subjects. The route he took to a career in bioethics exemplifies how physicians of an earlier generation tended to rely on circumstance and coincidence rather than on traditional pathways to achieve their career goals. An all-consuming interest in a subject took precedence over the certainty of obtaining the best training and guidance.

Harlan Krumholz, Jeffrey R. Bender, Fred Gorelick, and Perry L. Miller are all medical school professors and successful physician-scientists of recent vintage. We learn from them about the advantages and disadvantages of being a physician who conducts biomedical research. They experience both the immediate gratification of making a sick person well as well as the long-term gratification of contributing to advances in biomedical science. They worry, however, about the years it took to achieve their goals, and they cope with the challenge of being simultaneously competent at the bedside and in the research setting. The consensus seems to be that advancement requires spending more time as a researcher than as a clinician. Nevertheless, the four leading physician scientists reporting here feel comfortable in their dual roles.

This section also illustrates the limitless variety of research that is available to physician-scientists. Krumholz uses medical records and other patient-centered information to study the quality of medical care. Bender and Gorelick use isolated tissues and cells to learn about disease processes in blood vessels and cellular trafficking in the pancreas. Miller uses computer science to promote medical care in the operating room and to advance understanding of the human genome. They all find a dual career remarkably rewarding and too much fun to seem like a job. Physician-scientists not only care for patients and head up research laboratories, they also teach young clinicians and investigators.

You certainly need not, however, endure the lengthy process of becoming a physician to feel the joy of making important discoveries in medical science while teaching that science to graduate students and medical students. Susan Hockfield depicts the excitement of biomedical research carried out by those who do not wish to be practicing physicians.

The message of this section is clear: although the road to a successful career in biomedical research is both long and difficult, the journey can take many forms and can be extraordinarily exciting and rewarding.

LEON**ROSENBERG**

On Being and Becoming a Physician-Scientist

Each autumn some 16,000 young people—now about half men and half women—begin their medical studies in the United States at one of 125 medical schools. The vast majority of these future physicians intend to spend most of their professional lives in clinical medicine as clinicians, that is, working directly with patients. Only about 10 percent say they plan to be physician-scientists, that is, medical doctors who devote most of their time to research. Nearly half the latter group enrolls in joint M.D./Ph.D. programs designed to confer both degrees in 7 or 8 years.

These demographics have changed dramatically in the nearly 50 years since I began medical school at the University of Wisconsin. There were only 81 medical schools in the United States then, and the entering class contained just under 7,500 students—more than 95 percent of whom were men. I don't know how many of us expected to become physician-scientists, because M.D./Ph.D. programs didn't exist and no data on this career choice had been collected. But I do know that I would not have been among them. I saw science as a means to an end, not as a way of life. I intended to practice medicine— probably in Madison, Wisconsin, where I was born and raised.

To me, medicine meant taking care of sick people, and I cannot remember ever wanting to do anything else. This manifest destiny was molded in large part by my immigrant, self-educated Jewish parents, who expected their three sons to be "professional men." And so we are: two doctors, one lawyer. But that isn't all my parents wanted. We were to excel academically—preferably near home—and to be unending sources of parental pride (a pale translation of the Yiddish word "nachas"). The scorecard on this goal reads two "yes," one "no."

I was beyond dutiful. I lived at home during college and escaped only by marrying at age twenty-one and moving into an apartment two miles away. I was one of those creatures referred to as a "p.c." (perfect child), whose grades throughout high school, college, and medical school did not deviate even once from the first letter of the alphabet. This compulsion for academic overachievement delighted my parents, particularly my father, whose approval was of paramount importance to me.

No one encouraged my being exposed to research during college, and in the absence of such mentoring I skimmed merrily across the surface of science and the humanities and entered medical school after my junior year. During medical school, my introduction to research began. I spent the summers after my first and second years doing research—one year spent with a cardiovascular surgeon, the other with a pathologist. Both experiences were positive, but neither was life changing. I moved unswervingly toward clinical medicine.

And then, in a burst of delayed maturation, I used medical school graduation to finally uproot myself from home and parents. I came to Columbia-Presbyterian Hospital in New York as an intern in the specialty called internal medicine. The chief of the department was Robert Loeb, an accomplished physician-scientist and, arguably, also the most distinguished clinician and teacher of his day. Loeb viewed his interns and residents as disciples, and I felt honored to be among them. I learned how to be a physician from Loeb, his faculty colleagues, and my fellow residents. Loeb's knowledge was encyclopedic, his bedside abilities inspirational. His teaching style was far from gentle, however, and like many in his flock, I was burned twice by his withering criticism and public scoldings. (Such behavior was tolerated, even expected, of "medical giants" then.) These insults, the first I had ever suffered, were as close to war wounds as I would get. They caused great pain, but only temporarily. They punctured my pride and injected some humility in its place.

As I moved through my internship, I noted that many of my colleagues were preparing to go to the National Institutes of Health (NIH) in Bethesda, Maryland, for research training. You see, these were the days when the NIH budget was increasing by leaps and bounds, the NIH internal (or intramural) program was burgeoning, and a well-paid opportunity to do research was beckoning those physicians with the "right stuff." The lure was too powerful to resist, so I applied even though I had no idea what area of research interested me. I merely went with the flow, knowing that time spent at NIH would also satisfy my obligation to serve in the armed forces (hence the nickname "yellow berets" for those who ended up at NIH during the Korean War era).

I came to Bethesda in 1959 as a clinical associate in the metabolism division of the National Cancer Institute. Things began badly. My supervisor suggested a nonlaboratory project. He proposed that I analyze ten years' worth of data on chemical analyses of blood, urine, and stool of cancer patients in the hope that I could tell him what the results revealed about whole-body metabolism in patients with malignancy. This seemed like a mindless and hopeless "fishing expedition," so I refused, thereby quickly coming to an impasse with him that nearly resulted in my leaving NIH. The chief of the service rescued me. He reminded me that I was a novice in research, urged me not to jump to conclusions, and generously allowed me to seek a more suitable research mentor and setting.

I wandered about intellectually for several months until I became responsible for the care of an eight-year-old boy with a previously undiagnosed disorder that ran in his family. The illness was characterized by progressive skeletal muscle wasting and a selective amino acid transport defect in his kidneys. He died two years later, just as his two older brothers had, leaving behind a host of questions about the cause, pathophysiology, and mode of inheritance. After reading everything I could about medical genetics (which wasn't much in those days) and about amino acid metabolism (which was in vogue), I developed a hypothesis to explain the family's inherited illness. I needed a place to test my theory, which turned out to be the laboratory of Dr. Stanton Segal. He was an ideal mentor for me.

Segal was a young, talented physician-scientist interested in the biochemical basis of inherited metabolic disorders. He was also smart, tireless, and nurturing, and loved doing experiments. I will never forget the thrill I felt the first time I conceived, planned, conducted, and interpreted an experiment to test our hypothesis. We measured the uptake of radioisotopically labeled amino acids by rat kidney slices. Although, in retrospect, the findings were hardly earth-shattering, the sense of wonder and well-being they engendered was so intense that I knew I must direct my career toward medical research and follow the tiny band of pioneers who called themselves medical geneticists. And so I did, and have done ever since. I did the equivalent of a doctoral degree at NIH, taking courses in physical chemistry, biochemistry, and calculus, and working in Segal's laboratory on mechanisms of amino acid transport and its disorders.

After six years I moved to Yale University School of Medicine, where for twenty-six years I moved freely among the departments of internal medicine, pediatrics, and human genetics and, as freely, among the core functions of a university: research, teaching, clinical care, and administration. But there was one constant: my laboratory. It was my port in any storm. It was where I felt most excited and complete. Exploiting the rapidly increasing knowledge of genetics and of cell and molecular biology—but always starting at the bedside of a sick child with a life-threatening metabolic disorder—my graduate students, postdoctoral fellows, technicians, and I sought to figure out the cause of the condition and to use that understanding to improve our means of diagnosis, treatment, and prevention. We were well supported by peer-reviewed grants awarded by NIH and had the good fortune to make a couple of important discoveries. We conducted laboratory and patient-oriented investigation, moving comfortably back and forth across the bridge between the bedside and the laboratory.

The personal rewards from this research have been unexpectedly large. They have included invitations to speak all over the world; publications in diverse books and journals; election to prestigious professional organizations; friendships with colleagues whose common denominator is the pursuit of knowledge through research; and opportunities to lead organizations, large and small, in academia and industry. But no reward approaches the one offered by the palpable thrill of discovery. The excitement of being somewhere no one has been before, knowing that this "place" is special because it goes beyond personal attainment to affect the health and lives of others.

So much for the "being" a physician-scientist part of my essay's title. What about the "becoming" aspect? Let me offer a few ideas about becoming a physician-scientist in the twenty-first century, but do not expect a prescription. Most important, persist in your inclination toward medicine. Don't be driven off course by complaints about managed care, by disillusioned medical practitioners, or by the profit-making seduction of the dot.coms or Wall Street. No other profession or way of life offers medicine's richness of opportunity or ways to make a significant difference. I am certain this will be true in the century of your adulthood, as it has been in mine.

For those of you whose aspirations as physician-scientists are clear, the M.D./Ph.D. programs are attractive and efficient vehicles. These very competitive programs have economic advantages. Your tuition to medical school and graduate school will be covered by institutional grants, relieving you of the considerable debt now saddling most graduates of medical schools. For those of you who may want to combine medicine and science, let me suggest that serious research experience before medical school will test that inclination. For those who are not drawn to research, I say, "not so fast." Find an opportunity to work in a laboratory before or during medical school—during summers or, better still, by taking a year off from school. Surveys reveal that the earlier the positive research experience, the more likely the enduring commitment. The more research-intensive the medical school you attend, the more opportunities you will have to be "turned on." This is particularly true for women, whose involvement in research has lagged behind that of men, and whose participation must be encouraged as their proportion swells among physicians. My own unpublished results show that women at the most research-intensive schools retain their initial interest in research careers to a greater degree than do those who attend less research-intensive schools.

Finally, and most important, remember that you are not locked into a career when you receive the M.D. degree. Be open to the surprises that await you during subsequent training in a specialty residency or subspecialty fellowship. Don't be afraid to strike out on your own or stumble onto unmarked paths. My experience tells me they may be the very ones that lead to joy and fulfillment.

ROBERT J.LEVINE

A Bioethicist Concerned with Research Involving Humans as Subjects

All persons, living and dead,
are purely coincidental,
and should not be construed.
—Kurt Vonnegut, Jr.

As an undergraduate at Duke University, I knew I wanted to be a general practitioner (now they're called family practitioners or primary care doctors). I even had a sketch of the home I planned to build with my office in it. The first big change in my thinking concerned becoming an academic physician instead of going into private medical practice. This process began during my second year at George Washington University School of Medicine with a microbiology professor who persuaded me that I could multiply my contribution to medical practice by teaching medical students. The process was completed during my third and fourth years, when I found that I was so thorough (I prefer "thorough" to "compulsive") in my history and physical examinations that I could not complete them in less than two hours. I made more than my share of esoteric diagnoses, an accomplishment that specialists in internal medicine and neurology value highly. However, with the realization that a career pursued at this "thorough" pace would result in an income about 5 percent above the poverty line, I decided on an academic career as a specialist in internal medicine.

I was an intern at the Peter Bent Brigham Hospital in Boston at a time when virtually all young male doctors were required to serve in the military. Many of us competed for a very small number of positions at the National Institutes of Health (NIH). There, one would have a very high quality postdoctoral fellowship as a commissioned officer in the United States Public Health Service (USPHS). Although this was a "uniformed" rather than a "military" unit, it satisfied the requirement for military service. We were called the "yellow berets." (At the time, the U.S. Army Special Forces Units wore "green berets"; "yellow" was a term applied to cowards who dared not risk exposure to combat.)

Fortunately, I secured a position at NIH in the Experimental Therapeutics Branch of the National Heart Institute. I chose this in part because it had a large clinical service and I was not confident I would enjoy working in a scientific laboratory. (Clinical services at NIH were devoted to providing medical care for patients and normal volunteers who were serving as research subjects.) When I arrived at NIH, I thought I hated science. But once I became involved in it I found that I loved science; what I hated was the way it was taught in the 1950s. I was quite successful. I concentrated on the study of the biochemical processes (enzymes) involved in the biosynthesis (creation in the living animal) of histamine and serotonin, two compounds that have multiple and diverse hormone-like activities. I also studied the biological effects of administering to animals (including humans) drugs that blocked the enzymes involved in the biosynthesis of histamine and serotonin.

I moved to Yale, where I soon became Chief of the Section of Clinical Pharmacology, Associate Editor of *Biochemical Pharmacology*, and a member of a prestigious society for clinical investigators. A senior professor nominated me for an award for being the leading young pharmacologist in the nation. I was troubled to learn that he found it necessary to write a lengthy defense of my apparent lack of focus in studying two chemicals rather than just one. He told me he was concerned that the award committee might think I was a dilettante. I did not win the award, but I did get tenure.

I was still, by inclination, a generalist. My pharmacology professor-sponsor (for the pharmacology award) notwithstanding, I took several steps to ensure that I would continue to be active in a broad spectrum of medical and scientific arenas. Two of these steps are important in the further development of this story. First, I became a member and then Chairperson of the Institutional Review Board (IRB) at Yale–New Haven Medical Center. An IRB reviews all proposals to conduct research involving human subjects in the institution; no such research can be done without the board's approval. This step put me in touch with the then scanty literature of medical ethics as well as with the entire range of research in all clinical departments at a major medical center. Second, I accepted the editorship of *Clinical Research,* the journal of the American Federation for Clinical Research (AFCR), on the condition that I could expand it to include articles in what I then called the "social, political, and economic ecology" of clinical research. Before long, it was the preferred medium for leading authors on the topic of research ethics, and many academics referred to it as the "Journal of Medical Ethics."

In the early 1970s, the U.S. government began proposing regulations to "safeguard the rights and welfare of human research subjects." The preamble to the regulations stated that these proposals were grounded in considerations of ethics. I considered the ethics presented in these regulations faulty in several respects. Believing that enforcement of these regulations would be highly destructive to the field of research involving humans as subjects, I responded by writing polemics, editorials (in my position at *Clinical Research,* I had a bully pulpit), and the AFCR's position statements on the new regulatory proposals.

In 1974 the U.S. Congress established the National Commission for the Protection of Human Subjects of Biomedical and Behavioral Research. The commission was directed to identify the ethical principles that should underlie the conduct of research involving human subjects and to recommend guidelines to ensure that research would be done according to those principles. To this date, the entire system of regulations for the protection of human research subjects is based on the recommendations of the commission. I was recruited to serve as the commission's "special consultant" and to write its "background theoretical essays," which meant that every sentence in the general mandate to the commission became the title of a paper I wrote. The titles included: "The Nature and Definition of Informed Consent in Various Research Settings," "The Role of Assessment of Risk/Benefit Criteria in the Determination of the Appropriateness of Research Involving Human Subjects," and "On the Relevance of Ethical Principles and Guidelines Developed for Research to Health Services Conducted or Supported by the Federal Government."

These background theoretical essays were sent to experts and scholars in diverse relevant fields, along with a request for their criticism. My work was evaluated and criticized by leaders in such fields as ethics, law, philosophy, theology, surgery, and other medical specialties. They gave me advice for improvement of my analytical techniques or my fund of relevant empirical knowledge. They argued for or against my conclusions. It is hard to imagine that anyone could have designed a better postdoctoral fellowship in the field of research ethics.

When I signed on as the National Commission's consultant, I thought I would spend two years defending my profession. When Congress extended the commission's term to four years, I renewed my contract to continue with them. Much to my surprise, I found that I liked this work every bit as much as I did pharmacology; it also appealed to my basic tendency to be a generalist. I never returned to the laboratory. In the process of defending my profession I had discovered a new one.

I would like to conclude with some advice to those who would like to follow in my footsteps, as it were, to have a career like mine. But first I need to know what you mean by a career like mine. If your goal is to become an academic bioethicist, the path I followed is forever closed. In the late 1960s, when I made the first moves that culminated in my becoming a bioethicist, the word "bioethics" had just been invented. In the early 1970s it was said that a person of average intelligence and energy could read the entire literature of bioethics in one month and in the next month could become a contributor to that literature. Now that the field has had some time to mature, one must have credentials to enter it. A physician who wishes to pursue a career as a scholar in bioethics should either get an additional degree in a field such as philosophy, law, history, or ethics or find some other way to have an equivalent experience. The goal of this exercise is to learn how to think about the subject matter as a scholar in the humanities. This will help you appreciate the subtleties of philosophical or legal analysis and thereby become a better critic of and contributor to the literature of your field. As a physician-ethicist you will begin with an advantage over the typical philosopher. The philosopher may know well how to analyze the problems of medicine but not necessarily know which problems are worthy of analysis or what it is about those problems that physicians find problematic. There are, of course, some noteworthy exceptions. Many of them have spent a good deal of time immersing themselves in the experience of medicine.

I want to distinguish the career of a scholar in bioethics from that of a teacher of or consultant in bioethics. One can become a very good teacher or consultant with much less formal preparation. There are excellent one- or two-year postdoctoral fellowships at several medical schools that are designed to prepare health care professionals for such a career.

If, on the other hand, what you mean by a career like mine is to follow the leads life offers to engage in some of the most exciting medical developments of your time, something different is required. You must have confidence that the path you have chosen will be exciting and important. (Yes, in the 1960s, clinical pharmacology was that exciting and important.) You must be willing to make commitments that some of your colleagues won't understand. In the 1970s, in the academic medical setting, philosophy and history were generally regarded as activities pursued by emeritus deans or department chairs. My age peers in the 1970s expressed concern that I was aging prematurely. I have no regrets about having chosen bioethics when I did; it was the right choice for me at the time. Now it's a different time in a different world. If I were thirty years younger today I might have a go at anthropology.

Conducting Patient-Centered Research

B y the time I was a Yale undergraduate I knew I would be a doctor. My father is a physician, and from a young age I accompanied him to the hospital on Sunday mornings when he visited his patients. From those experiences I became familiar with the rhythm of the patient–doctor relationship—its special intimacy and the opportunity it afforded a physician to make a positive difference for someone who needed help.

Teachers told me that the path to medicine was through science, and I gained the usual experiences. I majored in biology and spent summers in research laboratories. Although I enjoyed asking questions and finding answers, I also found that my interest in medicine naturally took me beyond basic science. I took classes in psychology, sociology, philosophy, history, religious studies, and English literature. I wondered whether I could find a medical career that would allow me to explore all my interests.

In my junior year, as part of a Yale internship program, I spent my spring term living in a rural community in western North Carolina where I worked on a research project for the Office of Rural Health Services. I evaluated the impact of community clinics staffed by nurse practitioners in medically underserved areas. I tried to gauge the effect these clinics had on the people of Clingman, North Carolina, by surveying patients, clinic staff, and the people who lived in the area. I also tried to determine whether this model was viable and generalizable (that is, applicable to other areas; other sites throughout the state had begun similar efforts to combat the doctor shortage in rural areas). I learned that the most important advances made in biomedical laboratories would not be of help to these people if they had no access to care.

At graduation, I received a Yale traveling fellowship to study rural health services in England, Sweden, India, and China. I had been accepted to medical school but decided that the opportunity to travel was worth my having to reapply to medical school the following year. Because the traveling fellowship was as much about my personal development and broadening my perspective as it was about producing scholarly work, I felt free to improvise. In England and Sweden I visited general practitioners in rural practices and interviewed them and their patients about the quality of care. In India and China I focused on one region and examined different strategies to improve population health. The year taught me about the immense variation in medical practice and health care delivery, with important implications for the health of a population. Again, I saw that the way medicine is organized and medical care is delivered makes a difference.

In medical school, in the midst of the basic science curriculum that characterizes the first two years, I developed an opportunity to work in a neighborhood health clinic in Roxbury, one of the most economically depressed neighborhoods of Boston. In the middle of Boston, a medical Mecca, I found an underserved community that suffered many of the same problems one finds in underdeveloped countries or in rural counties of the United States. The best medical science and care was not finding its way to those living in Roxbury. I wondered how I might find a place in medicine in which I could improve the care and outcomes of vulnerable and underserved populations.

After my initial experiences on clinical wards, I attended a class that helped me find my niche. At that point, I was looking for a way to combine my interest in medicine, health care, and research in order to make a difference. The monthlong course covered a wide range of topics about applied clinical research. This discipline employed the rigorous and evolving methodology of clinical epidemiology and health services research, was directed toward improving clinical decision making and health care delivery, and was about identifying opportunities to improve care. The teachers of the course had a deep understanding of the medical literature; they knew the strength of the evidence and its relevance to individual patients. One teacher who particularly inspired me was Lee Goldman, a cardiologist, who later became my medical school advisor.

Here in the field of applied clinical research, I realized, was the way to be a "triple threat" in today's era of specialization. The research was about better patient care and health care delivery. And both contribute to making one a better teacher and an even better clinician.

During my residency I devoted myself to becoming the best clinician I could be. Although I pursued a couple of research projects in my last two years as a resident, I focused primarily on patient care. Subsequently, during my cardiology fellowship, I earned a master's degree in health policy and management and began to acquire the methodological skills I needed to do applied clinical research. After my fellowship, Yale University offered me an opportunity to develop a position that would allow me to see patients, conduct research, and teach—and particularly to enjoy the freedom to define the research questions I believed were important to pursue.

I found no shortage of important topics. Although advances in medical care are extending our ability to prevent disease and cure illness, our health care system is under stress. Far too many Americans lack health insurance, and many others encounter barriers to the care they need. The current system of payment for medical services has evolved to address acute disease, and lacks the proper incentives to optimize the care of patients with chronic disease, conditions that afflict an increasing number of Americans. The cost of care is rising rapidly, but the benefit of the additional investments is marginal. Perverse financial incentives put the economic interests of individuals and institutions in conflict with those of patients and society. We know far too little about the effectiveness of clinical and public health strategies to promote the health of populations.

In addition, decisions for individual patients rarely incorporate precise estimates of risk and benefit. Studies document a staggering variation in the quality of care that results in marked disparities in the outcomes of patients. Large gaps exist in translating best practice to

392   CONDUCTING BIOMEDICAL RESEARCH

the bedside. Medical errors occur far too commonly, and too little effort has been directed toward creating a safe health care system that optimizes health and compassionately treats patients at the end of life. Thus, at the cusp of a dramatic expansion of the power of medicine, we are challenged by the realization that health care delivery has not kept pace with the contemporary needs of our society. And yet, if we ask the right questions and apply the appropriate methods, we can generate knowledge that can directly improve the practice of medicine and the care of patients.

As I began my research, I realized that I wanted to do work that would improve the practice of medicine in these areas. As a rule, I do not see the publication of a paper as the end product of my work. I see papers and research projects as a means to understand how we should achieve positive change and disseminate knowledge that may help others. The potential of my work, I believe, will be realized only if health care professionals or policy makers incorporate it into practice.

So I searched for and found a perfect place for myself, where I have had many perfect days. These days are filled with interactions with colleagues, patients, and students. The collaborative research often involves investigators from various backgrounds. In some cases we find novel uses of existing data; in other projects we need to collect currently unavailable information. Good research requires us to question conventional wisdom often and to generate, always, knowledge that matters. For me, applied clinical research—generating knowledge that makes a difference for people whom I will never know—is immensely gratifying. Seeing individual patients and helping people I *do* know is also a privilege. My familiarity with the margins of uncertainty in medical evidence has committed me to a style of practice that is participatory and seeks to engage patients in the important decisions concerning their care. Finally, these days commonly provide the chance to mentor or teach others at important junctures in their professional development. In that process, I can share my perspectives and learn from others.

Most days I can't believe that I get paid for this work. I am never aware that what I am doing has anything to do with receiving compensation. Like most physicians, I find that my biggest and most important challenge is to find a balance in my life. I am married and have four children. Although I am fully engaged in my career, my family is my priority—and it is their love and support that is essential to my success.

As you embark upon your careers, do not compromise on the goal of finding the place where you can make the best contribution— where your effort produces good work—and where you can feel that the days are never long enough.

JEFFREYR.BENDER

A Career as Physician-Scientist
Is It Worth the Effort?

I have become fascinated by the reasons medical school applicants offer for wanting to dive into the medical profession. It seems some unique aspect of our developmental years has driven each of us in that direction. For me, two factors motivated my thinking about professions in college. First, I always liked science; I suppose it appealed to my intellectual curiosity, as well as to my sense of logic. Second, as we all do, I had a life experience that dictated, in part, my future endeavors. My mother died from breast cancer when I was fourteen. This, of course, did not fit with my logical impressions of the world.

While in college, I thought that a career in "medical research" would give me a chance to provide new information that might help fight human disease, while allowing me to be involved with something I seemed to enjoy. I thought about going to graduate school and developing a career as a scientist. Although not particularly knowledgeable about the differences between graduate and medical school, my father reasoned that if I were truly interested in medical research, why not go to medical school? I would gain the perspective of medicine and would not exclude the possibility of entering the world of science. He thought this would provide a greater breadth of options and opportunities. Although I have come to know that a career as a scientist with a Ph.D. can be very productive and exciting, my father was, in fact, correct: my opportunities as a physician-scientist have been diverse and nearly unlimited.

I had the good fortune to attend medical school at University of California, San Francisco, a school that not only conducts premier research but also emphasizes the highest level of clinical expertise and humanistic qualities in training its students. It was at that time that I began to understand the ways in which medicine and science complement each other, and that a career based on the best of both could be incredibly fulfilling. I started to believe that I could have an impact on people's lives, both in the short term, by providing direct patient care, and in the much longer term, by contributing to medical science. My choice of clinical specialty and research training disciplines also required the merging of seemingly disparate approaches. I chose internal medicine and cardiology because I had enjoyed them during school and residency. I chose, on the basis of a smoldering intellectual interest, to do my research training in basic immunology. I understood that there was little precedent for combining immunology with cardiology, but I thought I could find a creative way to do it.

By the time I finished my training in clinical cardiology and immunology research, several things had become clear. First, I knew I was enthralled with both clinical cardiology and immunology research. Second, some early, developing general interest in the effects of inflammation and immunity on the vascular wall appeared fertile ground for career development. Third, I realized it was not necessary for me to choose between patient care and basic research. If well trained, I could work in both arenas. This would require focusing on priorities and working within an extremely supportive department.

I was fortunate to be offered a faculty appointment in such an environment. I was told I could maintain my "identity" as a trained cardiologist by being a member of a cardiology division, continuing to deliver patient care, albeit on a limited basis, one day a week and one or two months a year as an attending physician in the hospital. I was also told—in no uncertain terms—that the basis for my recruitment was my research program, which I would be given the opportunity to develop. This unequivocal message certainly helped me focus early on my academic faculty career. I realized that to conduct research at the highest level and to obtain grants, I would need to devote most of my time to research. I accepted this conceptually, although not without a struggle with the "concept."

I feared a loss of identity and that others might perceive me as not "clinically competent." Through hospital rotations, I assumed responsibility for various patients and wondered whether, because of my focus on research, I would be available to provide the highest level of patient care. I also wondered, naturally, whether I could be a successful, independent medical scientist. These insecurities and fears conspired against my peace of mind. However, my love of both patient care and research, as well as my sense of excitement about pursuing a combined career, have always sustained me and diminished my insecurities and negative feelings.

Another advantage, I found, of choosing to be a physician-scientist is the location required to pursue such a career. Although there are exceptions, the most favorable environment is within a university medical center, at a medical school. I am not sure what the best definition of "professor" is, but my career in medicine and medical science has allowed me to take a professorial approach, one that has been very fulfilling. I interact with colleagues who are leaders in their fields of clinical medicine and/or biomedical research. I am in constant contact with students and trainees at all levels while teaching in the classroom, the hospital, or the laboratory. The common devotion to generating new information founded on creative ideas and novel approaches generates an aura of unity within my university medical center. I cannot think of a more fertile and exciting place to develop and maintain a career.

The career of a physician-scientist carries with it several advantages. Some of these relate to the independent, positive aspects of being a physician or a scientist. Physicians have opportunities to become personally involved in the lives of their patients and patients' families. Each patient can and should be cherished, and our approach should be as empathic as possible. Amid serious acute or even terminal illness, a physician who holds these values can have a positive impact on a patient's life. In many ways, it is a privilege to be in such a position, and the immediate personal rewards are immense. Beyond "the diagnosis," or the technical aspects of clinical medicine, I would miss these personal interactions if I did not have them.

For a scientist, the daily rewards are quite different. They include the tremendous satisfaction derived from generating a new hypothesis, designing a new experiment, obtaining experimental results that promote further development of that hypothesis, and interacting with colleagues on an intellectual basis. Furthermore, the training of future physician-scientists (and Ph.D. scientists) carries with it many interpersonal rewards. In general, the greatest accomplishments are achieved not on a daily basis but over years, if not one's entire career. Many of my friends who are not in science ask, "When are you going to get the Nobel Prize?" I always laugh and tell them that although our goals are set high, small but consistent contributions to understanding human biology and disease are the norm. Although most of these small contributions will not win a Nobel Prize, they are important and rewarding. Overall, one needs to have long-term vision and patience. Science is intellectually stimulating, conceptually and practically exciting, but the rewards are gained at a much slower pace than the daily feedback one receives in other areas of medicine. The opportunity to experience both types of rewards is, in essence, an indulgence.

Each component of a physician-scientist's career contributes to the other, continuously. That is, scientists are trained to think in a very critical and analytical way, and their problem solving skills are heightened. These skills are enormously useful in approaching difficult clinical situations, those that require interpretive analysis. Conversely, involvement in patient care provides a scientist with continued insight into key problems and questions in human biology, those that can be formulated in such a way as to be addressed in the basic laboratory. Thus, one's fundamental research can always be performed in a directed, clinical context. Furthermore, we have recently entered the era of "molecular medicine." Efforts are expanding to apply basic, molecular discoveries to patient care. The term "translational research" has been proposed, which means that molecular and genetic discoveries will be translated into clinical studies, usually with animal models as intermediaries. Physician-scientists, who understand both basic research and clinical medicine, are the ones best equipped to lead these exciting new translational efforts.

In addition to all these positive aspects of a combined career, some disadvantages exist. The first difficulty one encounters both practically and emotionally is the training time required to become proficient and independent both in clinical medicine and in science. Today, one can independently practice clinical cardiology after medical school and six years of residency and fellowship training. My post–medical school training, which included an internal medicine residency, a clinical cardiology fellowship, and basic immunology research training, consumed nine years. With some of the progressive, streamlined, and individualized training programs available today, this nine-year period could be as "short" as seven years, not terribly different from the training period for a clinical cardiologist or a Ph.D. scientist. Certainly there are no true shortcuts, as training in two related but different disciplines necessarily takes longer than either alone. This "no shortcut" mentality is important to embrace, because it would be the greatest disservice to pursue a dual career but be inadequately trained and/or prematurely independent. Although long in duration, my training was actually an extremely enjoyable and rewarding phase of my professional career. After all, the decision to enter the world of academic medicine is based, in part, on a love of learning and on a constant desire to challenge intellectual limits. Those attributes defined the years I spent in both clinical and research training.

Going into debt, however, can be a major concern. I did incur some debt, but I was fortunate to attend a state university medical school, and this minimized the debt load. Fortunately, after medical school, the training years were compensated by salaries that prevented me from accumulating further financial burden. This advantage is sometimes offset by family responsibilities, as it is common for marriage and children to come along during the later stages of training. In fact, the last couple of years of rather protracted training can seem suspended in time in relation to the normal progression of adult life. To deal with these added responsibilities, trainees commonly "moonlight" at this stage, spending some of their off-hours each month working in a local emergency room or clinic. This work generally pays well, and the benefits of the extra monthly income can be substantial. Although this extended training period sounds burdensome, it is really a small price to pay for the opportunity to have such an exciting career. Of course, one's family must concur with this "cost-benefit analysis" and provide the emotional support and encouragement to complete the necessary training.

Another consideration for the potential physician-scientist is the demand on time. As you might imagine, being either a physician or a scientist is a full-time endeavor. Being both requires tremendous dedication if you are to perform at the highest level. It has become clear to me that life requires important choices and prioritization. I am now convinced that it is possible to function effectively as a "part-time physician" if you have been trained properly and participate in a strong clinical department. Through reading and interacting with your colleagues, staying current in clinical practice is possible. The basic instincts in delivering patient care, including empathy and concern for patients and their families, are never lost. These qualities define the core of an outstanding physician.

Furthermore, the challenges of being a productive scientist are great. They include developing, running, and continuously funding a research laboratory, all of which requires an emphasis that goes beyond the "50–50" approach. However, a variety of paradigms can work, and the "right" one depends upon the individual and the exact nature of his or her efforts and goals. The bottom line is that many hours are required, and difficult choices must be made continually. Most of us start our faculty careers at a time when we have young families. I have always given my family a high priority, and my decisions about hours spent must include time on the Little League field or at a school play. Despite the heavy demands on a physician-scientist's time, you can and should continue to place priority on your personal life.

A major disadvantage to a physician-scientist's career is more specific to science. When a physician achieves a level of excellence, his or her talents are generally accepted, often in perpetuity. In contrast, the peer review system requires that physician-scientists provide continuing evidence of their ability. They do this by submitting scientific manuscripts for publication and receiving favorable reviews of grant applications. This is part of the system, one to which we become accustomed and that makes good sense. However, a level of personal confidence is necessary to this process, especially during the early period of a career.

A career as a physician-scientist is as rewarding and exciting as any I can imagine. The goals are high, and the rewards are great. The amazing spectrum of opportunities allows you to make choices that fit best with your talents and desires. The diversity of daily experiences is phenomenal. If you possess the motivation, ability to focus, self-confidence, and patience to develop such a career, your life can be truly exciting. For me, a fascination with science, the death of a parent at a young age, and some good advice from a father who was not in the field all contributed to my decision to become a physician-scientist. As a result I am in the best professional place I can imagine. Yes, it is worth the effort, and the future is bright.

FRED**GORELICK**

The Path to Laboratory Research

P aths in life are formed like the weather: sometimes we are guided by the contours of the landscape, as when we are influenced by the actions of others; and sometimes we are pushed forward by our own internal forces.

My father was a physician. He had a deep respect for life, but as a pathologist he often dealt with that issue in retrospect. Presented with individuals at life's end, he read the map of their medical sojourn by examining the color, shape, and distortion of their organs. I first saw him conduct an autopsy when I was twelve. The patient was a middle-aged man who had died of pneumonia. As soon as the chest was opened the story was told. Mixed with the uniform pale pink colors of the lungs were discreet black deposits. The largest was the size of a pepper seed. The colors and textures were remarkable to my eye (I've used their combination more than once for the backgrounds of paintings I've done as an adult). My father guided my gloved forefinger across the surface of the lung. Its volume was easily compressed except in one area where it felt like a bone lay just below the surface. "Another coal miner with lung cancer," he said. He confirmed that diagnosis a moment later as he cut into the hardened region. Although that particular case was not among the most challenging my father saw, I knew he thrived on solving mysteries. And for him, the most irresistible mystery was why a life had ended.

The mission of the medical school I attended was to produce

physicians who would take care of patients. I think it did quite well at this task. Though research was a respected activity, it was not included in our curriculum. After a medical residency, I began a gastroenterology fellowship at Yale University, intending to return to the Ozark hills in two years to care for patients. Two insights gained during my second year of fellowship changed that goal. First, research was given a very high priority in my new environment. Second, a good friend several years my senior was frustrated by the boredom and lack of stimulation he found in private medical practice. The opportunity to experience a new aspect of medicine, solve novel forms of mystery, and avoid the possible monotony of private practice was an irresistible draw; I signed up for a third year of fellowship, just to do research. Once that decision was made, I faced the classic first question in an investigative career: What kind of work will I do?

The initial decision in a research career is choosing between research involving human subjects and research that excludes them—often called basic science. I chose the latter based upon my reading of scientific manuscripts and interacting with faculty. The "Methods" section of scientific manuscripts reveals the fundamental differences between the two types of research. Humans are not uniform; variations in human physiology make it very difficult to reliably compare groups. Furthermore, differences in diet, use of over-the-counter medications, and myriad environmental and social factors are difficult to control. Finally, the mechanics of organizing human studies can be daunting. In contrast, basic science studies can be performed under highly controlled conditions. Rats, mice, or cells in culture are bred on a defined genetic background, fed the same diet, and grown under uniform conditions. Enzymes can be purified and removed from the influence of other molecules. Thus, a fundamental difference between human investigations and basic science is the ability to control study conditions and to generate reliable results. Weighed against this ability, however, is the questionable relevance to humans of studies focusing on rodents or transformed cells. Uncomfortable with the uncertainty that accompanies human studies, I chose the path of basic science. That decision brought only momentary comfort, because I then needed to select a laboratory and a subject.

Trainees who achieve success early in their laboratory investigations are more likely to continue their careers in research. One's initial studies should not be too ambitious—begin with a low-risk project that has well-defined end points and requires no technical development. Although addressing a question in a relevant field is desirable, it is not essential early in a career. The methods and tools of science have now spread across most scientific disciplines. What is learned in one type of cell or tissue system is generally applicable to another. The goal is excellent training. A good training environment has several essential elements: the laboratory should be focused, experienced, successful, and supportive. There must be opportunity for close contact with either the primary investigator or other trained individuals in the laboratory. Basic science research should be a major focus there, with regular laboratory meetings and scientific seminars. A research project must be carefully outlined and time-dependent goals established when the trainee enters the laboratory. Since many trainees enter research six to eight years after learning basic science in medical school, some direct teaching is necessary. The best environment for consistently successful training is probably in a basic science department. However, some laboratories in clinical departments are excellent. On the advice of my first mentor, I left his laboratory in a clinical department and spent the next four years in a basic science department laboratory.

The idea that one can achieve at the highest levels as both clinician and investigator is unrealistic. It arose at a time when research was evolving more slowly, competition for research support was less, and clinical responsibilities were more limited. Both clinical practice and research are worthy enterprises, but it is difficult and even self-defeating to pursue both at the highest levels. After six years of struggling to fill both clinical and research roles, I resolved to give up the goal of being a consummate clinician. This was a difficult and risky decision; not only would it disappoint some of my advisors, but I was leaving the safe haven of clinical care, where the rewards are more predictable and frequent than those of research.

For me, the answer was to reframe the issue. I was able to find a path that allowed me to remain in clinical medicine and, similar to my research, to become focused on a single organ and topic: the pancreas and the role of a particular kind of cell in pancreatitis. That decision allowed me to become an expert in a clinical area without the weight of heavier expectations. As a result, I was appointed to the pancreatic section of my professional society's research council and to editorships on two biomedical journals for studies related to the pancreas. The decision also made my clinical role manageable and allowed me time for research. A successful and enjoyable research career comes with careful planning. Although clinical practice has great rewards, they can be sampled only in moderation if one is to thrive doing research.

Where did this research take me, and what did I learn along the way? My early work identified an enzyme in the pancreas that we thought was important for regulating secretion. The same enzyme was also found in the brain, but in concentrations a thousandfold higher. This made studying the function of the enzyme potentially much easier, so I moved to studies of the central nervous system. Our laboratory spent the next seven years examining the brain enzyme. During this period, tools were developed for studying the enzyme in the gastrointestinal tract, and this is the topic we now pursue. The lesson I learned during this period was that scientists appreciate good science independent of the system being examined. My grants were funded, I was asked to speak about my work, and I brought knowledge of an emerging research area back to gastroenterologists.

Another lesson I learned was to stay on target. Successful research requires a tightly focused project. A common concern among young investigators is the fear that they will have no ideas. Soon after embarking on a research path, however, they realize there are multitudes of questions; with scientific maturity comes the understanding that one cannot pursue everything that is potentially important, fruitful, or engaging. Taking on too many projects is a common pitfall for many young investigators. With scientific maturity also comes the realization that some hypotheses may be plausible but can't be proved—learn when to stop pursuing a topic and change direction.

Research prospers through communication. The exchange of ideas among peers and more seasoned investigators is a crucial part of the experience. Exchanges take place at the lab bench, in lab meetings, during visits to other institutions, at conferences, and through the written word. Although large conferences often attract the greatest attention, small, focused meetings hold the greatest value. Limited conference size, remote location, and allocation of free time make these settings ideal for meeting senior investigators. The importance of such encounters extends beyond the exchange of ideas. Establishing networks and exchanging valuable probes are critical outcomes of these conversations.

The importance of verbal and writing skills to successful research cannot be overstated. These talents do not come naturally and require careful development. Two mistakes commonly made in oral presentations are failing to provide a clearly stated hypothesis or adequate background, and presenting too much data. Slides must be simple and should provide one message at a time with smooth, sensible transitions. The audience can take away only a few facts; if they are confused or overwhelmed, they will remember little or nothing. Finally, an audience cannot absorb information for more than forty-five minutes, and in a one-hour talk the presenter must leave time for questions.

Attending scientific seminars is an important part of the scientific process. I always enter a conference with two goals. The first is to broadly advance my understanding of science. The second is to find connections or applications of others' work to my interests. Science now moves very rapidly; it is important to be aware of the latest techniques and concepts.

Skillful writing is integral to the scientific process; it is the major mechanism for communicating ideas and obtaining grants. Prose should be concise, precise, and compelling. Scientific papers are read for their content. The reader's time is limited, and wordy monologues will be ignored. Successful papers also provide recipes; research must be reproducible, and the methods and observations must be described with this goal in mind. Finally, the text should convince readers that the findings are important and valid. For most, the effort required to generate a sound scientific manuscript is considerable. A two-page manuscript we once published in the journal *Nature,* for example, was revised twenty-eight times before it was submitted.

Requesting support for one's research is often viewed as one of the drawbacks of basic science research, but it has some advantages. Work plans and research goals must be carefully considered over the long range. Achievements are weighed in the granting process and serve as a reminder that work must be published. However, I never spend more time on scientific text than I do when applying for a grant. (Lack of clarity, poor organization, and grammatical errors cause many grant applications to be rejected.) Other factors that lead to success are learned through experience. I advise our junior faculty to read several successful grant applications; their structure and verbiage are remarkably similar. Ask senior investigators to review your proposals. Common problems, such as an overambitious plan or lack of controls, can be easily corrected. When taking the long view, try to ask important research questions, especially ones that others are not working on.

The future of basic biomedical research looks very bright. One great advantage of entering a basic science career at this moment is the prospect for funding. In the 1990s, the National Institutes of Health was funding only between 5 and 10 percent of applications. During the first decade of 2000, that funding rate has doubled or tripled, and the prospects are good for continued increases. This fact ameliorates an onerous burden of research: obtaining financial support. To take full advantage of these advances in support, however, the clinical loads now being placed on many investigators must decrease.

A successful scientific career can provide great satisfaction. My path has been driven by curiosity, a reverence for life, and, as was true for my father, the joy of solving mysteries. These rewards are different from those that come from patient care, and they come less frequently. A passion for research and patience are required to stay the course. Among those exhilarating intellectual moments in science, much can be gained from its aesthetic. Take time to appreciate the beauty inherent in your field of science—from the complexity of its finely tuned interactions to its visual and artistic appeal. Research leaves no time for boredom.

PERRYL.MILLER

Medical Informatics
Computers and Patient Care

When I was growing up, modern computers were just being invented. As a result, I did not have a chance to learn about them when I was young, the way my children have. I took a short course in Fortran (an early computer language) as part of a summer job, and then took my first full computer course as a senior in college. It took me a while to decide what I wanted to do with my life. I liked science but didn't want to spend my life inside a research laboratory. I wanted to work with people in the real world. At the same time, there was something appealing about the computer. The computer is a laboratory for exploring ideas, for taking a difficult problem and working first to understand it and then to solve it.

In the process of exploring how these interests might all fit together, I went to graduate school for a Ph.D. in computer science, and then went to medical school and did my residency training in anesthesiology. Since that time, my main activity has involved combining computers and medicine in various ways while working in an academic medical center. I currently serve as director of the Yale Center for Medical Informatics, which I helped found.

Medical informatics is an emerging field at the intersection of medicine, computer science, and the information sciences. My first approach to medical informatics involved exploring how the computer might help the physician with patient care. When people think about the computer helping with patient care, they tend to think about diagnosis. The aspect of patient care that most interests me, however, is treatment. When a patient is in the hospital, for example, the doctor typically sees that patient once or twice a day for fairly brief periods of time. In between, the doctor is seeing many different patients with many different medical problems. It is hard for the doctor to keep a sharp focus on all the possible issues involved in each patient's care, and there is a real opportunity for the computer to help in this process. The computer is good at being methodical. Human beings have trouble keeping all aspects of a problem in mind at all times, particularly when they have to switch rapidly from one problem to another. At the very least, the computer can help prevent a doctor from overlooking certain aspects of a patient's care.

When I started working on these problems, a particular interest of mine was developing computer programs that *critique* a physician's plan for patient care. Most clinical advice systems being developed at that time tried to tell the physician how to practice medicine. Yet, with most medical problems there is seldom one and only one way to proceed. Different doctors have different practice styles and preferences, even when they are experts in a field. For example, the Yale expert and the Harvard expert may have very different approaches to certain medical problems. With this in mind, I felt it would be better to let the doctor first describe a patient and the plans for that patient's care. Then the computer could indicate, as politely and constructively as possible, what is positive about that approach and what might be done differently.

A second interest of mine involves access to network-based information. As more and more clinical materials—including textbooks, journal articles, and multimedia teaching units—are being made accessible over the Internet, it would be useful for the computer to be able to lead the physician to network-based information in the context of a particular patient's care. Ideally, the computer could look at a patient's electronic medical record and produce a list of clinical topics relevant to that patient's care. If the physician is interested in a particular topic, the computer could then lead the doctor to very specific material about that topic. This idealized scenario contrasts with the problems anyone currently faces when trying to retrieve information via the Web. We are deluged by a flood of information of variable quality that for the most part is not relevant to the problem at hand. I and my colleagues are currently developing a program we call ClinQuest, which will provide topic-driven retrieval for use within Yale's anesthesiology training program. When a patient is going to have surgery, for example, this system will list information important to that patient's anesthetic management. When an anesthesiology resident clicks on a topic, ClinQuest will produce a summary of the issues involved, followed by a set of Web pointers to preselected material discussing aspects of that particular topic in more detail.

Although my clinical specialty is anesthesiology, my work in medical informatics permits me to collaborate with doctors in many other fields, including internal medicine, surgery, pathology, laboratory medicine, diagnostic radiology, and psychiatry. Because I have training in both medicine and computer science, and intuitions about a problem from both a clinical and a computing point of view, I can serve as a "translator" between the two fields. The dual backgrounds, I believe, not only help me identify clinical problems to solve but also give me a sense of how best to use the computer to solve them in a clinically useful way.

In the past fifteen years, I have worked extensively with bioscientists as well as with clinicians. One bioscience project involved collaborating with computer scientists at Yale to explore the use of parallel computation in various bioscience applications. Parallel computation involves breaking a computation down into pieces that can be run simultaneously ("in parallel") on different machines, so computation is done more quickly.

There's been a dramatic explosion of work that applies informatics in the biosciences. In particular, several major projects related to the genome are going on at Yale right now. The human genome is essentially the blueprint of the human species. It contains all the genes that make us what we are. Once the human genome is fully sequenced and we know what all the genes are, however, the challenging problems will be just beginning. We need to understand what all the genes do, both in normal life processes and in disease. Major breakthroughs in biomedical computing research and massive amounts of computing will be required simply to begin to achieve this understanding. As a physician in the field of medical informatics, I will feel particularly ful-filled when we are finally able to relate all this information and under-standing to clinical medicine and, specifically, to the diagnosis and treatment of disease.

In addition to working in *clinical* informatics and *genome* in-formatics for the past seven years, I have been collaborating with neu-roscientists as part of the national Human Brain Project, in the newly named field of *neuro*informatics. People are doing research within neuroscience at many different levels ranging from the genetic, molec-ular receptor, and neuronal levels all the way up to the levels of brain pathways, systems, and behavior. The research includes imaging a cell's microanatomy and the brain's gross anatomy under many experi-mental conditions. It includes neurophysiology, pharmacology, and biochemistry. At each of these levels, scientists are generating large amounts of experimental data that can be stored in the computer. To understand a neuroscience phenomenon fully, however, one needs to link information tightly at many different levels so that it can be ana-lyzed in an integrated way. A particularly interesting way of analyzing the information involves using computer models that employ experi-mental data to make predictions that can then be tested by experiments in the laboratory. The results of these further experiments can then serve to refine the model, and so on. We are exploring these issues at Yale in the SenseLab project using the sense of smell as a model domain.

Informatics fascinates me because it intersects with virtually all areas of clinical medicine and the biosciences. Depending on a person's interests, informatics provides the opportunity to delve into one area very deeply, or to collaborate broadly with many different people in many fields, exploring all sorts of very different problems. I try to keep a fairly deep level of involvement in informatics projects in clinical deci-sion making. At the same time, though, I enjoy being involved in a wide range of other projects where other people do most of the work, but where I can help keep things moving in interesting directions.

A major activity at the Center for Medical Informatics involves training young physicians and bioscientists who want to enter the field. In general, these are people who have always been intrigued by com-puters but who have made the decision to go to medical school or into the biological sciences. They then decide that they would like to combine their interests in computers and biomedical science. Being part of the training program gives them the opportunity not only to learn about informatics but also to share their interests with like-minded fellow trainees and faculty. The National Library of Medicine, which currently supports much of this training in medical informatics, also organizes a number of seminars and courses. These provide one way to learn more about the field. Another resource is the American Medical Informatics Association.

The following Web links provide a good starting point for people interested in learning more about medical informatics:

Yale Center for Medical Informatics: *http://ycmi.med.yale.edu/*
SenseLab: *http://senselab.med.yale.edu/senselab/*
Human Brain Project: *http://www.nimh.nih.gov/neuroinformatics/ index.cfm*
National Library of Medicine: *www.nlm.nih.gov*
American Medical Informatics Association: *www.amia.org*

SUSAN**HOCKFIELD**

The Rewards of a Life in Science

From the time I was a very young child, I've been fascinated by the mystery of how biological systems work. A
modestly greater natural ability in science and math, relative to language arts and history, propelled me toward
medical school. And, much as the biological side of things
fascinated me, aspects of medicine appealed less. I was enormously
fortunate to approach a professor in an advanced cell biology course
in college (the most exciting course I had ever taken) with a question
about how one might determine the structure of a particular subcellu-
lar structure he had described in class. His startling answer was, "Why
don't you do that experiment?" It had never before occurred to me
that the frontiers of science were advanced by people like me. In my
view at the time, scientists were almost mythical figures. I hadn't understood that scientists were, in fact, my teachers and that my university was brimming with discoveries made by a large community of mere
mortals, which I might aspire to join.

Instead of applying to medical school, I found a position as a
starting-level technician in a neurobiology laboratory in a medical
school anatomy department. The laboratory experience was simply in-
toxicating. The ideas discussed every day in the lab provided intellectual stimulation beyond any I had encountered in any course; the techniques I learned created miraculous windows into the workings of cells
in the brain; and the literature was filled with new ideas and new ways
to think about fascinating problems. And perhaps most encouraging

of all was that the community of the laboratory—technicians, graduate students, postdoctoral fellows, and faculty—provided a perfect combination of support, challenge, and humor. I found another near-perfect balance in the combined demands for advanced technical and intellectual competence. The two years I spent as a research technician prepared me in critical ways for a Ph.D. program in graduate school and for my future career as a neuroscientist. I encourage young people who are thinking about a career in science to seek out an opportunity for a real-life experience in a lab before entering graduate school. The time is rarely wasted; valuable skills can be readily learned, and the experience can help you make decisions about future research directions.

Graduate study for a Ph.D., like many kinds of advanced study, can be exceedingly challenging. Over the course of doctoral education, you learn to learn in new and independent ways. You learn to read, interpret, and use primary literature in written papers and in experiments. You also learn to present ideas in published manuscripts, in the classroom, and in seminars and other public settings. Perhaps the most challenging aspect of doctoral study is the degree of independence required. Independent thought can be exhilarating, but it can also be a lonely enterprise! Most doctoral programs in the biological sciences require from four to six years, which can seem a very long time to still be in school when your college friends have already started jobs. But for many, the years in graduate school are golden years, the time in which self-definition and self-understanding reach new levels, and a period during which you can indulge your intellectual curiosity with near-monomaniacal intensity.

If you've decided that graduate study is for you, it is important to choose a program that suits your interests and needs. Some programs require that you know your research area with some precision at the start, others provide a year or two to select a laboratory for a dissertation project. An increasing number of programs offer considerable flexibility among the subfields in the biological sciences. These programs are usually receptive to students who already have well-formed ideas of their research directions as well as to students who would like to explore a range of possibilities.

I had the very good fortune to conduct my thesis research in a large research group at the National Institutes of Health. Here again, the community of scientists was central to the richness of the intellectual experience. My Ph.D. advisor was a neuroanatomist, but we had almost daily conversations with neurophysiologists, psychologists, pharmacologists, and clinicians in our group. At least several times a week a few of us would gather for lunch in the cafeteria, where we would informally and spontaneously discuss our latest results, papers we had read, or seminars we had attended. This experience set in place an important pattern for me: to seek out other scientists, no matter what their field or their stature, as I design and then interpret my own studies. I encourage young scientists to engage other scientists in discussion; it will expand your range of thought and also your community of peers.

Although graduate study was challenging for me, it was also a time of immense personal satisfaction. I learned topics that seemed beyond me at first, completed new and difficult experiments, wrote papers and had them accepted for publication, and presented my work at local and national meetings. A doctoral program transforms a student into a colleague and a scholar. Meeting and discussing science with local colleagues, and also with scientists from other institutions and countries whose work I have read and respected, remains among the greatest joys of scientific life.

"Where to go next?" must be answered at many junctures over the course of a scientist's life. A wise senior colleague advised me to choose each position based on where I could do my best work. Each individual will have a different optimal set of conditions for doing his or her best work. "Where to go next?" must be answered when you choose a graduate program. Once in a program, you will need to choose a laboratory for a dissertation project; you will then select a laboratory for postdoctoral study; and then you will decide where to continue your career. Most young scientists have more than a single option at each of these choice-points. My senior colleague's advice is worth heeding, but each individual needs to determine the significant variables at each juncture. Do you enjoy working with a small group or a large group? Do you prefer to work on your own or in closely knit teams? Do you enjoy a competitive environment or do you prefer a more collegial style? Do you flourish when you can concentrate on a limited set of topics or do you prefer to have access to a wide range of ideas? For example, you may enter a graduate program that permits you to carry out "rotations," brief (one- to three-month) research projects in several labs to help you choose a lab for your dissertation research. During the rotations, you should look for a lab that is intellectually stimulating and that has a "personality," or patterns of interaction, with which you feel comfortable.

Currently, a Ph.D. degree in the biological sciences can lead to a variety of exciting careers. The more classical academic routes, which lead to a research university or to a medical school or to a four-year college, continue to attract many scientists. However, the burgeoning pharmaceutical and biotech industries now offer additional, fresh possibilities. Beyond these, Ph.D. recipients now have the opportunity to enter less traditional career paths, such as publishing, investment banking, and consulting. Many graduate schools have offices and programs designed to help graduate students learn about different career options.

My career has unfolded in several kinds of academic settings, each of which has afforded distinct opportunities. During graduate school, I took my courses and had teaching opportunities in a basic science department of a medical school, while I carried out my research in a national science laboratory that was independent of a university. Serving as a teaching assistant alongside experienced faculty members taught me an enormous amount about the subject matter, about teaching, and about communication. As I've described, my research skills and style were honed in the laboratories at the NIH. After a postdoctoral year in a basic science department of a medical school that was not connected to a research university, my first position as an independent scientist was at the Cold Spring Harbor Laboratory, a private research laboratory. The environment for research at CSHL is conducive to a kind of concentrated effort that one finds at only a few places in the world. Ideas germinate fast because one can concentrate on science with only modest administrative or teaching demands. Scientific visitors to CSHL for courses, seminars, workshops, symposia, and meetings provide continual exposure to the latest discoveries. For those who thrive on an intense, focused approach to science, I can think of no better setting in which to begin an independent career.

After several productive years at CSHL, I moved to a basic science department of a medical school that is part of a major research university. Working in a research university affords many wonderful opportunities to teach and to work with young scientists. Not only is the quality of the science here as high as it is anywhere, my colleagues in other disciplines further enrich my intellectual life.

A career as a Ph.D. in the biological sciences is among the most rewarding imaginable. The challenges and demands are great, but the rewards are ample. The challenges include the competitive pressure of continual grant renewals and of publishing research in top-ranked journals. Securing funding and publishing the results of your research are requirements for maintaining a research laboratory. But the joys are unparalleled. There is the awe in discovering a new gene or protein that plays a critical role in brain function or in observing a structure that has never been seen before. There's also the deep satisfaction that comes from helping a student understand a complex concept or leading a graduate student to think independently. And one has the deep sense of community that comes when sharing with junior and senior colleagues the discoveries that advance the frontiers of knowledge. Research science combines the thrill of discovery with a life in a community of scholars.

PART EIGHT

Becoming a Physician-Executive

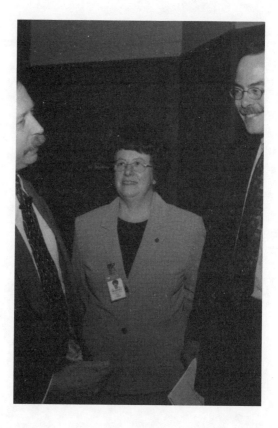

n the past, physicians remained physicians for life, though there have always been exceptions. A few noble souls left medicine to join the clergy, and some even became medical missionaries, like Schweitzer in Lambarene or Grenfell in Greenland. A few became lawyers. But unlike their "noble" counterparts in the clergy, in a time when the "conspiracy of silence" prevented lawyers from discovering evidence of mistakes or malfeasance by physicians, these few ran the risk of being regarded by their erstwhile medical colleagues as hired guns.

For the majority, however, medicine was the passion, and its practice was not lightly abandoned. As medicine has become a commodity, though, much in that ethos has changed. The practice of medicine is now considered by society to be as much a business as a profession. Medicine's adoption of business practices, and the external pressures exerted by our economy and by a growing sense of prudence, changed that seemingly singular scene. It became clear that delivering medical care required understanding the economic principles and business ethic that began to permeate medicine. Physicians began to take courses at business schools, and more went to law school. The "bottom line" implied more about finances than about the prognosis of disease. Many older physicians became discouraged enough to retire early, while other, usually younger, physicians chose to try to develop the new system.

The two writers in this section chose to contribute to this development in exciting ways. Each has formed a career as a physician-executive. Attilio Granata does much of his work analyzing patient outcomes and considers those outcomes alongside the quality, cost, and availability of the care offered. He describes the new definition of "quality" in health care that has developed and the "evaluative clinical sciences" used to measure it. As a physician, he is at the core of this new science in his role as a physician-executive. E. Paul MacCarthy is a pharmaceutical executive trained in academic medicine and research, experienced in institutional review boards, and now deeply involved in the day-to-day work of drug development. He conveys his overview of the development of a drug, through its investigational stages to marketing, in his role as head of medical sciences for a major pharmaceutical corporation. Both physicians describe the benefits they believe that these new careers in business may bring to medical practice, to patients, and to the welfare of the nation.

ATTILIO**GRANATA**

The Role of the Physician-Executive in Health Care Management

What is happening to health care today? What are the implications of the rising costs of health care, technological advances, and the increasing influence of insurance companies? And how should medicine/health care respond? Should medicine employ an industrial management method in response to these changes? Or should medicine—that unique, complex, and intimate discipline—find another way?

Rapidly increasing health care costs during the 1980s and 1990s made the United States the world's leader in gross domestic product spent on health care. But those who pay for care—employers and government—wonder why such enormous spending doesn't buy us straight As in measurable health. Our infant mortality rates are poor compared to those in the rest of the developed world, our life expectancy is lower than that in most developed nations, and we fail utterly in providing universal health care for all citizens. As we devote more of our resources to paying for health care, how can it be that we continue to lag behind other nations in key outcome indicators, and that the number of uninsured or uncovered citizens continues to rise?

Quality, cost, and availability of care are related but highly variable. Almost thirty years ago, John Wennberg (at Dartmouth) and others observed that rates of medical procedures and treatments per unit of local population varied tremendously. They observed as much as five- to tenfold differences across states, counties, cities, medical groups, and even the same physicians within a group over time, even when corrected for the patients' severity of illness. They noticed that patients in Boston, for example, which has many more hospital beds per inhabitant than does New Haven, were much more likely to be hospitalized for the same degree of illness than their New Haven counterparts. Even more startling, they found that the patients in New Haven, who were hospitalized less frequently, were no worse off in terms of outcomes of recovery or mortality! As health costs continued to rise logarithmically, payors naturally began questioning the value of their expenditures.

It is easy to measure the cost but much more difficult to measure the outcomes and quality of health care. We are all too aware that managed care companies have been attempting to cap the health care spending gusher by imposing numerous requirements such as pre-approval of elective procedures, limited networks of doctors and hospitals, and daily micromanagement of hospital inpatients. This attempt was temporarily successful during the mid-1990s, effectively and finally ending the "blank-check" reimbursement for health care that had been in fashion for the previous sixty years. But quality of care continues to suffer—and some argue that the financial cure has been far worse than the disease.

During the last decade of the twentieth century and the first decade of the twenty-first, a new definition of quality has been evolving. This evolution was spurred in part by the same U.S.-based advances in statistical process control and operations management that led to the revitalization of Japan after World War II. Quality in health care now had to include better adherence to evidence-based guidelines, or, in the words of process control experts, there had to be reduction in *unnecessary* variation. Allowing for "necessary" variation in health care was, of course, critical because of the unique needs of every patient as well as incomplete knowledge of human pathophysiology. Yet, unexplained wide ranges in health care resource use implied there was much waste to trim.

Thus, a new field of health care evolved, called the "evaluative clinical sciences," which includes areas such as outcomes measurement, cost-effectiveness analysis, and evidence-based medicine. This new field has led to comprehensive efforts to better quantify physician and hospital performance in terms of outcomes and quality, as well as, simply, cost. And, it is necessary for the physician to be at the center of this process, in a new role called the "physician executive."

Why are physicians necessary in this role, and what do physician executives do? One of their major tasks is to ensure appropriate and necessary care by trying to focus on what works. For example, practice guidelines are being developed based on scientific evidence. Further, evaluation of the performance of physicians, hospitals, and other providers measures their outcomes and provides feedback to enable them to improve what they do. If noticeably wide variations in care can somehow be reduced, one might be able to provide an improved level of care while making available previously wasted resources to those without full coverage. Physician executives hope that by emphasizing appropriate and proven care practices, they can improve cost, quality, and access together.

In a thriving economy, that goal is centered in profits, individual aggressiveness, and competition, so valid questions remain about health care. Is health care becoming another commodity, something bought and sold only on the basis of price? Is access to even basic primary health care to be considered a luxury like a fine automobile, or a social necessity like education or police and fire protection? Why has the percentage of the population without comprehensive, basic health insurance coverage steadily increased, even during the thriving economy of the late 1990s? Physicians, as advocates for their patients, must maintain a strong presence in the regulation, resource deployment, and strategic planning of our health care system to ensure that these and other issues are not lost to a market mentality that considers long-term planning as looking two fiscal quarters ahead.

Managed care companies and other payors have consistently called upon physicians to do more with less. As a result, it has become essential for many physicians to learn the same language and skills as administrators and business leaders. This is so especially because *medicine is not just another business*—it involves deep mysteries of the body and mind, pain and suffering, vulnerability and loss of control, and reliance upon the expertise and compassion of others. Yet, because of its unique scope, any plan for and deployment of health resources across a population must involve some degree of scientific methodology. Patients, physicians, and payors must have full faith that precious resources are being used to their fullest possible extent to enhance the health of individual patients and the population.

The physician executive is a new kind of practitioner who specializes in a specific *population* of patients. We are physicians with clinical training and management experience who spend much or all of our time helping to manage and support the care of individual patients as well as groups of patients. This task might involve assisting in the operation and/or direction of medical groups, hospitals, multi-hospital systems, government health agencies, pharmaceutical and technology companies, insurance companies, and any entity concerned with *how one spends limited resources for the maximal benefit of patients, both individually and collectively.*

The tasks of the physician executive require familiarity with clinical medicine, business, public health, epidemiology, biostatistics, computerized information systems, as well as bioethics, patient satisfaction, and the public good. Daily activities involve a mixture of art and science similar to that required in the field of clinical medicine. The ability to confidently make decisions under uncertainty is a key prerequisite. In making such decisions, each physician executive must remember and follow every ethical principle pledged in the Hippocratic Oath.

The difficulty with simultaneously managing groups of patients rather than a stream of individual patients, as in a practice or on a hospital ward, is that resources to manage such groups tend to be fixed, or at least relatively limited. Therefore, to ensure the greatest health of the population and of the individuals who make it up, physician leaders must be familiar with measuring medical outcomes, connecting journal-based science with how patients are treated in the real world, and assessing the risks and benefits of spending resources on some things but not others. We cannot spend infinitely to meet every patient's demand; making resource allocation decisions requires strong input not only from patients themselves but also from those skilled in the clinical knowledge underlying such decisions.

At this moment, several factors guarantee the need for the skills of the physician executive for many decades to come. The aging of the population will greatly increase demand for medical services. Tremendous advances in biotechnology, including the genome project, will place great strain on a system trying to eliminate or control disease while trying also to achieve fiscal survival. The information and consumerism revolution brought on by the Web will make it routine for patients to choose and assess their physicians as if they were leafing through *Consumer Reports,* and to look up clinical information previously available only in medical journals or libraries. Rising anti–managed care sentiment will compel legislatures, and insurance companies, to relax restrictions on coverage. And, far, far down the political road, someone will finally ask the question, "Why does being covered for health care depend on where you work, or even *if* you work?"

It is not difficult to design an ideal health care system that will provide better, more comprehensive care for every U.S. citizen without breaking the bank. The complexities lie in navigating that journey, from the status quo to the goal, even as each component of that system—physicians, government, the pharmaceutical industry, hospitals, insurance companies, and others—continues to pull harder in its own direction at the expense of the whole. Entities that make up a collective for mutual benefit have never succeeded in maximizing or even improving the entire group's benefit by acting entirely in each member's self-interest. Every component must yield something to the whole in order for a system to work optimally; by keeping the needs of patients at the center, physician executives will have a key role in such a search for compromise.

E.PAUL**MACCARTHY**

The Role of the Physician-Executive in the Pharmaceutical Industry

My transition to a career in pharmaceutical medicine followed sixteen years of training and the practice of medicine in an academic setting in Ireland, Australia, and, finally, the United States. After completing an internship and residency in internal medicine in Dublin, I spent three years as a National Heart Foundation of Australia postgraduate scholar doing clinical research on patients with hypertension. Clinical research is research involving patients and nonpatient subjects. This was followed by a fellowship in nephrology at the University of Cincinnati Medical Center and then a position as head of the hypertension service at that institution from 1981 until 1989. In addition, from 1987–1989, at the university I directed a new drug development unit sponsored by the pharmaceutical industry.

My training and career in academic medicine was excellent preparation for my subsequent career as a physician in the pharmaceutical industry. I learned fundamentals of good clinical research such as the ethics of research, the obligations of the investigator, grant writing, trial design, protocol writing (a protocol is a detailed description of the objectives, design, and organization of a study), data collection and analysis, statistics, report writing, and the publication process. I also served on the institutional review board (IRB) at the University of Cincinnati and participated as a principal investigator on many clinical research protocols for several pharmaceutical companies. While in this role, I had many opportunities to learn from experienced pharmaceutical physicians. I also learned much about the pharmaceutical industry by serving as a consultant in the field of hypertension and in my capacity as director of a new drug evaluation unit.

For many physicians the decision to leave academic medicine for a career in the pharmaceutical industry is not an easy one. Many are concerned with losing contact with patients. Others are concerned with leaving the "academic" aspect of academic medicine, while yet others are concerned with losing contact with their medical subspecialty. I have encountered these concerns and many more from physicians while interviewing them for positions at Bayer Corporation over the past twelve years. I have reassured them that usually they can continue to have patient contact by working in a nearby outpatient clinic setting one morning or afternoon each week. This is what many physicians have chosen to do at Bayer and is also an option at most major pharmaceutical companies. I reassure them that the scientific skill-set they have developed in clinical research in an academic environment is readily applicable to the daily job of the pharmaceutical physician involved in drug development. In addition, physicians involved in drug development are often in close contact with the leaders in a particular field of medicine as they consult on drug development issues. They also present the results of research on new drugs at important academic meetings. Thus, the move to the pharmaceutical industry does not involve a complete break from the environment of academic medicine. Medical subspecialists who join pharmaceutical companies usually find work first in the field of their relevant subspecialty. However, as they gain experience and are successful in industry, they usually take on broader responsibilities outside their area of subspecialty expertise.

For me, the decision to leave academic medicine for a position in the pharmaceutical industry was not a difficult one. I had learned much about this area while involved in industry-sponsored research in an academic medical setting. My first position in industry was as director of cardiovascular clinical research, which was not a big change from

the work of clinical research I was conducting in the academic environment. Following the transition to industry, I learned about the practical aspects of conducting clinical trials and the advantages and disadvantages of different types of clinical trial design. I also learned a
considerable amount about the regulatory aspect of clinical research
and drug development, the business aspect of the pharmaceutical industry, and the details of how to be an effective manager and leader.
With time, as I gained experience in drug development, I assumed
responsibility for research in areas outside my subspecialty. Although
this was initially daunting, I was fascinated to learn about drug development for Alzheimer's disease, hemophilia, and erectile dysfunction.
The most satisfying and enjoyable aspects of my career in the pharmaceutical industry so far have been the acquisition of new management
skills and technical knowledge, working in a global organization, and
having an impact on the lives of millions of patients by helping to
bring innovative medicines to the marketplace.

Most physicians who enter the pharmaceutical industry tend to
have positions in clinical research and usually are involved in the development of one or possibly two drug development candidates. Drug
development is a multidisciplinary activity, and the physician is just
one of many members of the drug development project team. Other
team members are from disciplines such as discovery research, toxicol-
ogy, pharmaceutical technology, pharmacokinetics, marketing, regulatory affairs, clinical operations, and project management. The pharmaceutical physician in drug development is involved in formulating the
drug development strategy, in writing the medical section of the investigational drug (IND) application, in the design of individual clinical
trial protocols, in supervising clinical trials, and in the analysis, reporting, and publication of trials. In addition to these activities, the
physician presents background information on a new drug candidate
to investigators at meetings and also responds to queries from investigators regarding protocol inclusion/exclusion criteria. The physician
also reviews adverse events during the course of a study to ensure that
patient safety is not compromised. On occasion, the physician may
also be involved in presenting data on a new drug development candidate to the Food and Drug Administration in closed meetings or at
open FDA advisory committee meetings. At the end of a drug development program, the physician participates in summarizing the individ-

ual clinical trial results in the clinical section of a new drug application (NDA), which is submitted to the FDA for approval to market the new drug in the United States. The drug development process from IND filing to NDA approval takes several years, and only about one in ten development candidates survives the development process to market approval and launch.

Although most physicians in industry are involved in clinical research and drug development, a variety of industry career options are open to physicians. The physician may be a clinical pharmacologist and be involved in early clinical drug development to assess the safety, tolerability, and pharmacokinetics (i.e., the study of the relationship between the dose of a drug administered and the serum or blood level achieved) of new compounds in phase I clinical trials and in conducting drug interaction studies and studies in special patient populations, for example, those with renal failure. Another career option for the physician is in drug safety and pharmacovigilance (i.e., all methods for assessing and preventing adverse drug reactions). This career involves responsibility for the assessment and reporting of serious adverse events from clinical trials and postmarketing surveillance to regulatory authorities. Some training in epidemiology is helpful to those who make this career choice. Another career option for the pharmaceutical physician is in drug discovery. Physicians who pursue this career option are usually M.D./Ph.D.s who have been involved in laboratory research in an academic setting before joining the pharmaceutical industry. Another career option for the physician is in the marketing end of the organization or at the interface between marketing and medicine. This may involve giving advice on the design of clinical trials to support the marketing of new compounds, training the sales force on the medical aspects of new products, advising on draft marketing plans, and providing medical information to health care providers on marketed products.

Yet another career option for an M.D. in industry is in regulatory affairs. This involves formulating the regulatory strategy for a new compound to assure timely submission of registration dossiers and the successful registration of a new drug internationally. The physician in regulatory affairs also builds solid professional relationships with key staff in regulatory organizations, ensures that excellent summaries of clinical trial results are submitted to regulatory authorities, and manages the responses to queries from these authorities. A solid knowledge of drug development is a key ingredient in a successful career in regulatory affairs. In fact, many physicians make the transition to regulatory affairs after first learning drug development in the clinical research department. Another important career option for the industry physician is in the area of new business development. This involves identifying possible opportunities for in-licensing (i.e., purchasing or acquiring) new compounds from other companies or from academic institutions. It also involves managing the process of thoroughly identifying all possible weaknesses in a compound that is being seriously considered for in-licensing. The area of new business development has a potentially major financial impact on the pharmaceutical company.

Physicians frequently ask me how they should prepare for a career as a pharmaceutical physician. I usually advise that they complete a fellowship in a medical subspecialty and get some experience in clinical research in academia as either a fellow or a junior faculty member. Courses in statistics, epidemiology, and pharmacokinetics are helpful but not mandatory. A master's degree in business (M.B.A.) is helpful to those physicians who want to work in new business development or in marketing. The key factors for a successful career as a pharmaceutical physician are a solid scientific background and training, strong communication and problem solving skills, and an ability to work well in a team environment. The ability to work well on a team is a vital skill because the scope and complexity of drug development is handled by multidisciplinary project teams, typically with ten to twenty members. In my experience, physicians who have not made a good transition to industry have had one or more of the following: poor verbal or written communication skills, difficulty in problem solving and accepting setbacks, difficulty in working under time constraints, and poor appreciation/acceptance of the commercial goals involved in drug development.

As a physician, you will have a variety of career options within the pharmaceutical industry. These options, which range from a research focus (e.g., in drug discovery) to a business focus (e.g., in marketing), are interesting, challenging, and rewarding and have the potential to affect the health of millions of patients.

PART NINE

Thinking About Medical Writing

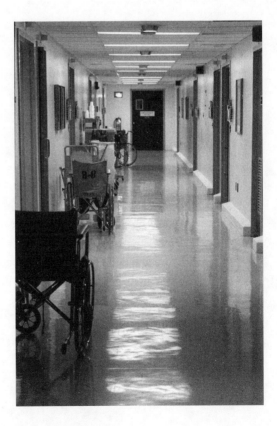

Over the past twenty-five years New Haven and Yale have seen the flowering of a literary movement composed largely of surgeons. While others have contributed much, Sherwin B. Nuland and Richard Selzer head the list of those who have made New Haven almost synonymous with literature and medicine. That they were surgeons who abandoned the scalpel for the pen will doubtless captivate graduate students looking for a Ph.D. dissertation.

Here we simply note another movement that has made the work of medical writing—and the humanities in medicine—particularly germane, and that is, as Thomas Duffy earlier reminded us, the recognition that narrative informs medical training almost as much as biology does. Patients are mind and body—or really, mind *in* body. They are more than a collection of organs or molecules, and physicians and health professionals should keep in mind that caring for disease is caring for people. That is hard to remember when hospitals have become intensive care units and when technical expertise is more important than character or compassion. But the patients lost by technology can be found again in anecdote and by contemplation.

And that is where literature has so much to offer—as Wordsworth put it, "emotion recollected in tranquility." Yet it is emotion that can re-energize the spirit, infuse us with understanding, and allow us to be present, listening, to our patients.

The thoughts expressed and advice given by Sherwin B. Nuland and Richard Selzer will generate your own musings, and the editors have no wish to guide your contemplation of these beautiful pieces.

SHERWIN B. NULAND

Excerpts from *How We Die*

Before there were two digits in my age, I had seen the hope (I choose the word deliberately) that a doctor's presence brings to a worried family. There were several frightening emergencies during my mother's long illness, even in the years before she had begun her descent to death. The mere knowledge that someone had gone to the drugstore phone to call the doctor, and the word that he was on the way, changed the atmosphere in our small apartment from terrified helplessness to a secure sense that somehow the dreadful situation could be made right. That man—the man who stepped across the threshold with a smile and an air of competence, who called each of us by name, who understood that beyond anything else we needed reassurance, and whose very entrance into our home conveyed it—that was the man I wanted to be.

My objective in becoming a physician was to be a general practitioner in the Bronx. In the first year of medical school, I learned how the body functions; in the second year, I learned how it gets sick. In the third and fourth years, I began to understand how to interpret the histories I elicited from my patients and to study the physical and chemical clues produced by their illnesses, that combination of overt and hidden findings that the eighteenth-century pathologist Giovanni Morgagni called "the cries of the suffering organs." I studied the various ways of listening to my patients and looking at them so that I might be able to discern those cries. I was taught to probe orifices, read X rays, and seek meaning in the state of blood and cast-off waste products of various descriptions. In time, I knew exactly which tests to order so that the more obvious clues might be used to lead me to the hidden changes that are part of sickness. That process is pathophysiology. Mastering its tortuous patterns is the means by which to understand the details of the way normal mechanisms of healthy life somehow go awry. To understand pathophysiology is to hold the key to diagnosis, without which there can be no cure. The quest of every doctor in approaching serious disease is to make the diagnosis and design and carry out the specific cure. This quest I call The Riddle, and I capitalize it so there will be no mistaking its dominance over every other consideration. The satisfaction of solving The Riddle is its own reward, and the fuel that drives the clinical engines of medicine's most highly trained specialists. It is every doctor's measure of his own abilities; it is the most important ingredient in professional self-image.

In one of his *Precepts,* Hippocrates wrote, "Where love of mankind is, there is also love of the art of medicine," and that is as true as it ever has been; were it otherwise, the burden of caring for our fellows would soon prove unbearable. Every medical specialist must admit that he has at times convinced patients to undergo diagnostic or therapeutic measures at a point in illness so far beyond reason that The Riddle might better have remained unsolved. Too often near the end, were the doctor able to see deeply within himself, he might recognize that his decisions and advice are motivated by his inability to give up The Riddle and admit defeat as long as there is any chance of solving it. Though he be kind and considerate of the patient he treats, he allows himself to push his kindness aside because the seduction of The Riddle is so strong and the failure to solve it renders him weak.

Every scientific or clinical advance carries with it a cultural implication, and often a symbolic one. The invention of the stethoscope in 1816, for example, can be viewed as having set in motion the process by which physicians came to distance themselves from their patients. Such an interpretation of the instrument's role was, in fact, considered by some medical commentators of the time to be one of its advantages, since not many clinicians, then or now, feel at ease with an ear pressed up against a diseased chest. That and its image as a visible evidence of status remain to this day unspoken reasons for the instrument's popularity. One need only spend a few hours on rounds with young resident physicians to observe the several roles played by this dangling evidence of authority and detachment.

Seen from the strictly clinical perspective, a stethoscope is nothing more than a device to transmit sounds; by the same kind of reasoning, an intensive care unit is merely a secluded treasure room of high-tech hope within the citadel in which we segregate the sick so that we may better care for them. Those tucked-away sanctums symbolize the purest form of our society's denial of the naturalness, and even the necessity, of death. For many of the dying, intensive care, with its isolation among strangers, extinguishes their hope of not being abandoned in the last hours. In fact, they *are* abandoned, to the good intentions of highly skilled professional personnel who barely know them.

This solitary death is now so well recognized that our society has organized against it, and well we should. From the wisdom of the legal documents called advance directives to the questionable philosophies of suicide societies, a range of options exists, and at bottom the goal of each of them is the same: a restoration of certainty that when the end is near, there will be at least this source of hope—that our last moments will be guided not by the bioengineers but by those who know who we are.

This hope, this assurance that there will be no unreasonable efforts, is an affirmation that the dignity to be sought in death is the appreciation by others of what one has been in life. It is a dignity that proceeds from a life well lived and from the acceptance of one's own death as a necessary process of nature that permits our species to continue in the form of our own children and the children of others. It is also the recognition that the *real* event taking place at the end of our life is our death, not the attempts to prevent it. We have somehow been so taken up with the wonders of modern science that our society puts the emphasis in the wrong place. It is the dying that is the important thing—the central player in the drama is the dying man; the dashing leader of that bustling squad of his would-be rescuers is only a spectator, and a groundling at that.

In ages past, the hour of death was, insofar as circumstances permitted, seen as a time of spiritual sanctity, and of a last communion with those being left behind. They dying expected this to be so, and it was not easily denied them. It was their consolation and the consolation of their loved ones for the parting and especially for the miseries that had very likely preceded it.

Sometimes a dying person's source of hope can be as undemanding as the wish to live until a daughter's graduation or even a holiday that has particular meaning. The medical literature documents the power of this kind of hope, describing instances in which it has maintained not only the life but the optimism of a dying man or woman for the necessary period. Every doctor and many laymen can tell of individuals who survived weeks beyond the most extreme expectations in order to have one last Christmas or to await the sight of a dear face arriving from some distant land.

The lesson in all of this is well known. Hope lies not only in an expectation of cure or even of the remission of present distress. For dying patients, the hope of cure will always be shown to be ultimately false, and even the hope of relief too often turns to ashes. When my time comes, I will seek hope in the knowledge that insofar as possible I will not be allowed to suffer or be subjected to needless attempts to maintain life; I will seek it in the certainty that I will not be abandoned to die alone; I am seeking it now, in the way I try to live my life, so that those who value what I am will have profited by my time on earth and be left with comforting recollections of what we have meant to one another.

The necessity of nature's final victory was expected and accepted in generations before our own. Doctors were far more willing to recognize the signs of defeat and far less arrogant about denying them. Medicine's humility in the face of nature's power has been lost, and with it has gone some of the moral authority of times past. With the vast increase in scientific knowledge has come a vast decrease in the acknowledgment that we still have control over far less than we would like. Physicians accept the conceit (in every sense of the word) that science has made us all-powerful and therefore the only proper judges of how our skills are to be used. The greater humility that should come with greater knowledge is instead replaced by medical hubris: since we can do so much, there is no limit to what should be attempted— *today,* and for *this patient!*

The more highly specialized the physician, the more likely is The

Riddle to be his primary motivation. To medicine's absorption with The Riddle we owe the great clinical advances of which all patients are the beneficiaries; to medicine's absorption with The Riddle we also owe our disappointment when we cherish expectations of doctors that they cannot fulfill and perhaps should not be asked to fulfill. The Riddle is the doctor's lodestone as an applied scientist; it is his albatross as a humane caregiver.

We bear more than pain and sorrow when we depart life. Among the heaviest burdens is apt to be regret, which deserves a word at this point. As inevitable as death is and as likely to be preceded by a difficult period, especially for people with cancer, there are additional pieces of baggage we shall all take to the grave, but from which we may somewhat disencumber ourselves if we anticipate them. By these, I mean conflicts unresolved, breached relationships not healed, potential unfulfilled, promises not kept, and years that will never be lived. For virtually every one of us, there will be unfinished business. Only the very old escape it, and then not always.

Perhaps the mere existence of things undone should be a sort of satisfaction in itself, though the idea would appear to be paradoxical. Only one who is long since dead while still seemingly alive does not have many "promises to keep, and miles to go before I sleep," and that state of inertness is not to be desired. To the wise advice that we live every day as though it will be our last, we do well to add the admonition to live every day as though we will be on this earth forever.

We do well also to avoid another unnecessary burden by remembering the caution of Robert Burns about the best-laid plans. Death rarely, if ever, acts according to our plans or even to our expectations. Nature has a job to do. It does its job by the method that seems most suited to each individual whom its powers have created. It has made this one susceptible to heart disease and that one to stroke and yet another to cancer, some after a long time on this earth and some after a time much too brief, at least by our own reckoning. The animal economy has formed the circumstances by which each generation is to be succeeded by the next. Against the relentless forces and cycles of nature there can be no lasting victory.

I am more concerned with the microcosm than the macrocosm; I am more interested in how a man lives than how a star dies; how a woman makes her way in the world than how a comet streaks across the heavens. If there is a God, He is present as much in the creation of each of us as He was at the creation of the earth. The human condition is the mystery that engages my fascination, not the condition of the cosmos.

To understand the human condition has been the work of my life. During that life, which is now into its seventh decade, I have had my share of sorrows and my share of triumphs. Sometimes I think I have had far more than my share of both, but that impression probably stems from the inclination we all share, which makes each of us see our own existence as a heightened example of universal experience—a life that is somehow larger than life, and felt more deeply.

A realistic expectation also demands our acceptance that one's allotted time on earth must be limited to an allowance consistent with the continuity of the existence of our species. Mankind, for all its unique gifts, is just as much a part of the ecosystem as is any other zoologic or botanical form, and nature does not distinguish. We die so that the world may continue to live. We have been given the miracle of life because trillions upon trillions of living things have prepared the way for us and then have died—in a sense, for us. We die, in turn, so that others may live. The tragedy of a single individual becomes, in the balance of natural things, the triumph of ongoing life.

Excerpts from *The Exact Location of the Soul*

L et us go. It is seven-thirty in the morning. The men's locker room is a scene of great activity. Surgeons, residents, interns, and students are dressing for the morning's work. There is a nervousness in the stalls, a nickering and stamping. These surgeons are neat; they hang their clothing in the lockers with precision; everything is folded along its creases. Paper boots are fitted over shoes with care, caps tied behind the head just so, the strings of the masks knotted and adjusted. Metal doors clang. The bodies of these men are like the furniture of your house; you have seen them every day for years. They seem beautiful and young, even the old ones. Their hands are pink and warm to the touch from so many scrubbings. Each fingernail is trimmed in a gentle curve. Their talk is all of football and baseball and gold. Surgeons love the notions of teams pitted one against the other, or of single combat. It is fitting that this be so. In the corridors the patients wait. They lie narcotized, silent, yet afraid, on stretchers, each one parked outside the room into which he will be taken. As each surgeon approaches his patient he, too, grows quiet. Who knows what dreams these surgeons have had?

The women surgeons dress with the nurses. Never mind. The inheritance of surgery is less a patrimony than a matrimony. "Male" is inspired tinkering, a knack for replacing the works. "Female" is a softness of touch, an intuition for planes and membranes. Like the poet, the surgeon must incorporate both. If pressed I should confess to the suspicion that women make better surgeons than men. Women know how to fold themselves about life. Women know blood, and they know pain.

The light in the operating room is no less important than the light in an artist's studio. It must be direct, cast no shadows, yet be free of glare. None of these has ever, to my knowledge, been achieved to perfection. It is to be expected then that a surgeon will complain of the poor light forced upon him by malicious electrical influences. But inferior light must not become the excuse behind which a nervous surgeon conceals his fumbling. Operating rooms must be of a certain size. Too small, and there is more likelihood of contamination by the collision of occupants and equipment. Too large, and the mind is distracted. Great empty spaces take away from the proceedings that lovely feeling of a close-knit team on an expedition. Of the two, I prefer small rooms which act to concentrate the thought and discipline the mind. Too much space smothers me. Being slight, I am able to insinuate myself among the material. Bulkier members of the species are less insertable. Let them have wider ranges.

You wheel the stretcher alongside the operating table and help the patient to slide himself from one to the other. Now you must keep in contact with your patient until he is asleep. Hold his hand if one is free of the anesthetist's use, or place your hand upon his chest, his shoulder. This will suggest to him that a protective spirit hovers over him. Speak quietly, as though privately, to your patient. Dwell upon his awakening. Say the word "recovery." It is a winged word. The sight and sound of you at this time is balm in Gilead to him. No matter how kindly the others are, he does not know them. You are his doctor, the only one who has received his trust. These others are strangers. Tangency in the operating room is both given and received. Often the patient will reach out to touch you, taking comfort from the feel of your body, just as you draw strength from his. The patient is not a plant of the genus *noli me tangere*, whose seed vessels would burst at the slightest touch. He is frightened, feels himself to be alone in a green and clanking place where there are no windows and he cannot see the sky. Let him look into your eyes for whatever distance and space he can find there.

One day you, too, will be a surgeon and stand over a table upon which a patient lies. In a few minutes you will take up a scalpel and lay open his body. Your patient may be, like the man I operated on today, old, wasted, his bowel obstructed by a tumor. All at once, before the induction of anesthesia, this man reached up his two hands. They trembled in the air like weightless dragonflies. The long papery fingers encircled my neck. His grip had a strength that surprised me. Not to strangle but to draw in through his hands all the blood and breath that coursed there. To this, you, too, will gladly submit, knowing that it is a greater offering than any mere surgery. It is only human love that keeps this from being the act of two madmen.

Take care not to get in the way of the anesthetist. During the induction of anesthesia, you have the chance to do small tasks that might assist him—tearing strips of adhesive tape for him to use in securing a needle in a vein, or pressing, if he should request it, the larynx of the patient to ease the passage of his tube into the trachea. It is a privilege to attend to the needs of an anesthetist.

If the anesthetic is to be spinal, help the patient to turn to one side and to curl his body. Now cradle and steady him until it is done. Never fear to be thought unmanly because of such service. Now your patient is ready to go to sleep. To wish each other luck is neither inappropriate nor insensitive. It is honest. The injection of Pentothal is given. You continue to soothe him with your touch and voice. Is there no hidden cabin of the brain, I have wondered, some dark sulcus where he will hold these words you say to him: "Relax. Go to sleep. Pick out a nice dream"?

"That's right, give in. Don't fight it," you say. And he submits. Perhaps one day he will summon these words forth to the blazing courtyard of consciousness. Then he will hear them again and think of you, and smile. Never doubt that he has heard you. Sounds are intensified during the induction of anesthesia. Now he is asleep and hears nothing. Anesthesia is an imitation of death, uninhabited even by dreams.

Like all ceremonies, washing the hands has a wisdom beyond mere practical worth. Like the donning of clean, loose-fitting clothing, it is an act of supplication. It goes without saying that the fingernails are kept short and straight and clean. There must be no sharp points to snag flesh. Nothing sets a patient's pulse to hammering like the sight of a cache of dirt beneath his surgeon's fingernails, for it implies carelessness with the flesh of others.

Take a pointed stick and wipe beneath each nail. Throw away the stick and take up the heavy-bristled brush. Drench it with soap and water. Proceed to scrub a finger at a time, then the thumb—front and back. Advance to the dorsum of the hand, firmly, and with ever-increasing circles. On to the palm. Flex the fingertips, back and forth, back and forth. Now in long, luxurious strokes, up and down the arm, to an inch above the elbow. Rinse, and do it again.

Poised above the patient the surgeon is like a priest guarding and preserving fire. He takes strength from this closeness. For the body of the patient is the sun, the whorl of light and heat that radiates life into this room. It is the patient's heat that foments this work, his light that makes it visible and possible. Without the patient this world is dead. He is the nucleus, all the rest, the cytoplasm. He, the seed; the rest, the fruit about him.

When the incision is made, the surgeon gazes though the aperture, and even as he does, something marvelous happens. He himself shrinks to accommodate the dimensions of this unexplored place. Once, while studying a group of tiny bonsai trees in a tray, I knelt to peer upward into their branches from below. Suddenly it was I who was small and the trees that were large. I was a pygmy in a towering forest. Such is the magic of bonsai, and such is the magic of Surgery.

The abdomen at the same time expands to incorporate him. He descends, reliving his childhood fears. He is once again in a mad, dark cellar with, high above, the fading light of earth.

Once inside, every artery is a red river to be forded or dammed up; every organ, a mountain to be skirted or climbed. The surgeon is a trekker in a land of mystery and beauty. Beneath his feet he feels the throbbing of a great engine. About his head a warm wind breathes. No less than the one he has just left, this new world holds all there is of good and evil. An intimate warmth encloses him. It has the humidity of his mother's unremembered womb. Nor does he once look back at what recedes outside. From the moment of his entry he is totally engaged. He is in a state of *topophilia*, wherein his vision changes. He sees vast dripping caverns, escarpments, lofty ranges. Pink and salmon and maroon creatures drowse in their beds. These creatures are friendly; the surgeon approaches them with affection. But there are fumes, too, a sluggish trickle. Far in the distance a stony gray crater presents itself. One, and then another, and another for as far as the eye can see. These are the very plains of Hell.

For years, the surgeon has dreamt of this place, conjured it in his mind, imagined all of its marvels. And now he is there. Unlike the poet's travels, which are figments and phantasms, this is real.

At first it seems that sound, too, has shrunk. There are only vast silences. Soon these silences are violated by the whoosh of blood coursing through hidden passageways and the throbbing of an engine far below. The surgeon experiences systole and diastole, not his own, but a rhythm absorbed from the landscape. A distant wind blows to and fro, folding and unfolding the fine linen that hangs between the flanks. But wait awhile and there are other sounds—whispers, giggling, murmurs, ticktocks retrieved from beyond the auditory threshold.

Once having shucked the outside world, the surgeon's mind has been set free. He is once again a child gazing with the liberated eyes of childhood. But a wise child, for he brings here all the reason and logic and knowledge of that other life. Like a mountaineer who must bring along his own food and oxygen, the surgeon feeds upon his past experience. It sustains him throughout his journey. But he must be certain to bring enough. Otherwise he will surely die in this unterrestrial place. Who would visit this awful place must be like a deer, gifted with presentiment. He must stand as the deer stands—motionless, breathless, quivering, to feel the distant sounds come nearer, the sounds that no one else can hear. He lays his ear to a kidney to hear its soft watery machinery. He listens to the filtration and extraction of the liver, the muddy slide of the gut, the ceaseless chewing of a tumor. He hears the whole cavern of the belly reddening.

For the surgeon, the distance between the lips of his incision and the prize he seeks, and for which he has been dispatched by his patron, is no more than twelve inches. Still there are gorges to be crossed on narrow swaying filaments, precipices to be scaled, Fate to be placated. All the while on his trek, the surgeon's mind urges toward that tumor. His eye is fixed upon its gray stony parapets. From the moment of incision he is already laying siege to it, tying off its supply routes, burning off the foliage that protects and conceals it, tightening his grip on it, even dwelling within it like a spy, gathering information, taking measurements, looking for signs of weakness. The surgeon hates and loves this tumor that both resists and offers itself to him. It is the object of his dreams. At last, he retrieves the tumor from this dream and holds it up to the light. Hunter and prey have met in one. A man among men in one world, he is a man alone and lonely in this other. Here within, he shares none of his terror or exhilaration. There is only the solitude of terrible works.

Now the expedition is completed. In jubilation or despair, the abdomen is closed. A line of sutures like the lashes of a closed eye marks the passageway. Already the scar begins to form across the entrance—blood, serum, a jelly of fibroblasts and tissue juice gathers, all the cellular throng that will barricade with boulders and walls of flesh.

Safe outside, the surgeon turns to gaze at the abdomen, imagining still the maroon and humid walls, the bare gray crags, the moment of victory or defeat. And the pulse beats faster at his wrist. Now the wound is dressed. How quickly an incision becomes a wound! The unbandaged eyes of the surgeon see beyond the sealed gate to the garden within where once, like Adam, he walked in high discovery. This sealed and silent abdomen, this, too, will never be the same as it was. For the surgeon has left his mark hewn into a remote trunk. All about the tumor he has built an altar of metal clips arranged under auspices.

His fingerprint is on the wall. And he has left his dreams behind to glide among the viscera, mute witnesses to what has transpired. The abdomen is closed; the surgeon's dreams remain within. Nor are the organs of this abdomen ever wholly forgotten. They have become part of the surgeon's past. And these organs have imparted to him a certain knowledge, whispered to him secrets that he will pass on to others. Much as a jewel box contains the dreams of a vain woman, or a casket of bones the dreams of a widow, inside this closed belly flit the fitful dreams of the surgeon.

CONTRIBUTORS

SUSAN S. ADDISS was commissioner of health for the state of Connecticut from 1991–1995. She has also served as president of the American Public Health Association (1984) and chair of the board of Planned Parenthood of Connecticut (2000–2002). She is vice-chair of the Connecticut Health Foundation, is a founding board member of Environment and Human Health, Inc., and serves on the board of the Watershed Fund of the Regional Water Association.

RAMIN AHMADI, M.D., M.P.H., is program director for internal medicine at Griffin Hospital in Derby, Connecticut, and assistant clinical professor of medicine at Yale University School of Medicine. His commitment to human rights has taken him to many countries, most recently Chechnya and East Timor. He is the founder of the Griffin Center for Health and Human Rights and the Iran Civil Society Institute. He is the author of three books and writes on the subject of human rights for several publications.

SANDRA ALFANO, Pharm.D., FASHP, is coordinator of the Investigational Drug Service at Yale–New Haven Hospital and vice-chair of the Human Investigation Committee at Yale University School of Medicine. She has held a variety of pharmacy practice and management positions over a twenty-five-year period. Alfano is on the faculty of the Yale School of Nursing and the University of Connecticut School of Pharmacy, where she teaches courses and provides experiential rotations. She is president-elect of the Connecticut Society of Health Systems Pharmacists.

DANA K. ANDERSEN, M.D., is board certified in both internal medicine and surgery. He was the chief of general surgery at the University of Chicago and at Yale University before joining the University of Massachusetts, where he is Harry M. Haidak Professor and chairman of the department of surgery at the University of Massachusetts Medical

School and chief of surgery at UMass Memorial Health Care. He specializes in pancreatic surgery and pancreatic disease.

NANCY R. ANGOFF, M.D., is assistant professor of internal medicine and associate dean for student affairs at Yale University School of Medicine. She cares for patients with HIV/AIDS and is interested in ethical and end-of-life issues in medicine, as well as the emotional and professional development of medical students.

RICHARD BELITSKY, M.D., is associate professor of psychiatry and the deputy chair for education in the department of psychiatry at Yale University School of Medicine. He is active in both undergraduate and graduate medical education, serving as the department's director of residency training, as well as director of medical student education. He also has remained active in clinical practice and has a strong interest in mental health services at prisons and jails.

JEFFREY R. BENDER, M.D., is professor of medicine and immunobiology, the associate chief of cardiovascular medicine, and the director of the Cardiovascular Laboratory at Yale University School of Medicine. He is an attending physician on the Cardiology Service at Yale–New Haven Hospital, and he directs a laboratory that studies molecular mechanisms in atherosclerosis and transplant rejection. He has been a member of Study Sections at the National Institutes of Health and the American Heart Association, and he serves on several AHA committees. He has been elected to the American Society for Clinical Investigation, the Interurban Club, and the Association of University Cardiologists.

FRANK BIA, M.D., M.P.H., is professor of medicine (infectious diseases) and laboratory medicine (clinical microbiology) and co-director of the International Health Program at Yale University School of Medicine. Bia received his bachelor of science degree from Fordham University and his medical degree from Cornell University Medical College. He obtained his master of public health in microbiology and tropical health from the Harvard School of Public Health. He moved to Yale as a fellow in infectious diseases in 1976, ultimately joining the medical faculty. While working in such countries as Haiti, China, and Thailand he followed his interests in tropical medicine and health.

PEGGY BIA, M.D., is professor of medicine, director of Clinical Skills Training, and director of the Doctor-Patient Encounter course at Yale University School of Medicine. After nephrology training at the University of Pennsylvania and Yale, she joined the Yale faculty in nephrology in 1978. She self-trained in transplant nephrology and gradually became the main medical caretaker of renal transplant patients at Yale, as well as the main teacher of renal transplantation for the nephrology training program. She has worked diligently as a clinician, teacher, and author of many clinical studies; in 2000 she began teaching the Doctor-Patient Encounter course at the medical school, and within a year she became the director of clinical skills training. She now divides her time between the medical school and outpatient care.

JOHN BLANTON, M.D., received his B.S from Purdue University and his M.D. from Yale University School of Medicine. He is assistant clinical professor of pediatrics at Yale and a fellow of the American Academy of Pediatrics and a member of the Ambulatory Pediatric Association.

MALCOLM B. BOWERS, JR., M.D., is professor of psychiatry at Yale University. He graduated from Southern Methodist University and received his M.D. from Washington University at St. Louis. He has been a full-time faculty member since 1965.

KELLY D. BROWNELL, Ph.D., is professor of psychology and epidemiology and public health at Yale University. He is also the director of the Yale Center for Eating and Weight Disorders. He served from 1995–99 as director of clinical training, and he is currently director of graduate studies in the department of psychology. In 1994 he became master of Silliman College at Yale; he served until 2000. He has been president of several national organizations, including the Society of Behavioral Medicine, the Association for the Advancement of Behavior Therapy, and the Division of Health Psychology of the American Psychological Association.

GERARD N. BURROW, M.D., is Dean Emeritus and David Paige Smith Professor of Medicine Emeritus of the Yale University School of Medicine. He is currently President and CEO of the Sea Research Foundation, which encompasses the Mystic Aquarium and the Institute for Exploration.

JULIE CANTOR, J.D., a lawyer and a student at Yale University School of Medicine, teaches two undergraduate seminars in Yale College: "Reproduction, Bioethics, and the Law" and "Medical Ethics, Law, and Literature." Cantor received her undergraduate and master's degrees from Stanford University and her law degree from University of California, Berkeley. After becoming a physician she hopes to engage the public and policy makers in issues of medicine and law.

HERBERT CHASE, JR., M.D., is deputy dean for education and professor of medicine at Yale University School of Medicine. After training in internal medicine and nephrology, and completing a post-doctoral fellowship, he established a laboratory at Columbia University, where he explored cellular signaling in epithelial tissues. Chase then turned his attentions to medical education and was involved in developing and participating in numerous courses at Columbia. He has received numerous teaching awards, including the Charles W. Bohmfalk Award for Distinguished Contributions to Teaching and the Presidential Teaching Award from Columbia University.

DEBORAH CIBELLI, C.N.M., M.S.N., is assistant clinical professor at Yale University School of Nursing. She has worked in the same private practice in New Haven for more than twenty years. She is chair of the Connecticut Chapter of the American College of Nurse-Midwives. In 1998 she received the American College of Nurse-Midwives Regional Award for Excellence for her contributions to the profession of midwifery.

MICHAEL COCCO is a certified chiropractor, a diplomate of the American Board of Chiropractic Neurology, and a certified acupuncturist. He is a member of the Connecticut Chiropractic Association and the American Chiropractic Association. He treats many nationally ranked track and field athletes. Cocco received his undergraduate degree from Southern Connecticut State University.

CHRISTOPHER P. COPPOLA, M.D., is a pediatric surgery fellow at the Children's National Medical Center in Washington, D.C. He is a major in the U.S. Air Force.

ANGELA DELISLE, PA-C, M.H.S., has been with Connecticut Gastroenterology Consultants since 1999. She provides hepatologic-based academic lectures for physicians' assistant programs at Quinnipiac and Yale Universities.

VINCENT DELUCA, JR., M.D., FACP, attended Fordham, Cornell, and Long Island College of Medicine. He is clinical professor of medicine at Yale University Medical School. He recently retired from Griffin Hospital in Derby, Connecticut, where he was chairman of medical education and chief of gastroenterology.

ROBERT M. DONALDSON, JR., M.D., received his training at Boston University. He is the David Paige Smith Professor of Medicine (Emeritus) at Yale University School of Medicine. Since 1959 he has been on the faculty of six medical schools across the United States. He headed a research program in gastroenterology until 1987, when he became a general internist and a physician to AIDS patients. As deputy dean of the Yale medical school, he played a leading role in the development of the AIDS Care Program at Yale.

JONATHAN A. DRANOFF, M.D., is an assistant professor of medicine in the department of internal medicine at Yale University School of Medicine. He works in the section of digestive diseases, where he studies signaling via extracellular nucleotides in the liver. His clinical activities include both hepatology and lumenal gastroenterology, although his greatest clinical interest is cholestatic liver disease.

THOMAS DUFFY, M.D., is professor of medicine and director of the Program for the Humanities in Medicine at Yale University School of Medicine.

ROSEMARIE FISHER, M.D., is professor of medicine and director of Graduate Medical Education at Yale–New Haven Hospital and Yale University School of Medicine. She is an internist/gastroenterologist. Previously she was director of the Internal Medicine Residency Program at Yale–New Haven Medical Center.

GERALD FRIEDLAND, M.D., is director of the AIDS Program and professor of medicine and epidemiology and public health at Yale University School of Medicine and Yale–New Haven Hospital. He has provided and organized HIV care and clinical and epidemiologic research in New York and New Haven since 1981. He has also developed local, national, and international programs to educate health care providers in HIV care.

CATHERINE GILLISS, D.NSc., is dean and professor at Yale University School of Nursing. Her scientific interests include the family and chronic illness. She has edited two books on family care and received the book of the year award from the *American Journal of Nursing*. Elected a fellow of the American Academy of Nursing in 1990, she now serves on the academy's board of directors. She is a past president of the National Organization of Nurse Practitioner Faculty and the Primary Care Policy Fellowship Society. Gilliss is a member of the national advisory committee for the Robert Wood Johnson Foundation's Partnership for Quality Education program. From 1993–2000 she was a trustee at the University of Portland, Oregon. She was a founding editorial board member of *Families, Systems & Health*, and she serves on the editorial board of the *Journal of Family Nursing*. She received her B.S.N. from Duke University, her M.S.N. from the Catholic University of America, and her D.N.Sc. from University of California at San Francisco.

CYNTHIA A. GINGALEWSKI, M.D., F.A.A.P., is assistant professor of surgery and pediatrics at the University of Massachusetts. She is a fellow of the American Academy of Pediatrics and an associate fellow at the Association of Women Surgeons, the American College of Surgeons, and the Association for Academic Surgery. Her research interests include necrotizing enterocolitis.

FRED GORELICK, M.D., is professor of medicine and cell biology at Yale University School of Medicine. He is chair of the pancreatic section of the American Gastroenterology Association and past president of the American Pancreatic Association. His research interests focus on pancreatic acinar cell function related to pancreatitis, as well as the regulation of vesicular movement in epithelial cells. He received his M.D. and completed his internal medicine residency at the University of Missouri, Columbia.

ATTILIO GRANATA, M.D., MBA, CPE, is associate clinical professor of internal medicine at Yale University School of Medicine. A member of the Yale clinical faculty since 1980, Granata is board-certified in internal medicine, critical care, and geriatrics. He received his B.S. and M.D. from Yale, completed his internal medicine residency at Stanford, and has an MBA from the Wharton School. He is a consultant to numerous organizations on strategic planning, technology assessment, cost-effectiveness analysis, and quality of care. His teaching and research interests focus on clinical medicine, health economics, and public policy.

DYAN GRIFFIN, M.D., F.A.A.P., is a clinical instructor at Yale University School of Medicine. She is also an associate with Pediatric & Medical Associates, the oldest group pediatric practice in Connecticut. Griffin received her medical school training at the University of Connecticut School of Medicine and then continued on to Yale–New Haven Hospital, where she completed a residency in pediatrics. She served as the pediatric chief resident at Yale for a year before beginning her career in private practice.

NORA GROCE, Ph.D., is an associate professor in the global health division at the Yale School of Public Health. She received her Ph.D. in medical anthropology from Brown University. She works in the fields of international health and development and is interested in social and cultural issues of health and the integration of western and traditional health care systems. She has done research on disability, violence, and urban health issues. She is also director of the Yale/World Health Organization Collaborative Center.

PETER N. HERBERT, M.D., is clinical professor of medicine, Yale University School of Medicine, and senior vice-president for medical affairs and chief of staff at Yale–New Haven Hospital. He received his M.D. from Yale and completed his residency at Yale–New Haven Hospital. He spent eight years at the National Institutes of Health and fourteen years at Brown University. For nine years he was chief of medicine at the Hospital of St. Raphael in New Haven.

BJÖRN HERMAN graduated from Yale University in 2001 and is doing a research fellowship at Beth Israel Medical Center's Advanced Medical Technology Institute in New York City. He aspires to be a surgeon and plans to enter medical school in 2003.

SUSAN HOCKFIELD, Ph.D., is the William Edward Gilbert Professor of Neurobiology and dean of the Graduate School of Arts and Sciences at Yale University. Her laboratory has been studying the molecular substrates of mammalian brain development.

ANGELA R. HOLDER, LL.M., is professor of the practice of medical ethics at the Center for the Study of Medical Ethics and Humanities, Duke University School of Medicine. Previously she was clinical professor of pediatrics (law) at Yale University School of Medicine. Holder has been president of the American Society of Law and Medicine, a member of the board of trustees of the Educational Commission for Foreign Medical Graduates, a member of the board and executive Committee of Planned Parenthood, and a member of the ethics committee of Leeway (the AIDS hospice in New Haven). She is a member of the Board of Visitors of the National Cathedral School. She was selected by the 1988 graduating class to be Yale medical school's commencement speaker that year.

JAMES JAMIESON, M.D., Ph.D., is professor of cell biology and director of medical studies, department of cell biology, at Yale University School of Medicine. He is also director of the M.D./Ph.D. program at Yale and director of the cell biology program at the Yale Comprehensive Cancer Center. He has received awards and been honored for his professional achievements and teaching excellence. He has served as president of the American Society for Cell Biology and as president of the American Pancreatic Association. He has written numerous articles and currently serves on the editorial board of the journal *Biochemical and Biophysical Research Communications.*

ALBERT R. JONSEN, Ph.D., is professor emeritus of ethics in medicine, University of Washington School of Medicine. He is a member of the Institute of Medicine, the National Academy of Sciences, and author of *A Short History of Medical Ethics.*

D. GEORGE JOSEPH, M.Phil., is a doctoral candidate in the history of medicine at Yale University School of Medicine. His interests are in the history of disease and public health, and he is researching American efforts to control leprosy and the medical-religious activities of missionaries in British India. He received undergraduate degrees in biology and history from the Washington University before coming to Yale for his master's and doctoral work.

JULIE JUNG KANG graduated from Yale College, class of 2002, with majors in molecular biophysics and biochemistry, and religious studies.

BOBBY KAPUR, M.D., is a resident in emergency medicine at Yale University Medical School. He is affiliated with the Society for Academic Emergency Medicine, the American College of Emergency Physicians, and the National Association of EMS Physicians. His research interests lie in international medicine.

GAIL KORRICK, M.S.W., A.C.S.W., L.C.S.W., B.C.D., is a psychiatric social worker who has counseled children, families, and couples for more than forty years. She is a member of the National Association of Social Workers (Connecticut Chapter) and the Connecticut Society of Clinic Social Work. She is on the board of many organizations, including the Regional Visiting Nurse Association.

MIKHAIL KOSIBOROD, M.D., is a clinical fellow in the section of cardiovascular medicine at Yale University School of Medicine. After receiving his B.A. from CUNY Queens College, he studied medicine at Mount Sinai School of Medicine. His internship and residency training was at Yale New Haven Hospital, where he has received the Kushlan Faculty Award and the Stephen R. Shell Housestaff Award. In 2000-2001 he was chief resident at Yale–New Haven. His major research interest lies in cardiovascular medicine.

HARLAN KRUMHOLZ, M.D., is associate professor of medicine (cardiology) at Yale University School of Medicine. He received his B.S. from Yale College in 1980 and his M.D. from Harvard Medical School in 1985. He also has an SM degree from the Harvard School of Public Health. His research focuses on using the methods of clinical epidemiology and health services research to improve the health and healthcare of individuals with, or at risk for, cardiovascular disease.

THOMAS L. LENTZ, M.D., is associate dean for admission and professor of cell biology at Yale University School of Medicine. He has been chair of the Committee on Admissions since 1972. He teaches cell biology and microscopic anatomy courses for first-year medical students. Past research has focused on the nicotinic acetylcholine receptor and the neurotropic rabies virus. He wrote the book *Cell Fine Structure.*

ROBERT J. LEVINE, M.D., is professor of medicine and lecturer in pharmacology at Yale University School of Medicine; director of the Law, Policy, and Ethics Core at the Yale Center for Interdisciplinary Research on AIDS; and co-chair of the executive committee of Yale's Interdisciplinary Bioethics Project. He is the author of numerous publications and is preparing the third edition of his book *Ethics and Regulation of Clinical Research.*

EVIE LINDEMANN has been a licensed psychotherapist for twenty-five years. She is involved in research at the Yale University School of Nursing (concerning use of coping-skills training with chronic illness), and has been active in conducting trauma interventions since September 11.

KATHLEEN S. LUNDGREN, M.Div., earned a master of divinity degree from Yale University with a concentration in medical ethics. She interned at the Connecticut Mental Health Center, where she developed her interest in the ethics of clinical research with vulnerable populations, with a particular focus on ethics in psychiatry. She is an editorial fellow at the Yale University Institution for Social and Policy Studies, serves on the Human Investigation Committee at the Yale University School of Medicine, is on the Advisory Board for Humanities in Medicine, and she is a member of several Yale University Bioethics research groups doing work on justice and vulnerable populations.

E. PAUL MACCARTHY, M.D., is vice-president and head of U.S. medical science for Bayer Corporation (Pharmaceutical Division). He received his M.D. and FRCPI from University College, Dublin, and was formerly chief of the hypertension section at the University of Cincinnati Medical Center.

BRUCE MCCLENNAN, M.D., is professor and chair of Yale University School of Medicine's department of diagnostic radiology. He also is chief of diagnostic imaging at Yale–New Haven Hospital. McClennan is secretary of the American Roentgen Ray Society; vice-president of the New England Roentgen Ray Society; member of the board of directors, Academy for Radiology Research; and editor and author of *Clinical Urography.*He received his B.S. from Union College and his M.D. from SUNY-Syracuse.

CHARLES MCKHANN, M.D., is professor emeritus of surgery at Yale University School of Medicine. His clinical interest was cancer surgery, particularly for breast cancer. He is the author of two books: *The Facts About Cancer: A Guide for Patients, Families, and Friends,* and *A Time to Die: The Place for Physician Assistance.* He chairs a Yale University research group on medical futility. McKhann received his B.A. from Harvard and his M.D. from the University of Pennsylvania.

MAURICE J. MAHONEY, M.D., J.D., is professor of genetics, pediatrics, and obstetrics and gynecology at Yale University School of Medicine.

He is director of the medical genetics unit at Yale. He also directs the Human Investigation Committee at Yale medical school.

MIKE MANN received a B.A. in 2002 in biology and Spanish from the University of Notre Dame. He has been a summer genetics research student at Yale University School of Medicine and has studied emergency medicine at the University of Panama School of Medicine. He was co-founder and coordinator of the International Student Bioethics Initiative at Notre Dame.

DAVID B. MELCHINGER is associate clinical professor of medicine at Yale University School of Medicine. He also practices internal medicine in New Haven. He enjoys teaching smallpox epidemiology to middle-schoolers throughout the country.

LAURA R. MENT, M.D., is professor, department of pediatrics and neurology, at Yale University School of Medicine. She works in a newborn special care unit at Yale–New Haven Hospital. She studies very low birthweight preterm infants and an animal model for the same.

JUANITA MERCHANT, M.D., Ph.D., is associate professor of internal medicine and physiology and is on the faculty for molecular and cellular biology at the University of Michigan at Ann Arbor. She is also an assistant investigator at the Howard Hughes Medical Institute. Merchant received her B.S. from Stanford University and her M.D. and Ph.D. (cell biology) from Yale. Her research focuses on the molecular mechanisms regulating gastrointestinal growth and transformation. She is an active member of American Gastroenterological Association and sits on several scientific review boards.

ALAN C. MERMANN, M.Div., M.D., is clinical professor of pediatrics and chaplain at Yale University School of Medicine and associate minister, Church of Christ Congregational in Norfolk, Connecticut. He is the author of three books and some fifty articles for professional journals.

PERRY L. MILLER, M.D., Ph.D., is professor of anesthesiology and of molecular, cellular, and developmental biology. He is also director of the

Center of Medical Informatics at Yale University. He received his A.B. from Harvard University (physics and chemistry), his M.S. from University of California-Berkeley, his Ph.D. in computer science from M.I.T., and his M.D from the University of Miami. Miller has worked in a variety of areas of computer science and biomedicine. He currently works on informatics projects in diverse areas, including clinical medicine, genomics, and neuroscience.

MARY JANE MINKIN, M.D., is clinical professor of obstetrics and gynecology at Yale University School of Medicine and a partner at Gynecology and Infertility, P.C., in New Haven. She received her Sc.B. from Brown University in biology and her M.D. from Yale.

VIVEK MURTHY is a fourth-year student in Yale School of Medicine and Yale School of Management's joint M.D./MBA program. He received his B.A. from Harvard and in 1995 co-founded VISIONS Worldwide, a nonprofit organization dedicated to HIV/AIDS prevention and general health promotion in the United States and India. He has received awards from the Soros Foundation, the AMA Foundation, and the *Chronicle of Philanthropy.* He is interested in integrative medicine, a field that seeks to combine allopathic medicine with complementary and alternative therapies.

SHERWIN B. NULAND is clinical professor of surgery at Yale University School of Medicine, and the author of numerous books and articles.

DOUGLAS P. OLSEN, RN, Ph.D., is associate professor, Yale School of Nursing, and associate director, Center for Health Policy and Ethics, at Yale University School of Medicine. His clinical specialization is psychiatric nursing, but most of his academic career has been devoted to the study of health care ethics. His particular areas of interest are the use of influence and responsibility in the clinical relationship, and ethics in mental health treatment. He is the assistant editor of *Nursing Ethics.* His publications have appeared in *Psychiatric Services,* the *Journal of Clinical Ethics,* and *Advances in Nursing Science.*

LYDIA PACE graduated from Yale College in 2001. She was a pre-med English major who worked for the Yale Interdisciplinary Bioethics Project. She is spending 2002 working in medical settings in Nepal and with the Population Council in South Africa. She plans to apply to medical school when she returns to the United States.

DENA RIFKIN, M.D., is an internal medicine resident with a strong interest in writing and reading about medicine. In 2000 she taught an undergraduate seminar at Yale College on literature, medicine, and the doctor-patient relationship. Rifkin received her A.B. from Harvard and her M.D. from Yale.

JULIE ROTHSTEIN ROSENBAUM, M.D., is a Robert Wood Johnson Clinical Scholar at Yale University School of Medicine. Rosenbaum majored in biomedical ethics at Brown University and completed her M.D. at Yale; she trained in internal medicine at Cornell Medical Center. Her work has focused on understanding critical events in residency training that have an impact on the professional and moral development of young physicians.

STANLEY H. ROSENBAUM, M.D., is professor of anesthesiology, medicine, and surgery, as well as the vice-chair for academic affairs in the department of anesthesiology at Yale University School of Medicine. He is an anesthesiologist with a major clinical interest in critical care medicine who spends his clinical time alternating between operating room anesthesiology and the care of patients in surgical and medical intensive care units. He also chairs the ethics committee of the Society of Critical Care Medicine, as well as the Health Professions Advisory Board of Yale College, which oversees the pre-medical advising system for Yale students and graduates.

LEON ROSENBERG, M.D., has been a professor of molecular biology at Princeton University since 1998. From 1991 to 1998 he was the chief scientific officer of Bristol-Myers Squibb Company. Rosenberg was a member of the faculty of Yale University School of Medicine, serving in several capacities—researcher, clinician, teacher, department chair, and dean. He is a past president of the Association of American Physicians and of the American Society of Human Genetics. He has been elected to the National Academy of Sciences, the Institute of Medicine, and the American Academy of Arts and Sciences.

D. A. ROSS is a third-year M.D./Ph.D. candidate at Yale University's Interdepartmental Neuroscience Program. He graduated from Yale College in 1999. His research focuses on the neural substrates of musical processing and includes a series of experiments that examine absolute or "perfect" pitch.

MICHAEL ROWE, Ph.D., is associate clinical professor of sociology, Yale University School of Medicine, department of psychiatry. He is a medical sociologist whose research interests include homelessness and mental illness, the organization of public mental health services, and alternatives to coercive mental health practices.. He is the author of *Crossing the Border: Encounters Between Homeless People and Outreach Workers,* and a memoir, *The Book of Jesse.*

PETER SALOVEY, Ph.D., is the Chris Argyris Professor and chair of psychology at Yale University. He is also professor of epidemiology and public health; director of the Health, Emotion, and Behavior Laboratory; and deputy director of the Center for Interdisciplinary Research on AIDS. Salovey completed his B.A. and M.A. at Stanford University. He received his graduate training in clinical psychology at Yale University. His research concerns two general issues: the psychological significance and function of human moods and emotions, and the application of social psychological principles to motivating health-protective behaviors. Salovey edits the Guilford Press series on Emotions and Social Behavior, was an associate editor of *Psychological Bulletin,* was the first editor of the *Review of General Psychology,* and serves as associate editor of *Emotion.*

RICHARD SELZER, M.D., is emeritus professor of general surgery at Yale University Medical School, where he practiced and taught for twenty-five years. He is the author of eleven volumes of essays, memoirs, and short stories. Selzer received his B.S. from Union College and his M.D. from Albany Medical College before completing his residency at Yale.

ANN SKOPEK, M.D., is assistant clinical professor of medicine at Yale University School of Medicine. She received her B.A. from Smith College, her M.D. from University of Connecticut and she has been in private practice in New Haven for more than twenty years.

HOWARD M. SPIRO, M.D., is a gastroenterologist who spent forty-four years at Yale University Medical School, where he set up the gastrointestinal section in 1955. He now doubles as a flaneur, walking from his home at one end of Temple Street to his office at the other end, where he is happily engaged as a medical consultant. He established the Program for the Humanities in Medicine at the Medical School and, a perpetual student, spends his free time auditing courses in Yale's Graduate School and College.

FLORENCE WALD served as dean of the Yale University School of Nursing from 1959 to 1968. She left the deanship to become a caregiver and researcher. With other members of an interdisciplinary research team, she founded and implemented the first hospice in the United States. Wald holds six honorary degrees and has been inducted into both the Connecticut and the National Women's Halls of Fame. In 2001 she was honored as a Living Legend by the American Academy of Nursing. She continues her hospice work, having recently brought compassionate care of the dying into prison settings. She received her B.A. from Mount Holyoke College and her M.N. and M.S. from Yale.

MARLYNN WEI is a student at Yale University School of Medicine who plans to pursue a joint M.D./J.D. degree. Her goal is to enter academic medicine and law with research interests focusing on health care for the elderly. She is a 2001 graduate of Yale College with honors in philosophy and molecular biophysics and biochemistry. She received the Branford College prize for scholarship.

STEFAN C. WEISS, M.D., M.H.S., is a resident in dermatology at Stanford University. After graduating cum laude in philosophy from Yale University, Weiss received his M.D. and M.H.S. from Duke University, where he created the Program for Humanities in Medicine. He was a fellow in the department of clinical bioethics at the National Institutes of Health and editor of MS/JAMA, the student section of the *Journal of the American Medical Association*. He currently sits on the governing council of the American Public Health Association.

MORRIS WESSEL, M.D., is clinical professor of pediatrics, Yale University School of Medicine, and consulting pediatrician at the Clifford Beers Child Guidance Clinic. He practiced primary pediatrics in New Haven from 1951 to 1993 and has a long history of involvement with programs serving children in the greater New Haven area. He received the Practitioner Research Award from the American Academy of Pediatrics and the C. Anderson Aldrich Award in Child Development from the Section on the Developmental and Behavioral Pediatrics of the American Academy of Pediatrics.

BRIAN WEST, M.D., FRCPath., is professor of pathology and director of anatomic pathology at New York University. West graduated in medicine from the University of Dublin, Trinity College. At Yale University Medical School he directed the section of gastrointestinal pathology and the digestive disease module in the medical student program. He was director of Surgical Pathology at the University of Texas before joining NYU. His professional interests are in gastrointestinal, hepatic, and infectious disease.

STEVEN WOLFSON, M.D., is associate clinical professor of medicine at Yale University School of Medicine. He received his B.A. from Columbia College and his M.D. from the New York University School of Medicine. He was formerly director of the Cardiac Catheterization Laboratory at Yale. He is founder and current president of Cardiology Associates of New Haven, P.C., a thirteen-member group cardiology practice. He is medical director and vice-chairman of the executive committee of the Yale Cardiology Network.

INDEX

Academic bioethicist, 162, 384–388
Academic medicine: bioethicist, 384–
388; career in, 110–114; inner-city
student's career path, 193–198;
pressures of, 212–213; women in,
189–192. *See also* Research
Acupuncture, 367, 371
Admissions. *See* Applying to medical
school
Advanced nurse practitioners, 33,
286, 289
Advisors: at medical school, 115–120;
premedical, 38–42
Affirmative action programs, 41, 193–
198
Aging population, effect on health
care system, 80–81
AIDS. *See* HIV/AIDS
Ainley, Marjorene, 192
Aldrich, C. Andrew, 238
Alternative medicine, 364–368, 369–
373
AMCAS. *See* American Medical Col-
lege Application Service
American Medical Association (AMA),
formation of, 155
American Medical College Application
Service (AMCAS), 39, 47
American medicine's obligations,
357–358
American Psychiatric Association, 255
Anatomic pathology, 265–268
Anthropologist turning to practice of
medicine, 343–348
Applied ethics, 316–320. *See also*
Ethics
Applying to medical school, 31–48;
acceptance rate, 38; admission pro-
cess, 38–42; advice by admissions

committee chairman, 43–48;
applying after third year of undergraduate college, 39; appropriateness for practice of medicine, 40–
41; background information, 43–
44; character and, 159–160; dean's
letter, 38, 40; deferred application,
36–37, 39–40; extracurricular activities, 35, 46; foreign medical
schools, 42; former medical school
dean's perspective, 78–82; four-year
plan toward admission to, 64–68;
hobbies, 227; interview, 39, 40–41,
65, 201; minority applicants, 199–
204; nontraditional paths to, 95–
96, 115–120; rejected applicants,
47–48; social component of admission process, 40–41; stress and,
103, 201; type of undergraduate education, 45, 64–65, 75–77, 226–
227; women applicants, 186–187.
See also College majors; Financial issues; Medical College Application
Test (MCAT)
Assertive mental health outreach,
321–326
Asylums, 255
Attorneys. *See* Lawyers
Autopsy pathologists, 268

Basic science research, 268–269
Behavior related to health and illness,
359–363
Bell, John, 174
Biller, Eunice, 284
Bio-psycho-social model, 172
Bioethics. *See* Ethics
Biomedical advances, effect on medi-
cal profession, 157

Biomedical model of disease, 170–172
Biomedical research, 379–416. *See also* Research
Blackwell, Frances Smith, 288
Brand, Stephen, 198
Brody, Baruch, 316

CAM (complementary and alternative medicine), 369–373
Camus, Albert, 178
Cardiologists, 74–77
Careers, health care. *See specific profession*
CAT scanning, 262
Center for Medical Informatics, 407–411
Certified nurse midwives (CNM), 298–302
Character of physician. *See* Ethics
Chechnya, physician's experience in, 183–184
Chiropractors, 364–368
Civil rights and medicine, 199–204; affirmative action programs, 193–198
Clinical pathology, 265, 268–269
Clinical pharmacy, 308
Clinical social workers, 332–336
College majors, 5–25; anthropology, 343–348; computer science, 407–411; English, 8–12; history, 5–7; importance of broad undergraduate, 34–35, 45; for midwifery, 300; pre-med, 18–21; science and bioethics, 22–25; science and humanities, 13–17. *See also* Applying to medical school
Complementary and alternative medicine (CAM), 369–373
Computer technology: medical informatics, 407–411; use in medical school, 93–94

Computerized transverse axial tomography, 262
Conflicts of interest, 93
Connecticut Hospice, 240
Costs of health care, 421–422; containment, 157
CT scanning, 262
Cytopathologists, 267

Deafness, hereditary in Martha's Vineyard, 345–347
Deans: former and present nursing school deans, 283–292; former medical school dean's perspective, 78–82; letter by undergraduate dean, 38, 40
Deferred application to medical school. *See* Applying to medical school
Deferred matriculation to medical school, 39–40
Deutel, Oscar, 219
Diagnostic imaging, 261–264
Diversity in medical school, 41, 193–198, 201–202
DNA fingerprinting, 274
Duff, Ray, 286

East Timor, physician's experience in, 181–183
Emergency Medical Technician (EMT), 61–62
Emergency room, resident's experience, 127–133
Engel, George, 172
Essay for medical school application, 36, 40, 65
Ethics: applied, 316–320; bioethicists, 384–388; genetics and, 274–275; medical, 159–163; physician's character, 159–165; problems in medicine, 172–173; undergraduate ma-

jor in, 22–25. *See also* Institutional Review Board (IRB)

Evaluative clinical sciences, 422–423

Exact Location of the Soul, The (Seltzer), 441–446

Faculty. *See* Medical school

Faith. *See* Religion

Family life and career, balancing, 112–113; 188; 193–194; 242–247, 310–311, 319, 399

Farley, Margaret, 318, 319

Fellowships, 140–141, 142–148

Financial issues: managing debt load of career choice, 398; M.D./Ph.D. programs, 52; medical school, 41–42; military scholarship, 62–63; research grants, 53–54, 147, 405–406; supporting salary in academic setting, 111

Fine needle aspiration (FNA) biopsy, 267

Flexner, Abraham, 170–171

Flexner Report, 170–171, 370

Ford, Loretta, 290

Foreign medical schools, 42

Fox, Renee C., 139

Functional MRI (fMRI), 101, 102, 263

Funding. *See* Financial issues

Genetics and medicine, 80, 271–275

Gesmonde, Gary, 365

Gifford, Robert, 118

Goldman, Lee, 391

Gortner, Susan, 290

Grades, 35–36, 40

Graduate studies. *See* Research

Grants, research, 53–54, 147, 405–406

Grey, Margaret, 291, 330

Griswold, A. W., 286

Grover, Joseph, 235

Gynecology and obstetrics, 248–253

Haslam, Kathleen, 192

Health care management, physician-executive role in, 421–425

Health professions, 283–373. *See also specific profession*

Health psychologists, 359–363

Heller, Renu, 196

Hemopathology, 268

Henderson, Virginia, 286

Herbal medicine, 371–372

Hewlett, Sylvia Ann, 310

History of medicine, lessons from, 349–358

HIV/AIDS: behavioral changes and, 359–360; development of youth programs and, 56, 57; physician's experience working with, 120, 178–180

Holistic medicine. *See* Complementary and alternative medicine (CAM)

Homeless, outreach to, 321–326

Horta, Jose Ramos, 181

Hospice programs, 240, 286–287

Hospital lawyer, 312–315

Hounsfield, Godfrey, 262

How We Die (Nuland), 435–440

Human rights and international health, 181–185

Humanities, 170–175, 435–446; as college major, 13–17

In vitro fertilization, 315

Information technology: medical informatics, 407–411; use in medical school, 93–94

Institutional Review Board (IRB): academic bioethicist, 384–388; ethicists and, 320; lawyers and, 314–315; pharmacists and, 311; physician-executive's career path, 427. *See also* Research

Internal medicine, future of, 219–225

International health and human
rights, 181–185
Interview for medical school. *See*
Applying to medical school
Inventory, personal, 34
IRB. *See* Institutional Review Board

Jackson, Edith, 237–240
Johns Hopkins Medical School, as educational standard, 170

Kean, Benjamin H., 113
Kessler, David A., 119
Kissick, Bill, 337, 341

Laboratory medicine, 268–269
Laub, Dori, 324
Lawyers: becoming physicians, 95–96;
in medical environment, 312–315
Leonard, Robert, 286
Letters of recommendation, 38, 39,
40, 66
Lippard, Vernon, 81–82
Loeb, Robert, 380
Ludmerer, Kenneth, 170

Magnetic resonance imaging (MRI),
10; 262–263
Majors. *See* College majors
Malpractice. *See* Medical malpractice
Mausksch, Ingeborg, 290
May, William F., 156
MCAT. *See* Medical College Application Test
M.D./Ph.D. programs: advantages of,
383; application procedure and prerequisites, 51; careers of graduates,
52–54; choosing, 49–54, 99–104;
director of, 49–54; enrollment in,
379; in pharmaceutical industry,
429; residency and, 53; sources of
support, 52. *See also* Physician-scientists; Research

Medical College Application Test
(MCAT): admission process and,
39–40; admission to M.D./Ph.D.
programs, 51; basic science courses
and, 45; described, 46–47; preparation for, 65; taking of, 46–47
Medical decision-making, 92
Medical informatics, 407–411
Medical malpractice, 157, 252, 313–314
Medical school: affirmative action programs, 41, 193–198; alternatives
to, 33; bio-psycho-social model,
172; biomedical model, 170–172;
clinical study, 90–91, 105–109;
comparison with law school, 95–
96; diversity and, 41, 193–204; ethics education, 159–165; Flexner
Report, 170–171, 370; former medical school dean's perspective, 78–
82; future trends, 78–82; hospital
chief of staff's perspective, 31–37;
humanities in, 353–354; lessons
from history of medicine, 349–358;
medical decision-making curriculum, 92; minority students, 193–
204; nontraditional paths to, 95–
96, 115–120; overview, 89–94;
patient-centered approach, 92–93;
personal growth and medical training, 55–58; preclinical experience,
89–90, 97–98; problem-based approach, 90; professional responsibility, 92–94; Russian system of, 134–
135; teaching of medical students,
110–114; themes in curriculum,
92–94; use of information technology, 93–94; women faculty members, 189–192; women students,
33–34, 186–187; "Yale system,"
79. *See also* Applying to medical
school; College majors; M.D./
Ph.D. programs

Medical School Admissions Requirements: United States and Canada, 2003–2004 (AAMC), 43–44
Medical sociologist, 321–326
Medical writing and the humanities, 435–446
Medicine: certifying boards and professional societies, 157; contemplating career in, 5–25; effect of biomedical advances on, 157; ethical problems, 172–173; genetics and, 271–275; history of, 154–155; humanities and, 170–175; international health and human rights, 181–185; as a profession, 153–158. *See also* Academic medicine; Physicians
Men: careers in obstetrics and gynecology, 293–297; careers in nursing, 293–297; surgery as male stronghold, 187
Mental health: health psychologists, 359–363; outreach workers, 321–326; psychiatric nursing, 285–286, 289–290; psychiatric research, 318–319. *See also* Psychiatrists
Mentors: importance of, 197–198; nursing career and, 286, 288, 290; pharmacy and, 309–310; research fellows and, 144–145
Midwives: alternative to medical school, 33; career as, 298–302
Military scholarship for medical school, 62–63
Minister as physician, 166–169
Minority students, 193–204
MRI. *See* Magnetic Resonance Imaging

National Institutes of Health (NIH). *See* M.D./Ph.D. programs
Nursing: advanced nurse practitioners, 33, 286, 289; careers of two leaders in, 283–292; identity crisis in, 295; men as nurses, 293–297; modern midwifery, 298–302; psychiatric, 285–286, 289–290

Obstetrics and gynecology, 248–253
Orlando, Ira, 286
Osler, William, 207, 208
Osteopaths, 42
Outreach workers, 321–326

PA program. *See* Physician assistants
Pap smears, 267
Pathologists, 265–270
Patient-centered approach, 92–93
Patient experience as influential, 8–12
Patient-physician relationship, 207–209
Patient's rights, 314
Pediatricians, 235–241; value as career choice, 203–204
Pellegrino, Edmund, 286
Peplau, Hilde, 286
Pepper, Max, 286
Personal inventory, 34
Personal statement in medical school application. *See* Applying to medical school
Pharmaceutical industry, physician-executive working in, 426–430
Pharmacists, 307–311
Pharmacogenomics, 274
Ph.D. programs, as alternatives, 33, 140; biological sciences, 412–416
Ph.D./M.D. programs. *See* M.D./Ph.D. programs
Physician assistants, 33, 303–306
Physician-executives: role in health care management, 421–425; role in pharmaceutical industry, 426–430
Physician-patient relationship, 92, 156–157, 162–165, 167, 169, 173–174, 207–209, 259–260

Physician-scientists: becoming, 379–383; career as, 394–400. *See also* M.D./Ph.D. programs; Research

Physicians: aging, 210–214; balancing family life and medical career, 32, 242–247; careers of, 219–275; character of, 159–165; future trends, 354–357; lessons from history of medicine, 349–358; minister physician's perspective, 166–169; obligations of profession, 156; personal growth of, 55–58; pharmaceutical industry, role in, 426–430; professionalism of, 155–156, 158; pros and cons of career, 37; religious faith and, 166–169; self-knowledge, 75; social commitment and, 176–180; society's view of, 31–32; training for, 89–148; transitions in life of, 205–209; type of practice, 212–213; women as, 186–192. *See also specific specialties;* M.D./Ph.D. programs; Research

Physicians for Human Rights, 184

Pierrel, Rosemary, 186

Powers, Grover, 235

Premedical advisors, 38–42

Primary care: and older physicians, 212–213; internal medicine as, 222

Privacy of genetic information, 275

Professional responsibility, 93. *See also* Ethics

Professionalism, 158

Psychiatric nursing, 285–286, 289–290

Psychiatrists, 69–73, 254–260; history of psychiatry, 255–256. *See also* Mental health

Psychologists, health, 359–363

Public health: career in, 176–180, 337–342; studies in medical school, 93

Publishing research, 146–147, 405

Quality of care, 422–423

Radiologists, 261–264

Religion: and physicians, 166–169; divinity degree and bioethics, 318

Relman, A., 158

Research: ethics and, 164, 311, 318–320, 386–387, 318; balancing with medicine, 142–148; basic science, 268–269; conferences and seminars, benefits of, 404–405; experiments, 145; fellowships, 140–148; grants, 53–54, 147, 405–406; on human subjects, 384–388; inspiration of medicine and, 137–141; laboratory career, 401–406; medical informatics, 407–411; on medical school application, 66; mentors, 144–145; patient-centered, 139–140, 389–393; physician-scientist's role, 379–383; publishing, 146–147, 405; rewards of life in science, 412–416; writing skills and, 405. *See also* Institutional Review Board (IRB); M.D./Ph.D. programs; Ph.D. programs

Residency: challenges of, 32, 121–126; chief resident's perspective, 134–136; chief resident's role, 126; emergency room experiences, 127–133; fellowships, 140–148; historical development of, 31; and M.D./Ph.D. programs, 53; medical resident's perspective, 64–68; pathologists, 266–270; surgical resident's perspective, 59–63; women in, 187–188

Robinson, Mary, 184

Roentgen, Wilhelm Conrad, 261

Rooming-in for infant care, 238–239

Rural health care services, 389–390

Rush, Benjamin, 256

St. Christopher's Hospice, 286–287
Saunders, Cicely, 286–287
Scarry, Elaine, 318
Scholarships, military, 62–63. *See also*
Financial issues
Scientists, physician. *See* Physician-
scientists
Segal, Stanton, 381–382
Self-knowledge of physicians, 75
Settlement houses, 332
Shem, Samuel, 122
Sign Language, Vineyard, 346
Smith, Lloyd H., 79
Smoking, effects of reducing, 359
Social workers, 327–336
Soelle, Dorothee, 318
Spanish, benefits of familiarity with,
59–60
Specialties. *See specific type*
Spinella, Giovanna, 192
Spock, Benjamin, 238
Starr, Paul, 154
Students. *See* Applying to medical
school; College majors; Medical
school
Surgeons, 226–234; *The Exact Loca-
tion of the Soul* (Selzer), 441–446;
as male specialty, 187

"Talk to the Doctor" column, 252
Tanner, Kathryn, 318
Techne, 225
Tennant, Elizabeth, 286
Terrorism, specter of, 80, 356–357
Thompson, John, 338

Time management. *See* Family life and
career, balancing
Transitions in medical life, 205–209

Underserved communities, 389–390

Volunteer activities and medical
school application, 66–67

Waxman, Merle, 192, 319
Web sites: M.D./Ph.D. programs, 51,
52; medical informatics, 411; medical schools, 44
Wennberg, John, 421–422
Winternitz, Milton, 79, 236
Women, 186–192; balancing family
life and medical career, 33–34,
242–247, 310–311, 319; career
choices of, 187–189; medical school
and, 33–34, 186–187, 250; as medical school faculty members, 189–192;
modern midwifery, 298–302; obstetrics and gynecology, 248–253; residency programs and, 187, 188
Writing, medical: excerpts from, 435–
446; publishing research, 146–147,
405

X-rays, 261–262

"Yale system" of medical education, 79
Yamada, Tadataka, 198
Year off from school prior to M.D./
Ph.D. programs, 53
Yellow Berets, 381

CREDITS

Photographs on part title opening pages:

Pages 1, 27, 83, 215, 375, and 431: photos by Michael Marsland, Yale University, Office of Public Affairs.

Page 149: Courtesy of Cushing/Whitney Medical Library, Yale Medical School (*N.B.: photo of John P. Peters, M.D. Dr. Peters spent his entire faculty career at Yale University where he was chief of the Metabolic Division in the Department of Medicine from 1922–1955. His enduring scientific contributions paralleled his intense commitment to the care of the fervent mission to ensure that the physician was an advocate of the patient.*)

Page 277: EyeWire/Getty Images. All rights reserved.

Page 417: photo by Anita Tellier. Courtesy of ITS Med—Media Services, Katherine Krauss, Yale–New Haven Hospital.